50 STUDIES

every

Plastic Surgeon Should Know

50 STUDIES

every

Plastic Surgeon Should Know

EDITOR

C. Scott Hultman, MD, MBA, FACS

Ethel F. and James A. Valone Distinguished Professor
of Plastic and Reconstructive Surgery;
Division Chief and Program Director, Plastic Surgery,
University of North Carolina School of Medicine;
Founder and Executive Director, University of North Carolina
Burn Reconstruction and Aesthetic Center;
Associate Director, North Carolina Jaycee Burn Center,
Chapel Hill, North Carolina

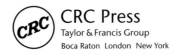

CRC Press
Taylor & Francis Group
Boca Raton London New York

CRC Press is an imprint of the
Taylor & Francis Group, an **informa** business

CRC Press
Taylor & Francis Group
6000 Broken Sound Parkway NW, Suite 300
Boca Raton, FL 33487-2742

© 2015 by Taylor & Francis Group, LLC
CRC Press is an imprint of Taylor & Francis Group, an Informa business

No claim to original U.S. Government works

Printed on acid-free paper
Version Date: 20140903

International Standard Book Number-13: 978-1-4822-4082-5 (Pack - Book and Ebook)

**Visit the Taylor & Francis Web site at
http://www.taylorandfrancis.com**

**and the CRC Press Web site at
http://www.crcpress.com**

To my wife Suzanne,
who would agree that our three greatest contributions
are Chloe, Hank, and Timothy

Cover artwork:
"The Knife Thrower," Plate XV from Jazz. Henri Matisse, 1946.
©2014 Succession H. Matisse/Artists Rights Society (ARS), New York.
Digital image: Archives H. Matisse, all rights reserved.

PUBLISHER   Karen Berger
ASSOCIATE EDITOR   Megan Fennell
PROJECT MANAGER   Idelle Winer
VICE PRESIDENT OF PRODUCTION AND MANUFACTURING   Carolyn Reich
DIRECTOR OF GRAPHICS   Brett Stone
GRAPHICS TECHNICIAN   Ngoc-Thuy Khuu
ILLUSTRATORS   Brenda L. Bunch, Jennifer N. Gentry
LAYOUT ARTISTS   Elaine Kitsis
PRODUCTION   Chris Lane, Linda Maulin

Contributors

Reviewers

Anne E. Argenta, MD
Resident, Department of Plastic Surgery, University of Pittsburgh Medical Center, Pittsburgh, Pennsylvania

Saif Al-Bustani, MD, DMD
Resident, Division of Plastic and Reconstructive Surgery, Department of Surgery, University of North Carolina School of Medicine, Chapel Hill, North Carolina

Paul DiEgidio, MD
Resident, Department of Surgery, University of South Carolina School of Medicine, Columbia, South Carolina

S. Tyler Elkins-Williams, MD
Resident, Division of Plastic and Reconstructive Surgery, Department of Surgery, University of North Carolina School of Medicine, Chapel Hill, North Carolina

Rafi Fredman, MD, FACS
Resident, Division of Plastic and Reconstructive Surgery, Department of Surgery, University of North Carolina School of Medicine, Chapel Hill, North Carolina

Jonathan S. Friedstat, MD
Resident, Division of Plastic and Reconstructive Surgery, Department of Surgery, University of North Carolina School of Medicine, Chapel Hill, North Carolina

Ryan M. Garcia, MD
Hand Surgery Fellow, Department of Orthopaedics, Duke University School of Medicine, Durham, North Carolina

Kimberly S. Jones, MD
Resident, Division of Plastic and Reconstructive Surgery, Department of Surgery, University of North Carolina School of Medicine, Chapel Hill, North Carolina

Daniel J. Krochmal, MD, FACS
Resident, Division of Plastic and Reconstructive Surgery, Department of Surgery, University of North Carolina School of Medicine, Chapel Hill, North Carolina

Yuen-Jong Liu, MD
Resident, Division of Plastic and Reconstructive Surgery, Department of Surgery, University of North Carolina School of Medicine, Chapel Hill, North Carolina

H. Wolfgang Losken, MD, MBChB, FCS(SA), FRCS(Ed)
Craniofacial Surgeon (retired), Division of Plastic Surgery, University of North Carolina School of Medicine, Chapel Hill, North Carolina

Patrick Mannal, MD
Resident, Division of Plastic and
Reconstructive Surgery, Department of
Surgery, University of North Carolina
School of Medicine, Chapel Hill, North
Carolina

Shiara Ortiz-Pujols, MD
Resident, Division of Plastic and
Reconstructive Surgery, Department of
Surgery, University of North Carolina
School of Medicine, Chapel Hill, North
Carolina

J. Megan M. Patterson, MD
Assistant Professor, Department of
Orthopaedics, University of North Carolina
School of Medicine, Chapel Hill, North
Carolina

Michelle C. Roughton, MD
Assistant Professor, Division of Plastic
and Reconstructive Surgery, Department
of Surgery, University of North Carolina
School of Medicine, Chapel Hill, North
Carolina

David S. Ruch, MD
Professor, Director of Hand and Upper
Extremity Surgery, Duke University School
of Medicine, Durham, North Carolina

Amita R. Shah, MD, PhD
Resident, Division of Plastic and
Reconstructive Surgery, Department of
Surgery, University of North Carolina
School of Medicine, Chapel Hill, North
Carolina

Brandon S. Smetana, MD
Resident, Department of Orthopaedic
Surgery, University of North Carolina
School of Medicine, Chapel Hill, North
Carolina

Shruti C. Tannan, MD
Hand Surgery Fellow, The Hand Center of
San Antonio, San Antonio, Texas

Anna F. Tyson, MD, MPH
Research Fellow, Department of General
Surgery, University of North Carolina
School of Medicine, Chapel Hill, North
Carolina

Ida Janelle Wagner, MD
Resident, Division of Plastic and
Reconstructive Surgery, Department of
Surgery, University of North Carolina
School of Medicine, Chapel Hill, North
Carolina

Felicia N. Williams, MD
Assistant Professor of Surgery, North
Carolina Jaycee Burn Center, Chapel Hill,
North Carolina

Jeyhan S. Wood, MD
Assistant Professor, Division of Plastic
and Reconstructive Surgery, Department
of Surgery, University of North Carolina
School of Medicine, Chapel Hill, North
Carolina

Cindy Wu, MD
Assistant Professor, Division of Plastic
and Reconstructive Surgery, Department
of Surgery, University of North Carolina
School of Medicine, Chapel Hill, North
Carolina

Shunsuke Yoshida, MD, MS
Resident, Division of Plastic and
Reconstructive Surgery, Department of
Surgery, University of North Carolina
School of Medicine, Chapel Hill, North
Carolina

Study Author Reflections

Louis C. Argenta, MD, FACS
Professor, Department of Plastic and
Reconstructive Surgery, Wake Forest Baptist
Medical Center, Winston-Salem, North
Carolina

Stephan Ariyan, MD, MBA, FACS
Professor of Surgery (Plastic) and of
Dermatology, Yale School of Medicine;
Clinical Program Leader, Melanoma
Program, Smilow Cancer Hospital at Yale–
New Haven, New Haven, Connecticut

Burt Brent, MD
Associate Professor (retired), Stanford
University Medical Center, San Francisco,
California

David W. Chang, MD, FACS
Professor of Surgery, Section of Plastic
and Reconstructive Surgery, Department
of Surgery, The University of Chicago
Medicine & Biological Sciences, Chicago,
Illinois

Matthias B. Donelan, MD, FACS
Chief of Staff, Shriners Hospitals for
Children–Boston; Associate Clinical
Professor of Surgery, Harvard Medical
School; Associate Visiting Surgeon,
Massachusetts General Hospital, Boston,
Massachusetts

Loren H. Engrav, MD, FACS
Professor Emeritus, Division of Surgery and
Plastic Surgery, University of Washington,
Seattle, Washington

Leonard T. Furlow, Jr., MD, FACS
Clinical Professor, Department of Plastic
Surgery, University of Florida College of
Medicine, Gainesville, Florida

Ruth Graf, MD, PhD
Adjunct Professor of Plastic Surgery,
Federal University of Paraná, Brazil

James C. Grotting, MD, FACS
Clinical Professor, Division of Plastic
Surgery, The University of Alabama at
Birmingham; Clinical Professor, Division
of Plastic Surgery, The University of
Wisconsin, Madison; Private Practice,
Grotting & Cohn Plastic Surgery,
Birmingham, Alabama

Bahman Guyuron, MD, FACS
Chair, Department of Plastic Surgery,
University Hospitals Case Medical Center;
Kiehn-DesPrez Professor, Case Western
Reserve University, Cleveland, Ohio

David Herndon, MD, FACS
Professor, Department of Surgery; Professor,
Department of Pediatrics, The University
of Texas Medical Branch; Chief of Staff
and Director of Research, Shriners Burn
Hospital, Galveston, Texas

C. Scott Hultman, MD, MBA, FACS
Ethel F. and James A. Valone Distinguished
Professor of Plastic and Reconstructive
Surgery; Division Chief and Program
Director, Plastic Surgery, University of
North Carolina School of Medicine; Founder
and Executive Director, University of North
Carolina Burn Reconstruction and Aesthetic
Center; Associate Director, North Carolina
Jaycee Burn Center, Chapel Hill, North
Carolina

Yves-Gérard Illouz, MD, FACS
Professor, French Faculty of Medicine,
Paris V Descartes; Professor, Department of
Plastic Surgery, Hôpital Saint-Louis, Paris,
France

Donald H. Lalonde, MD, Hons BSc, MSc, FRCSC
Professor of Surgery, Department of Plastic Surgery, Dalhousie University, Saint John, New Brunswick, Canada

Graham D. Lister, MD
Honorary Professor of Surgery, University of Ljubljana, Slovenia

Susan E. Mackinnon, MD, FACS
Chief and Shoenberg Professor, Division of Plastic and Reconstructive Surgery, Washington University School of Medicine, St. Louis, Missouri

Paul Manson, MD, FACS
Distinguished Service Professor of Plastic Surgery, Johns Hopkins School of Medicine; Hansjoerg Wyss Distinguished Professor of Surgery, The University of Maryland Shock Trauma Unit, The University of Maryland School of Medicine, Baltimore, Maryland

David W. Mathes, MD, FACS
Professor of Surgery; Chief, Division of Plastic and Reconstructive Surgery, University of Colorado, Denver, Anschutz Medical Campus, Aurora, Colorado; Attending Surgeon, VA Eastern Colorado Health Care System, Denver, Colorado

Joseph McCarthy, MD, FACS
Lawrence D. Bell Professor of Plastic Surgery, Department of Plastic Surgery, New York University School of Medicine, New York, New York

John B. McCraw, MD, FACS
Emeritus Professor, Division of Plastic Surgery, Department of Surgery, The University of Mississippi School of Medicine, Jackson, Mississippi

Frederick J. Menick, MD
Private practice, Tucson, Arizona

Foad Nahai, MD, FACS
Professor of Surgery, Emory University School of Medicine, Atlanta, Georgia

Basil A. Pruitt, Jr., MD, FACS, FCCM, MCCM
Clinical Professor, Betty and Bob Kelso Distinguished Chair in Burn and Trauma Surgery; Dr. Ferdinand P. Herff Chair in Surgery, Department of Surgery, Division of Trauma and Emergency Services, University of Texas Health Science Center, San Antonio, Texas; Professor of Surgery, Uniformed Services University of the Health Sciences, Bethesda, Maryland

Oscar M. Ramirez, MD
Clinical Assistant Professor, Johns Hopkins University School of Medicine; Clinical Assistant Professor, University of Maryland School of Medicine, Baltimore, Maryland

Eduardo D. Rodriguez, MD, DDS
Helen L. Kimmel Professor of Reconstructive Plastic Surgery; Chair, Department of Plastic Surgery, New York University Langone Medical Center, New York, New York

Jack H. Sheen, MD
Surgeon (retired), Private practice, Santa Barbara, California

Maria Siemionow, MD, PhD, DSc
Professor of Orthopaedics; Director of Microsurgery Research, Department of Orthopaedics, University of Illinois at Chicago, Chicago, Illinois

Expert Commentary

Gregory M. Buncke, MD, FACS
Director, The Buncke Clinic; Chair, Division
of Microsurgery; Chair, Department of
Plastic Surgery, California Pacific Medical
Center, San Francisco, California

C. Scott Hultman, MD, MBA, FACS
Ethel F. and James A. Valone Distinguished
Professor of Plastic and Reconstructive
Surgery; Division Chief and Program
Director, Plastic Surgery, University of
North Carolina School of Medicine; Founder
and Executive Director, University of North
Carolina Burn Reconstruction and Aesthetic
Center; Associate Director, North Carolina
Jaycee Burn Center, Chapel Hill, North
Carolina

Albert Losken, MD, FACS
William G. Hamm, MD Professor of
Surgery; Program Director, Division of
Plastic Surgery, Emory University School of
Medicine, Atlanta, Georgia

**H. Wolfgang Losken, MD, MBChB, FCS(SA),
FRCS(Ed)**
Craniofacial Surgeon (retired), Division
of Plastic Surgery, University of North
Carolina School of Medicine, Chapel Hill,
North Carolina

Ernest K. Manders, MD, FACS
Medical Director, Facial Nerve Center,
McGowan Institute for Regenerative
Medicine, University of Pittsburgh School of
Medicine, Pittsburgh, Pennsylvania

Wyndell H. Merritt, MD, FACS
Associate Professor of Plastic Surgery,
The University of Virginia, Charlottesville,
Virginia; Assistant Clinical Professor
of Surgery, Division of Plastic &
Reconstructive Surgery, Virginia
Commonwealth University, Richmond,
Virginia

Anthony A. Meyer, MD, PhD, FACS, FRCS
Colin G. Thomas, Jr., MD Distinguished
Professor of Surgery; Chair, Department
of Surgery, University of North Carolina
School of Medicine, Chapel Hill, North
Carolina

Michelle C. Roughton, MD
Assistant Professor, Division of Plastic
and Reconstructive Surgery, Department
of Surgery, University of North Carolina
School of Medicine, Chapel Hill, North
Carolina

Robert L. Sheridan, MD, FAAP, FACS
Burn Service Medical Director, Boston
Shriners Hospital for Children; Division
of Burns, Massachusetts General Hospital;
Associate Professor of Surgery, Harvard
Medical School, Boston, Massachusetts

John A. van Aalst, MD, FACS
Associate Professor of Surgery; Director of
Pediatric and Craniofacial Plastic Surgery,
Division of Plastic and Reconstructive
Surgery, University of North Carolina
School of Medicine, Chapel Hill, North
Carolina

Preface

Five hundred years after this observation, Robert Hooke, writing to his rival, Sir Isaac Newton, in 1676 restated this as: "If I have seen further, it is by standing on the shoulders of giants." This metaphor for discovering truth by building on previous discoveries would become a guiding principle for scientific progress, serving as a model for inquiry and investigation.

As a student and educator of plastic surgery, I often wonder: 'Who are the giants in our field? On whose shoulders am I standing?'

This book, *50 Studies Every Plastic Surgeon Should Know,* represents an attempt to identify the most influential contributors of our discipline, who have laid the foundation for the modern practice of plastic surgery. My goals in compiling this book were as follows:
- To review and consolidate our collective working knowledge
- To demonstrate the vast depth and diversity of plastic surgery
- To highlight the importance of innovation as our core competency
- To teach trainees our origins and inspire practitioners to educate
- To provoke the reader into thinking about what studies were not included in this book, but should have been, because of error, personal perspective, or editorial discretion
- To inspire future leaders into making their own lasting contributions to our specialty

Selecting the 50 studies "every plastic surgeon should know" proved to be a formidable task. I knew that I wanted to start with skin grafting and end with face transplantation. However, identifying the 48 studies in between challenged me to assess critically and objectively which contributions have had the greatest impact on how we practice our craft.

To identify these papers, I created a set of rules that guided my selection process. Because I wanted to focus on the modern era (defined as within the past century), I necessarily excluded the Edwin Smith papyrus, the Sushruta surgical text, Vesalius' anatomic treatise, *De Humani Corporus Fabrica,* Tagliacozzi's "Italian method" of nasal reconstruction, and Barronio's skin transplantation in sheep—all monumental achievements, but beyond the scope of this book. Furthermore, I made the admittedly controversial decisions not to include Alexis Carrel's work on vascular anastomoses, Sir Peter Medawar's discovery of acquired immune tolerance, or Joseph Murray's kidney transplantation, because these accomplishments had far-reaching implications across so many other surgical disciplines. The desire to represent the breadth of plastic surgery also limited the depth of each subject area, so that no single subspecialty was neglected. Finally, some surgeons could have made the list more than once, but to provide a larger palette of papers, I included only those surgeons' most important contributions.

The 50 studies that emerged were based on the following:
1. Careful review of several reports that ranked publications by citation index and number[1-5]
2. Recently published surveys from members of the American Council of Academic Plastic Surgeons and the Southeastern Society of Plastic and Reconstructive Surgeons[6]
3. Interviews with multiple thought leaders in plastic surgery (John McCraw, Leonard Furlow, Wolfgang Losken, Luis and Henry Vasconez, Wyndell Merritt, Ernest Manders, and James Grotting)
4. Frank McDowell's *Source Book of Plastic Surgery,* which includes scores of original manuscripts from the nineteenth and early twentieth century[7]

These reviews were put into a more or less standard format so that the reader can become familiar with the methods, results, limitations, and implications of each paper. I have also added a short reference list for each review, to serve as a springboard for further inquiry. Additionally, I was able to obtain commentaries from 27 original authors, supplemented by expert reflections and editorial perspectives.

My only regret is that we could not include any more papers beyond our top 50, because the next 50 were almost as provocative, exciting, and/or influential. I would like to apologize specifically to Sir Archibald McIndoe, a professional hero of mine, who was inspired by the landmark advances in facial reconstruction developed by his cousin, Sir Harold Gillies, to devise multiple techniques of burn reconstruction for the treatment of pilots injured in World War II.

My own knowledge of the history of plastic surgery increased dramatically over the course of this project, and my belief that innovation is our core competency was only strengthened. However, I also learned that Sir Isaac Newton was partly wrong: Indeed, we do stand on the shoulders of giants, who have passed on information and insight to succeeding generations, but this only leads to incremental progress. Plastic surgery is largely driven, though, by disruptive innovation, which can stimulate radical and abrupt change. The development of modern plastic surgery has unfolded more like the punctuated equilibrium of Stephen Jay Gould than the glacial change of Charles Darwin's selective evolution. Our specialty is defined by, and dependent on, the paradigm shifts that Thomas Kuhn embraced in *The Structure of Scientific Revolutions*. Rather than progressing through the slow accumulation of knowledge, our specialty is propelled into the future by individuals with remarkable wisdom, courage, and insight. This book is about those individuals and their singular, visionary contributions to our collective body of work.

REFERENCES

1. Zhang WJ, Li YF, Zhang JL, et al. Classic citations in main plastic and reconstructive surgery journals. Ann Plast Surg 71:103-108, 2013.
2. Loonen MP, Hage JJ, Kon M. Plastic surgery classics: characteristics of the 50 top-cited articles in four plastic surgery journals since 1946. Plast Reconstr Surg 121:320e-327e, 2008.
3. Joyce CW, Kelly JC, Carroll SM. The 100 top-cited classic papers in hand surgery. J Plast Surg Hand Surg 48:227-233, 2014.
4. Eberlin KR, Labow BI, Upton J, et al. High-impact articles in hand surgery. Hand 7:157-162, 2012.
5. Joyce CW, Carroll SM. Microsurgery: the top 50 classic papers in plastic surgery: a citation analysis. Arch Plast Surg 41:153-157, 2014.
6. Hultman CS, Friedstat JS. The ACAPS and SESPRS surveys to identify the most influential innovators and innovations in plastic surgery: no line on the horizon. Ann Plast Surg 72:S202-S207, 2014.
7. McDowell F, ed. The Source Book of Plastic Surgery. Baltimore: Williams & Wilkins, 1977.

Acknowledgments

Unlike the singular achievements of many surgeons featured in this book, the book itself is the product of a large team of writers, contributors, editors, and publishers.

First and foremost, I am indebted to the plastic surgery residents of the University of North Carolina, who did most of the research and wrote nearly all of the text. As such, future royalties from this book will be applied to a resident education fund to enhance their learning.

Second, I am very grateful for and humbled by the willingness of our original study authors and subject matter experts to provide reflections on these top 50 papers. Their contributions added distinct value to the project and served to validate our choices regarding which papers to include.

Third, I would like to express my sincere appreciation to Karen Berger for her enthusiasm about publishing such a book, Sue Hodgson and Megan Fennell for managing the editorial process, Idelle Winer for transforming our manuscript into polished pages, Brenda Bunch for designing the cover, and Ted Hobgood for his expertise in helping to select the best fonts.

Finally, I need to thank my own professional giants who have lifted me up, to see the world from their perspective. George Sheldon taught me how to think three steps ahead; Maurice "Josh" Jurkiewicz showed me that plastic surgery really was "problem solving" and "general surgery done well"; and John Bostwick consistently demonstrated the interconnectedness of art and science, form and function, principles and techniques. Anthony Meyer, one of plastic surgery's greatest advocates, continues to represent the highest level of integrity any professional can espouse.

C. Scott Hultman

Contents

Section One Foundations

Section Two Hand Surgery

Section Three   Craniofacial Surgery

Section Four   Head and Neck Reconstruction

Section Five   Breast Reconstruction

Section Six   Microsurgery

Section Seven   Trunk Reconstruction

Section Eight   Burn Surgery

Section Nine   Aesthetic Surgery

Section Ten   Innovations

50 STUDIES

every

Plastic Surgeon Should Know

CHAPTER 1

The Use and Uses of Large Split Skin Grafts of Intermediate Thickness

Blair VP, Brown JB. Surg Gynecol Obstet 49:82-97, 1929

Reviewed by Paul DiEgidio, MD

> *Early, quick, and permanent surfacing of burns and other cutaneous defects conserves health, comfort, function, time, and money: while unnecessary waiting spells economic waste.*[1]

Overview   Blair and Brown reported that intermediate (split-) thickness skin grafts can be used successfully to treat a variety of tissue defects. The following is a review of their described techniques, the results of several cases shared by the authors, a discussion about the merits and shortcomings of these techniques, and finally an update on more recent articles and advances based on this original seminal article.

Research Question   What does split-thickness skin grafting contribute to the treatment of scars, cancer reconstruction, thermal, electrical, and radiation burns, large face and neck blemishes, and chronically granulating wound beds?

Funding   Unknown

Study Dates   Late 1920s

Publishing Date   January 1, 1929

Location   Department of Surgery, Washington University School of Medicine, St. Louis, MO

Subjects   Patients with functional or cosmetic deformity with the potential for improvement with or cured by split-thickness skin grafting

Exclusion Criteria   Patients with active skin infection either at the proposed site of harvest, grafting, or remote areas. Patients who had wounds inappropriate for split-thickness skin grafting had:

- Areas where thinner grafts may not provide sufficient protection to a weight-bearing surface
- Wounds with unequal and uneven surfaces where thinner grafts would not correct these inequalities
- Wounds with a movable edge where the graft could cause contraction and further deformity such as the base of the neck

Sample Size   Not applicable

Intervention   The authors used split-thickness skin grafting techniques on an array of pathologies that would benefit from this intervention.

Endpoints   (1) "Take," indicating the percentage of the skin graft surviving the transfer, (2) function, and (3) cosmetic outcome

Technique   The authors approached the description of their techniques in a chronologic fashion divided into seven distinct categories:

1. Preparation of the area to be grafted
2. Preliminary preparation of bare and granulating areas including indolent ulcers
3. Source of the graft
4. Cutting of the graft
5. Application of the grafts
6. Dressings and postoperative care of the graft
7. Dressing and postoperative care of the donor site

Preparation of the area to be grafted.   The first issue raised by the authors was the presence of a skin infection. They strongly recommended that the operation be abandoned not only if there was evidence of an infection at the site of proposed grafting, but also if there were distant infections including "pimples, boils, and impetigo." These pathologies were listed as a contraindication to performing their technique. For the preparation of noninfected areas, the authors concluded "ordinary cleansing care, the removal of all scurf or scales the day before operation, and the use of some antiseptic solution in the operating room are sufficient." Diverse conglomerations of preoperative conditioning techniques including ultraviolet radiation and blood transfusions were also described but are not currently used today.

Preliminary preparation of bare and granulating areas including indolent ulcers.   The recommendations to cleanse "sluggish or dirty" granulation tissue were performed with damp dressing changes "with some sort of an aqueous solution changed every 8 hours, by rest, and by postural control of the return circulation." Three key factors were identified in the preparation of granulating tissue: (1) that the dressing is damp and absorbent, not sloppy or allowed to dry in place; (2) that it is changed sufficiently often; and (3) that it is firmly and comfortably applied. For old granulation tissue or indolent ulcers, they recommended excision down to the deepest layers of the scar base before grafting.

Source of the graft.   The general principles identified for source selection consisted of the following: take the grafts from the areas without inflammation; that the hair-bearing quality of the source be considered because thicker cuts of graft may be likely to grow hair; and that the harvest site be in an area of low cosmetic profile. From these principles they identified "the inner and outer surfaces of the upper half or lower two-thirds of the thigh, the lateral surface of the buttock, and the front of the abdomen. In babies still in diapers, the abdomen is the site of choice."

Cutting of the graft.   Technical considerations included taking enough graft to cover the intended recipient area with a small amount to overlap the skin edges; making as few passes with the knife as possible to avoid grafts of uneven thickness; and holding tension on the skin above and below the knife.

Application of the grafts.   The two key principles identified in the application were to obtain adequate hemostasis and to suture the graft in place under approximated normal tension. The former included suture ligation of visible bleeding vessels and applying pressure with gauze both before and after graft placement to denuded areas with diffuse bleeding not amenable to suture ligation. (Note: this paper was published in 1929 and electrocautery was not in widespread use. Its first application in the operating room was just 27 months earlier on Oct. 1, 1926.[2])

Dressings and postoperative care of the graft.   Four factors emerged as essential in the discussion of dressings and postoperative care: (1) the absence of virulent infection, (2) fixation, (3) pressure, and (4) provision for drainage. The first factor has been discussed previously. The typical dressing for providing fixation and pressure included Xeroform impregnated gauze, then dry gauze, followed by a pressure dressing, including a "liberal" use of adhesive plaster. For uneven surfaces the addition of several large, flat, damp marine sponges were applied over the gauze pads. The first dressing applied in the operating room was left in place from 4 to 10 days with early removal if there was concern about underlying infection, blood clots, or failure of the graft. Wax forms were used for special situations including "within the mouth, on the eyelid, and on the lip" to obtain adequate graft-to-donor site fixation and pressure.

Dressings and postoperative care of the donor site.   The authors identified two factors that may cause pain in greater amounts than anticipated at the donor site: (1) infection and (2) movement of or pulling on the dressing. The authors used a standard dressing that included six layers of Xeroform gauze covered with a flat gauze pad, which was then strapped in placed by adhesive plaster. They believed that plastering the dressing in place would prevent sliding or pulling on the raw surface. An absorbent pad was then placed around this dressing to prevent leaking fluid from entering the wound bed to soak the dressing. They found that removal on the ninth day revealed a "healed" wound. For a dressing that had fallen off before then, they recommended replacement with a damp pressure dressing.

Results   Three specific applications of the technique were addressed in this article beyond the previously discussed general descriptions: the treatment of deep burns, roentgen-ray and radium burns, and large face and neck blemishes.

1. Treatment of deep burns. The authors recommended two treatment options for deep burns: (1) the former was early excision of the burned tissue with immediate grafting, and (2) the latter was early excision with delayed grafting to allow granulation beds to form. The authors advised against a practice of "allowing these wounds to become deeply infected and to granulate and suppurate for months and possibly years before the wounds are covered with hard, distorting, limiting scars which, without later help, cripple the victim throughout life and later are too often the site of cancer." In their experience early excision of deep burns allowed a granulation bed to form within a month, and grafting at this juncture led to healed grafts in place 2 weeks later.

2. Roentgen-ray and radium burns. Radiation burns were treated with excision beyond the areas of endarteritis, telangiectasia, and active keratosis, followed by grafting with full-thickness or split-thickness skin grafts. If deeper excision was required because of scarring, the authors recommended that the graft bed be prepared by excising the dermis down to a thin layer, followed by immediate grafting with split-thickness skin grafts.

3. Large face and neck blemishes. The technique for split-thickness skin grafting for large face or neck blemishes consisted of excision down to the subcutaneous tissue, followed by 3 weeks of granulation preparation. The grafting process was similar to that for burns. The authors described scenarios in which these cosmetically sensitive areas could potentially benefit from skin grafting: oil-filled or dirt-filled abrasions, large nevi or hairy moles, and scars from trauma, acid, or radiation. In addition, they advocated the use of grafting therapy to treat skin damaged from longstanding severe acne or smallpox, because great improvement could be expected from grafting the scar base after superficial excision of the lesions.

Criticisms/Limitations   Early descriptions of surgical techniques could be open to criticism based on what is now known about the topic. However, because Drs. Blair and Brown were pioneers in the field, it is difficult to compare their work with the standard of care at that time (as evidenced by the references in the 1968 reprint in which Dr. Blair was the first and sole author on each of the references[3]).

Relevant Studies   Although this article discusses fundamental principles of modern skin grafting, the use of skin grafts has been around for 2500 to 3000 years. Additional advancements in the field have occurred in the past several decades, including the power-driven dermatome in the 1940s,[4] the introduction of meshed skin grafts by Tanner et al in 1964,[5] and dozens of other innovations to date, making this a readily reproducible procedure with reliable outcomes. Continued research in the field has allowed further discovery and innovation. Medawar's work in immunology helped pioneer the study of acute rejection and second-set rejection of skin xenografts mediated by preformed antibodies.[6]

In 1981 the cultured epithelial autograft (CEA) was introduced as an option for major burn treatment. CEA can be applied as sheets or in an aerosolized liquid suspension commonly referred to as "spray on skin." Although both are limited by cost and time for the CEA to mature (3 to 4 weeks), it remains a viable alternative to allografts in patients with large body surface area burns. Furthermore, recent studies have found that a CEA contains higher levels of growth factors and matrix metalloproteinase when compared with allografts. This could theoretically potentiate better wound healing.[7]

Wound vacuum-assisted closure devices have also been used to assist with skin grafting. A recent review article[8] on their application to skin grafts concluded the following benefits:
- Active stimulation of epithelial mitosis; the authors concluded this was from mechanical stretch stimulating release of growth factors and increased microcirculatory flow and angiogenesis.
- Prevention of complications from shearing, hematomas, edema, and exudates; the review article also stated an average take rate of 95% compared with the 70% to 85% seen with traditional bolster dressings.

Temporary Dressings   Xenograft use in modern medicine focuses on porcine acellular dermal matrix. Used as a temporary dressing, the xenograft sloughs off as the dermis epithelializes underneath. The addition of silver nitrate adds an antimicrobial component to these dressings. The use of xenografts decreases the need for dressing changes. An allograft ordinarily refers to human cadaveric split-thickness grafts and can be used to cover large areas of excised burns or other wounds in which an autograft may not be available. An immune response to foreign tissue typically rejects the graft in 2 to 3 weeks, during which time dermal regeneration has taken place beneath. The allograft will rarely become incorporated into the host. Previously described benefits of an allograft include decreased length of stay, improved epithelialization, and decreased hypertrophic scars; however, its routine use is limited by availability.[9]

Although wound care of the donor site has been a topic of great debate ever since the publication of the initial articles on skin grafting, no dressing has proved superior in the healing rate and quality, pain, infection, and cost. Further research on the topic is needed.[10]

Summary   The basic principles described here still hold true today. Modern advancements provide a convenience; however, without these newer additions, the aforementioned techniques described by Drs. Blair and Brown still provide a good option to cover a variety of tissue deficits.

REFERENCES

1. Blair VP, Brown JB. The use and uses of large split skin grafts of intermediate thickness. Surg Gynecol Obstet 49:82-97, 1929.
2. Massarweh NN, Cosgriff N, Slakey DP. Electrosurgery: history, principles, and current and future uses. J Am Coll Surg 202:520-530, 2006.
3. Blair VP, Brown JB. The use and uses of large split skin grafts of intermediate thickness. Plast Reconstr Surg 42:65-75, 1968.
4. Ratner D. Skin grafting. From here to there. Dermatol Clin 16:75-90, 1998.
5. Tanner JC Jr, Vandeput J, Olley JF. The mesh skin graft. Plast Reconstr Surg 34:287-292, 1964.
6. Simpson E. Reminiscences of Sir Peter Medawar: in hope of antigen-specific transplantation tolerance. Am J Transplant 4:1937-1940, 2004.
7. Allouni A, Papini R, Lewis D. Spray-on-skin cells in burns: a common practice with no agreed protocol. Burns 39:1391-1394, 2013.
8. Azzopardi EA, Boyce DE, Dickson WA, et al. Application of topical negative pressure (vacuum-assisted closure) to split-thickness skin grafts: a structured evidence-based review. Ann Plast Surg 70:23-29, 2013.
9. Lineen E, Namias N. Biologic dressing in burns. J Craniofac Surg 19:923-928, 2008.
10. Voineskos SH, Ayeni OA, McKnight L, et al. Systematic review of skin graft donor-site dressings. Plast Reconstr Surg 124:298-306, 2009.
11. Reverdin JL. Greffe épidermique—expérience faite dans le service de M. le docteur Guyon, à l'hôpital Necker. Bull Soc Imp de Chir de Paris 10:511-515, 1869.
12. Lawson G. On the transplantation of portions of skin for the closure of large granulating surfaces. Trans Clin Soc Lond 4:49, 1871.
13. Ollier LXEL. Sur les greffes cutanées ou autoplastiques. Bull Acad Med Paris 1:243, 1872.
14. Thiersch C. Ueber die feineren anatomischen veranderungen bei aufheilung von haut auf granulationen. Verhandl Deutsch Gesellch Chir Berlin 3:69, 1874.
15. Wolfe JR. A new method of performing plastic operations. Br Med J 2:360, 1875.
16. Krause F. [The translation of large unpedicled skin flaps] Verhandl Deutsch Gesellch Chir Berlin 22:46, 1893.
17. Lanz O. Die transplantation betreffend. Zentralblatt fur Chirurgie 35:3, 1908.

EDITORIAL PERSPECTIVE

C. Scott Hultman, MD, MBA, FACS

Although Blair and Brown were certainly not the first surgeons to report on the use of skin grafts, this 1929 paper marks the beginning of the modern skin graft. The authors established unequivocally that large sheets of skin could be harvested to cover many types of complex wounds and provide definitive healing. The insight that Blair and Brown communicated is that donor areas from split grafts healed from the deeper epithelium that lines the sebaceous glands and hair follicles rather than from the remnants of surface epithelium. Such a discovery allowed the surgeon to harvest dermis with the epidermis, which forever changed how skin grafts were procured and improved the mechanical and biologic properties of transplanted skin.

Plastic surgeons should know the history of skin grafting partly because this procedure remains one of the most commonly performed methods to obtain stable wound closure. More important, however, the evolution of skin grafting represents a fascinating process of incremental innovation, marked by periods of intermittent refinement, relative stagnation, and sometimes failure, followed by bursts of creativity that advanced the technique.

For the record:

    1869: Reverdin reports on the use of epidermal grafts or "seeds of skin" to close a wound on the forearm.[11]
    1871: Lawson harvests full-thickness skin grafts from the brachial region to cover ulcers of the lower extremity and eyelid defects.[12]
    1872: Ollier publishes the first account of intermediate split-thickness skin grafting with large "dermoepidermal" strips.[13]
    1874: Thiersch stresses the importance of wound bed preparation, including the excision of scar and granulation tissue, before skin grafting.[14]
    1875: Wolfe notes that the removal of all fat from the undersurface of full-thickness skin grafts improves graft take.[15]
    1893: Krause demonstrates the ability to skin graft muscle, fascia, and bone and stresses the importance of graft compression and immobilization to optimize take.[16]
    1908: Lanz develops the process of meshing skin grafts to increase their potential surface area.[17]
Late 1930s: Padgett invents the rotary drum dermatome.

CHAPTER 2

The Theory and Practical Use of the Z-incision for the Relief of Scar Contractures

Davis JS, Kitlowski EA. Ann Surg 109:1001-1015, 1939

Reviewed by Yuen-Jong Liu, MD

The purpose of this communication is to again call attention to a maneuver which for many years has been most useful to us when dealing with contracted scars . . . The operative procedure of the Z-plastic is simpler than other methods for relaxing scar contractures; tissues are successfully utilized which would otherwise be discarded; . . . contractions can be permanently relieved by this method which would be difficult or impractical to correct by skin grafting.[1]

Background   The ideal soft tissue reconstruction starts with the removal of all scar tissue. However, this may be impractical in contracted scars, particularly in burn wounds and inner joint spaces, where the scar tissue may be so extensive that its excision would leave inadequate soft tissue for closure and the wound bed may not reliably support grafting. When a contracted band of scar tissue that limits the range of motion across a joint is present, the technique known as *Z-plasty* can release tension in the direction of the contraction by taking laxity from the orthogonal direction.[1]

Technique   The Z-plasty uses a Z or reversed-Z incision. Fig. 2-1 illustrates the steps of the tissue transposition, wherein the central axis of the incision CD is elongated at the expense of shortening the orthogonal axis AB.

The Z incision (*A*) is made with equal lengths, AC, CD, and DB and 60 degrees at X and Y. The incision may be flipped horizontally to make a reverse-Z incision. The central axis of the Z, between points C and D, lies along the contracted scar that is to be lengthened. The corners of the incision together ACBD make a rhombus. The incision is made in the skin (*B*), and triangular flaps are elevated under AXD and CYB. The corners X and Y should be rounded to avoid creating tissue ischemia at the very tip of the corners. The two triangular flaps are transposed (*C*), pulling points A and B closer

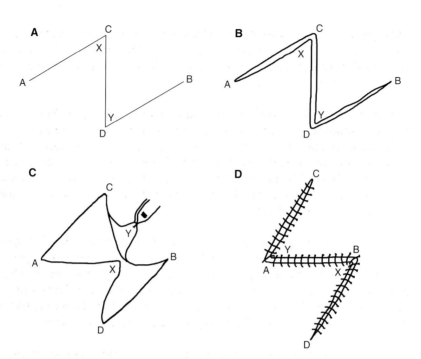

Fig. 2-1 Z-plasty technique. (Adapted from Davis JS, Kitlowski, EA. The theory and practical use of the Z-incision for the relief of scar contractures. Ann Surg 109:1001-1015, 1939.)

and releasing more distance between C and D. The wound is sutured (*D*) such that X has been transposed from C to B and Y has been transposed from D to A.

In theory, the Z incision should be made with equal length along each edge, AC, CD, and DB, and 60-degree angles at X and Y. The corners ACBD thus form a rhombus that consists of two equilateral triangular flaps AXD and CYB that are transposed. In practice, variations can be made depending on the surface contour and laxity of the tissue in the direction orthogonal to the contracted scar. As the angles at X and Y increase, more elongation can be achieved along the contracted scar CD while corners A and B are also pulled closer together with a degree of rotation.[1]

Anesthesia is best achieved if the patient is under general or regional anesthesia. Local infiltration of anesthetic solution risks the viability of the transposition flaps, which already bear scar tissue.

Results   The Z-plasty has optimal results in skin with normal texture in which there is congenital tethering or webbing, such as in the neck or popliteal space or in patients with syndactyly. However, unscarred skin webs are uncommon, and the Z-plasty is most frequently applied to heavily scarred tissues such as burn wounds.[1] The technique may also be used to reposition anatomic landmarks that have healed in poor alignment, such as the eyebrows, eyelids, and oral commissures.

Generally, the Z-plasty enjoys considerable success. In patients in whom the use of the Z-plasty has not sufficiently released the tissue along a contracted scar, the incision may be allowed to heal over 6 months. After the new scar heals and becomes revascularized, the Z-plasty may be reapplied. Massaging and stretching may encourage the scarred tissue to soften and facilitate additional transposition. In children the procedure may also be repeated along a contracted scar if it does not grow or stretch at the same rate as the surrounding native tissue.[1]

Discussion   The earliest reported use of the Z-plasty was by Denonvilliers[2] in 1856. In 1931 Davis wrote a thorough historical review of reported uses of the technique, which appeared to have been developed independently on multiple occasions.[3] In his index paper[1] Davis wrote the first systemic geometric analysis and popularized the technique. More recently, Rohrich and Zbar[4] proposed an algorithm for the implementation of the Z-plasty and integrated the concept of relaxed skin tension lines.

The Z-plasty is a versatile, local transposition flap that relieves tension along closed scarred wounds. In an existing or anticipated soft tissue defect, other local transposition flaps may be used. The rhombic flap, also known as the *Limberg flap,* is often useful when the simple fusiform excision of a skin lesion followed by primary closure results in excessive tension, particularly along the short axis.[5] Generalization of the rhombic flap with rounded corners results in the slide-swing plasty.[6]

These techniques are often used on the face, where the skin has less mobility and laxity. Local transposition flaps avoid the use of skin grafts, which are more visually apparent in such a cosmetically sensitive area. Whereas the rhombic flap and slide-swing plasty recruit skin by rotation, the V-Y advancement flap recruits skin by translation, with favorable outcomes on the forehead, nose, and cheeks.[7] Skin defects of the eyelid require special attention because of the importance of preserving coverage of the eye and avoiding or treating ectropion. Here the simplest reconstruction is a rotation flap, which either moves the skin medially from the lateral cheek or moves the skin laterally from the glabella.[8]

The Z-plasty is frequently useful to release contracted scars in the hand, where contractures limit mobility in the numerous joints. Burn scars in the web space and syndactyly can be treated with repeated application of the Z-plasty. Other techniques, such as the STARplasty, are also useful to relieve contracted web spaces.[9]

REFERENCES

1. Davis JS, Kitlowski EA. The theory and practical use of the Z-incision for the relief of scar contractures. Ann Surg 109:1001-1015, 1939.
2. Denonvilliers C. Blépharoplastie. Bull Soc Chir Paris 7:243, 1856.
3. Davis JS. The relaxation of scar contractures by means of the Z-, or reversed Z-type incision: stressing the use of scar infiltrated tissues. Ann Surg 94:871-884, 1931.
4. Rohrich RJ, Zbar RI. A simplified algorithm for the use of Z-plasty. Plast Reconstr Surg 103:1513-1517, 1999.
5. Borges AF. The rhombic flap. Plast Reconstr Surg 67:458-466, 1981.
6. Schrudde J, Petrovici V. The use of slide-swing plasty in closing skin defects: a clinical study based on 1,308 cases. Plast Reconstr Surg 67:467-481, 1981.
7. Zook EG, Van Beek AL, Russell RC, et al. V-Y advancement flap for facial defects. Plast Reconstr Surg 65:786-797, 1980.
8. Mustardé JC. The use of flaps in the orbital region. Plast Reconstr Surg 45:146-150, 1970.
9. Hultman CS, Teotia S, Calvert C, et al. STARplasty for reconstruction of the burned web space: introduction of an alternative technique for the correction of dorsal neosyndactyly. Ann Plast Surg 54:281-287, 2005.

EDITORIAL PERSPECTIVE

C. Scott Hultman, MD, MBA, FACS

Albert Einstein is often quoted as saying, "Compound interest is the most powerful force in the universe." I would argue that the Z-plasty is the most powerful force in plastic surgery.

CHAPTER 3

Surgical Replacement of the Breast

Gillies H. Proc R Soc Med 52:597-602, 1959

Reviewed by Anna F. Tyson, MD, MPH

This plea for the replacement of the breast contour after excision is presented for what it is worth to the surgeon and to the patient. It has for its object the removal of the tell-tale scar, a constant reminder of her disaster, and creation of a make-believe substitute. Reconstruction of the mammary prominence is indicated after local or radical removal, after atrophy following radiation, or when the gland has failed to develop. It is difficult to appreciate the amount of psychological trauma such a loss entails on the female outlook.[1]

Research Question   Can breast reconstruction be accomplished with the autologous tissue of tubed pedicled flaps, introducing new tissues from a distance?

Historical Context   Sir Harold Gillies,[2] one of the prominent pioneers of early reconstructive surgery, is in many respects the founder of the modern field of plastic surgery. Born in New Zealand in 1882, he was educated at Cambridge and received his surgical training at St. Bartholomew's Hospital in London.[2] Originally trained as an ear, nose and throat surgeon, his career trajectory changed dramatically with the onset of the First World War.[3] Gillies was sent to France with the Red Cross and placed into service with Auguste Valadier, an informally trained practitioner with a special interest in facial reconstruction.[2] Valadier's groundbreaking work with jaw reconstruction sparked Gillies' imagination. At the time, few resources and little energy were devoted to reconstructive surgery. However, Gillies persuaded the War Office to open the first hospital devoted to the treatment of facial injuries, even going so far as to distribute preprinted address labels to facilitate the delivery of patients to his hospital.[2,4]

Much of Gillies' early surgical work involved the treatment of complex burn and blast injuries sustained during the war. In particular, he popularized use of the tube pedicle flap.[2,5] Before antibiotics, the exposed surface of a flap almost invariably became infected, resulting in high complication and failure rates. By wrapping the flap into a tube and suturing the exposed edges together, surgeons were able to protect the exposed surface during the period of vascularization. The use of a tube pedicle flap was first described in the medical literature by a Ukrainian ophthalmologist, Vladimir Filatov.[5] However, Gillies likely discovered the tube pedicle flap independently because this previous report was published in a Russian language ophthalmology journal. Gillies[1] used tube pedicle flaps extensively in facial reconstruction and later expanded the technique to address the growing field of breast reconstruction.

Funding Not applicable

Study Dates 1942, 1946, 1951, and 1958

Publishing Date 1959

Location London, England

Overview of Design This highlighted case series describes a novel approach to breast reconstruction with the use of a tube pedicle flap from periumbilical skin and fat. The author first explains the necessity of the new procedure and outlines the limitations of previous procedures. He then answers several questions about the timing of reconstruction in the setting of mastectomy for breast cancer. He illustrates the procedure in a series of drawings, including the timing between intervals. Finally, he presents four case reports of female patients who underwent staged reconstruction with tube pedicle flaps from the periumbilical region.

Intervention Breast reconstruction with a tube pedicle flap begins at the initial mastectomy. In the initial stage the pedicle is prepared, creating a 6-inch by 3-inch straight flap that extends from the anterior axillary line toward the umbilicus. A circular "pancake" flap, measuring 6 inches in diameter, is drawn surrounding the umbilicus. The pedicle is raised, and the exposed edges are sutured together, forming a 6-inch long tube (Fig. 3-1). The donor site is closed primarily or grafted. The surgeon then allows 2 weeks for the pedicle to mature. During the second stage, the "pancake" flap is partially raised, leaving a 2-inch base at the medial edge (Fig. 3-2). After waiting 1 additional week, the surgeon returns to the operating room to complete the flap excision and implant the "pancake" flap at the breast site. The pedicle remains attached to its lateral mooring (Fig. 3-3). The abdominal defect is closed primarily or with a skin graft. The surgeon then waits 3 weeks for the flap to become well vascularized. During the final stage of the procedure, the pedicle is divided and the breast mound is constructed (Fig. 3-4). The excess pedicle may be used to enhance the breast mound if needed. With proper positioning, the umbilicus is fashioned into a nipple, with cartilage or other implantable material used to provide prominence. The full procedure takes 5 to 6 weeks to complete and leaves some secondary defect and scarring on the abdomen. However, the final product provides an acceptable restoration of the breast mound and a near-symmetrical chest.

A

B

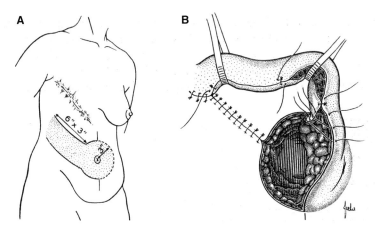

Fig. 3-1   A, Plan and incision. **B,** Pedicle tubed to midline. Donor area closed or grafted. *Wait two weeks.* (From Gillies H. Surgical replacement of the breast. Proc R Soc Med 52:597-602, 1959.)

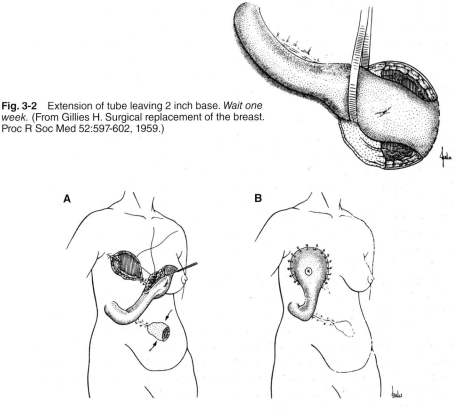

Fig. 3-2   Extension of tube leaving 2 inch base. *Wait one week.* (From Gillies H. Surgical replacement of the breast. Proc R Soc Med 52:597-602, 1959.)

A

B

Fig. 3-3   A, Freeing of medial end of flap. Excision of scar. **B,** Implantation in mammary position. *Wait three weeks.* (From Gillies H. Surgical replacement of the breast. Proc R Soc Med 52:597-602, 1959.)

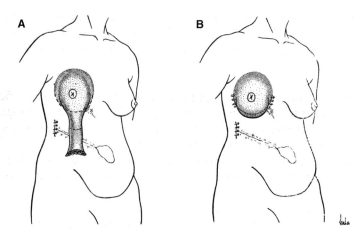

Fig. 3-4   A, Division of pedicle. **B,** Skin and fat fitted in. (From Gillies H. Surgical replacement of the breast. Proc R Soc Med 52:597-602, 1959.)

Endpoints   The management of breast cancer has changed dramatically over the years.[6] When Halsted first introduced the radical mastectomy in 1889, many surgeons feared that reconstruction of the breast would hide a recurrence.[6,7] Ultimately, these fears were unfounded, but these beliefs delayed the acceptance and advancement of breast reconstruction. Early surgeons obtained coverage with the use of split-thickness or full-thickness skin grafts or local advancement flaps, although these solutions often resulted in undue tension, contracture, and disfigurement.[5,6] In the early twentieth century, European surgeons attempted true reconstruction with musculocutaneous flaps from the latissimus dorsi or pectoral muscles.[7,8] Although effective to some degree, many of these procedures were extensive and deforming.[8]

Gillies' popularization of the tube pedicle flap after World War I led to multiple variations in pedicle flap reconstruction. In the 1940s and 1950s, surgeons used pedicle flaps from the contralateral breast, abdomen, or buttocks to create breast mounds, with mixed results.[5,8] Gillies' use of the tube pedicle flap from the periumbilical region allowed acceptable reconstruction with minimal secondary deformity.[8] Although still time-consuming and prone to flap failure, this work paved the way for future improvements in breast reconstruction.[7]

As breast reconstruction gained in popularity and acceptance, improved cosmesis became a top priority. Technologic developments beginning in the 1960s allowed silicone implants and tissue expanders to increase in size and improve symmetry. The 1970s saw the reintroduction of flap reconstruction with the latissimus dorsi muscle with much better results because of improved infection control and surgical technique.[7] Gillies' use of abdominal tissue for reconstruction was revisited in 1982 when

Hartrampf, Schlefan, and Black introduced the pedicled transversely oriented abdominal musculocutaneous (TRAM) flap.[7] The TRAM flap has remained popular, and advances in microsurgery have now allowed free TRAM flap reconstruction, further improving cosmesis.

Breast cancer remains one of the most common cancers in the world and affects thousands of women every year. Breast reconstruction affords the woman the opportunity for psychological recovery. Advances in the detection and treatment have allowed more conservative surgical management and improved cosmetic results. In the future we will continue to refine our technique, but we should not lose sight of the foundation of breast reconstruction, which was begun by the early pioneers of plastic surgery.

Summary   Sir Harold Gillies' work during the First World War and the years after was instrumental in the recognition of plastic surgery as a specialty. His introduction of the tube pedicle flap revolutionized the field of reconstructive surgery and set the stage for our current use of distant musculocutaneous flaps for breast reconstruction.

Implications   Sir Harold Gillies' contributions to the field of plastic surgery were not limited to technical innovation. His determination to achieve good cosmetic and functional results and his insistence that reconstructive surgery is important for a patient's psychological recovery opened many doors in the acceptance of plastic surgery as a bona fide specialty.[3] His collaboration with dentists, physicians, radiologists, and artists set the stage for the formation of the multidisciplinary team.[2] Gillies' dedication to his patients and enthusiasm about the art and science of plastic surgery made him a favorite among his students and peers.

Gillies was also instrumental in the initiation of international collaborative meetings. As early as 1923, he helped organize meetings between American, British, and French surgeons, and in the 1930s, he was one of the founding members of the society that eventually became the International Confederation of Plastic and Reconstructive Surgeons.[3] This collaboration between plastic surgeons across countries was invaluable in gaining official recognition of the specialty.[3]

In the years after Gillies death in 1960, former students and colleagues paid tribute to his many teachings. His "commandments," which outlined the principles of plastic surgery, are repeated, revered, and obeyed even today.[1,2] Among them he stressed the importance of careful observation, thorough planning, and meticulous postoperative care.[9] His adage "never do today what can honourably be put off until tomorrow" has proved sound not only in plastic surgery but also in other fields.[2,9] His instruction to "replace what is normal in a normal position and retain it there" has become a tenet of reconstructive surgery.[2,10]

REFERENCES

1. Gillies H. Surgical replacement of the breast. Proc R Soc Med 52:597-602, 1959.
2. Shastri-Hurst N. Sir Harold Gillies CBE, FRCS: the father of modern plastic surgery. Trauma 14:179-187, 2011.
3. Bamji A. Sir Harold Gillies: surgical pioneer. Trauma 8:143-156, 2006.
4. Matthews DN. Gillies: mastermind of modern plastic surgery. Br J Plast Surg 32:68-77, 1979.
5. Santoni-Rugiu P, Sykes PJ. Skin Flaps. A History of Plastic Surgery. New York: Springer-Verlag, 2007.
6. Losken A, Jurkiewicz MJ. History of breast reconstruction. Breast Dis 16:3-9, 2002.
7. Uroskie TW, Colen LB. History of breast reconstruction. Semin Plast Surg 18:65-69, 2004.
8. Edgerton MT. Breast reconstruction after radical mastectomy. South Med J 60:719-723, 1967.
9. FitzGibbon GM. The commandments of Gillies. Br J Plast Surg 21:226-239, 1968.
10. Millard DR Jr. Jousting with the first knight of plastic surgery. Br J Plast Surg 25:73-82, 1972.

EXPERT COMMENTARY

Michelle C. Roughton, MD

> *Plastic surgery is a perpetual battle of beauty versus blood supply.*
> —Sir Harold Gillies

This quote was a favorite of Dr. Larry Gottlieb during my plastic surgery training at the University of Chicago. He was an unabashed admirer of one of the founding fathers of plastic surgery, Sir Harold Gillies. Gillies was a surgeon during World War I, a war in which defensive trench warfare became prevalent. Heads exposed over the trench were at risk of injury. The wearing of helmets grew in popularity, which allowed improved survival. As a result, soldiers sustained and survived facial trauma in increasing numbers. Gillies described and popularized early head and neck reconstruction and the unmatched value of forehead flaps for nasal reconstruction. His tube pedicle flaps incorporate the fundamental principles of plastic surgery such as the "delay phenomenon" and "replacing like-with-like." Plastic surgery is a discipline that is known for problem-solving and progress. Improved survival in warfare even today has opened the door for innovation such as limb and face transplant and prosthetics that were just fantasy in the day of Sir Gillies.

CHAPTER 4

Clinical Definition of Independent Myocutaneous Vascular Territories

McCraw JB, Dibbell DG, Carraway JH. Plast Reconstr Surg 60:341-352, 1977

Reviewed by Shruti C. Tannan, MD

Compound muscle—skin flaps should, by derivation, be termed 'musculocutaneous' (L. musculus, L. cutis) flaps. The term 'myocutaneous' (Gr. mys, L. cutis) is used for the sake of brevity. Editorial Note [from journal author]: Editors are notoriously reluctant to admit a new hybrid word to their pages. This one was printed only after careful consideration of the pros and cons, and with no great sense of joy.[1]

Research Question What is the area of viable muscle and skin supplied by the dominant vascular pedicles of myocutaneous flaps? What anatomic areas can each myocutaneous flap reconstruct and how is this determined?

Funding Unknown

Study Dates 1970s

Publishing Date September 1977

Location Department of Plastic Surgery, Eastern Virginia Medical School, Norfolk, VA, and Division of Plastic Surgery, University of Wisconsin Medical School, Madison, WI

Subjects Patients with complex wounds with prior vascular insults requiring new blood supply, large defects requiring soft tissue bulk, or coverage of vital structures

Sample Size 161 patients

Design Observational study reporting the myocutaneous vascular territories, axis of rotation, and arc of each flap as observed during clinical applications

Results   This study very elegantly characterizes the vascular territories of the myocutaneous flaps listed in Table 4-1.[1]

In their results the authors systematically discuss each flap, with the typical cutaneous dimensions, pedicle entry point into the muscle, subsequent "axis of rotation" of the flap, and the anatomic areas that can be reconstructed with the flap within its "arc" or reach. Their table organizes a concise summary of their clinical findings, along with the authors' observations regarding the sensation of the flap after transposition and donor site functional loss.

Table 4-1   Myocutaneous Vascular Territories

Flap	Dimensions	Axis	Arc	Sensation	Functional Loss
Sternomastoid	6 × 24 cm	6-7 cm below mastoid	Midline lip, malar area, temporal fossa	Poor	Moderate
Upper trapezius	7 × 35 cm (one delay)	5 cm below mastoid	Anterior floor mouth, tonsil, nasolabial fold, temporal fossa, opposite shoulder, and mastoid	None	Minimal
Latissimus	12 × 35 cm	Posterior axillary fold	Sternum, clavicle, upper anterior, and posterior chest	Poor	Minimal
Lower sacrospinalis	10 × 20 cm	5 cm lateral to L4	Upper sacrum, T12 midline	Poor	None
Upper rectus abdominis (island)	3-30 × 28 cm	Xyphoid	Axilla, clavicle, sternum	None	Minimal
Thoracoepigastric	12 × 30 cm	Lateral rectus fascia at intercostal margin	Midsternum, anterior chest wall, axilla	Poor	None
Lower rectus abdominis (island)	4-15 × 20 cm	Pubic tubercle	Perineum, anterior spine, iliac crest	None	Minimal
Upper ½ sartorius	6 × 16 cm	8 cm below inguinal ligament	Pubis, anterior spine, iliac crest	Poor	None
Lower ½ sartorius	6 × 20 cm	Hunter's canal	Tibial tubercle, popliteal fossa	None	None
Rectus femoris	7 × 40 cm	7 cm below inguinal ligament	Umbilicus, greater trochanter, opposite pubic tubercle	Good	Moderate, terminal knee extension
Gracilis	6 × 24 cm	6-7 cm below pubic tubercle	Suprapubic, perineum, mid-sacrum, anterior spine iliac crest	Fair	None
Biceps femoris long head	12 × 35 cm	8 cm below ischium	Perineum, ischium	Normal	Minimal (except running)
Gastrocnemius (medial or lateral head)	8 × 30-35 cm	Tibial tubercle	Upper ½ calf, knee, popliteal fossa, lower femur	Poor	Minimal (except running)

From McCraw JB, Dibbell DG, Carraway JH. Clinical definition of independent myocutaneous vascular territories. Plast Reconstr Surg 60:341-352, 1977.

In addition to the systematic discussion of each flap's vascular territory and the potential clinical applications, the authors present three cases in which select myocutaneous flaps were used to reconstruct complex defects requiring well-vascularized tissue and durable skin coverage. A rectus femoris flap was used to reconstruct the abdominal wall, a sacrospinalis flap was used to cover a radiated back wound, and sensate biceps femoris flaps were elevated and used to successfully reconstruct a neovagina.

Criticisms/Limitations   This is an observational study and as such does not include postoperative follow-up or details regarding the clinical outcomes of the 161 flaps performed.

Relevant Studies   McCraw et al[1] published this article at a time when dissatisfaction with the unreliable results of random pattern cutaneous flaps and the inadequate bulk of axial cutaneous flaps of the day fueled an interest in a bulky, well-vascularized flap with a skin paddle. Although the concept of vascular inflow to the skin traveling through what are now known as musculocutaneous perforators was described by Dr. Tansini in 1906,[2] his work was largely passed over by the surgical community of his time.[3]

McCraw and Dibbell's dog[4] and cadaver injection studies and the paper reviewed in this section[1] revealed the vascular basis of myocutaneous territories. The results of their careful study serve as an anatomic guide for myocutaneous flaps that are critical components of the modern day reconstructive surgeon's armamentarium. Taylor and Palmer[5] subsequently delineated separate angiosomes or the vascular territories of more than 300 perforators, building on the fundamental findings of McCraw et al.

Muscle flaps for pedicled and subsequent free flap transfer were described by Mathes et al[6] and Mathes and Nahai[7,8] as Dr. McCraw was characterizing the cutaneous vascular territories of these muscle flaps. The combined efforts of these surgeons' cadaver and clinical studies[1,4-8] resulted in a comprehensive understanding of the vascular anatomy of muscle flaps and their myocutaneous counterparts, providing increased options for surgeons and their patients.

Summary   In this article the authors define the vascular territories of 13 clinical myocutaneous flaps and present cases in which select flaps were used to successfully reconstruct complex wounds.

REFERENCES

1. McCraw JB, Dibbell DG, Carraway JH. Clinical definition of independent myocutaneous vascular territories. Plast Reconstr Surg 60:341-352, 1977.
2. Tansini I. Sopra il mio nuovo processo di amputatzione della mammilla. Gaz Med Ital 57:141, 1906.
3. Santoni-Rugiu P, Sykes PJ. A History of Plastic Surgery. Berlin: Springer-Verlag, 2007.
4. McCraw JB, Dibbell DG. Experimental definition of independent myocutaneous vascular territories. Plast Reconstr Surg 60:212-220, 1977.
5. Taylor GI, Palmer JH. The vascular territories (angiosomes) of the body: experimental study and clinical applications. Br J Plast Surg 40:113-141, 1987.
6. Mathes SJ, McCraw JB, Vasconez LO. Muscle transposition flaps for coverage of lower extremity defects: anatomic considerations. Surg Clin North Am 54:1337-1354, 1974.
7. Mathes SJ, Nahai F. Classification of the vascular anatomy of muscles: experimental and clinical correlation. Plast Reconstr Surg 67:177-187, 1981.
8. Mathes SJ, Nahai F. Clinical Applications for Muscle and Musculocutaneous Flaps. St Louis: CV Mosby, 1982.

STUDY AUTHOR REFLECTIONS

The Search for Island Myocutaneous Flaps: Interview With
John B. McCraw, MD, FACS, by Shruti C. Tannan, MD, April 2014

Question   You designed and popularized the very first island myocutaneous flap and provided an extensive scientific basis for this concept. What prompted this line of study and research?

Answer   My pursuit of the island myocutaneous flap began in 1967 during my research time as a Duke orthopaedic resident. I was interested in limb replantation since medical school, and Dr. J. Leonard Goldner at Duke was interested in pursuing what is now called composite tissue allotransplantation as a method for the treatment of Volkmann's ischemic contracture. He had the laboratory already set up for me when I arrived, including collaborations with physiology. The physiologists wanted us to design a "sick flap model" in a frog. Interestingly, I raised a rectus femoris flap but it was healthy, and needless to say I was thrilled and the physiologists were upset. My job from then on was to become a muscle expert, and I have worked with many excellent surgeons along the way. I began dissecting cadaver limbs at Duke to learn every muscle and its supplying blood vessels. During this time I realized that these local muscle flaps could be a backup plan for Dr. Goldner's composite tissue transplantation idea, because I knew no institutional review board would ever approve of such an experiment. At Duke I found about 10 flaps I could use to treat the Volkmann's ischemic contracture, but then I realized that to pursue flap surgery, I would need to enter the plastic surgery field. I was introduced to Dr. Peacock and through him to Dr. Jurkiewicz and went on to train with him in Florida. I then followed him to Emory when he started a program there in July 1972. Steve Mathes was a third-year general surgery resident at the time, and he would obtain limbs that we would dissect together. I showed him the flaps that I had pursued years before. I still remember when I did the first myocutaneous flap and presented it to Dr. J on rounds. This lady had a bad radiation wound, and I used a gluteal myocutaneous flap to cover it, but the large back cut on the skin gave it away that the main blood supply was coming through the muscle. This was very contrary to the thinking at the time, and Dr. J immediately said there is something different about this flap, John. P.G. Arnold and I studied these flaps, and we then decided we would like to make a color atlas of the flaps, but we wanted to wait until we had more patients and more data. The Air Force Base in San Antonio is where I had that experience with most of the patients in the 1977 paper included in this book. Although I did all of the laboratory work, Dave Dibbell, with whom I worked in San Antonio, was equally responsible for developing the concepts and clinical use of these flaps. In the Air Force and for many years later, Dave and I had lengthy talks, in person or on the phone, almost every day. I have said many times that Dave Dibbell gave me a wonderful 1-year residency in myocutaneous flaps at Wilford Hall. Let me explain.

Tansini in 1906 did cadaver studies with the help of his pathologist to better understand the blood supply of the latissimus myocutaneous flap, which he first described in 1896. He completely understood the vascular distribution of vessels in and around the axilla. Although he did not create a pure "island" (dangling vessel) flap because he left a cutaneous bridge, he recognized that the latissimus dorsi muscle enhanced the viable length of the vertical, proximally based skin flap that he used, and he treated the vessels as island vessels.

Just as valuable to plastic surgery was his understanding of the fascia and network of vessels supplying this flap. It was commonly believed by practicing plastic surgeons until the arrival of myocutaneous flaps in the 1970s that the fascia acted as a "parasite" to skin flaps. The fascia was thought to contribute bulk to already fatty flaps and detracted from the blood supply of skin flaps. Tansini recognized the value of the fascia in skin flaps as an extra source of the blood supply, and he probably observed the small vessels on the surface of the fascia, if I had to guess.

In Tansini's paper you will see several "x's" in the distal skin flap. The skin distal to the x's would not have survived without the attached latissimus muscle. Tansini was clearly the "father" of myocutaneous flaps and the only other person to experimentally study the blood supply of a myocutaneous flap.

I am reasonably sure that no one else did what Tansini did with myocutaneous flaps or published it before our 1977 paper. As late as 1976, I know personally that Nick Georgiade, the originator of the thigh flap, thought that the thigh flap required a "broad base of skin" to survive. Krizek did a dog experiment to see if skin would support muscle. It did not.

Many surgeons in Europe and the United States used and reported muscle flaps— temporalis, sternocleidomastoid, pectoralis, gracilis, soleus, and gastrocnemius. These reports are cited in our atlas *(McCraw and Arnold's Atlas).* The most important paper on muscle flaps was Kanavel's report in *Surgery, Gynecology & Obstetrics* in 1921. He understood island vessels in most muscles, and he reported a variety of island muscle flaps, including the reversed vastus medialis, rectus femoris, pectoralis, and an inferior rectus abdominis transposed into the pelvis. This report is the first to show the usefulness of island muscle flaps in "rigid cavities," that is, the pelvis and chest.

Nick Georgiade described the total thigh flap in 1954, and Paul Weeks described the total leg flap in 1968. I was inspired by both of these reports, which made it clear to me that island vessels could support both muscle and skin. Orticochea's 1971 to 1972 gracilis myocutaneous flap, which was in actuality an island flap, had a similar effect on me.

Dave Dibbell and I popularized the general use of these myocutaneous flaps—in a sense "packaging" many previous observations into an orderly process. Dave was and is a genius at designing operations. He taught me to plan an operation both in step-by-step and rotational three-dimensions. What Dave found exciting about myocutaneous flaps was their capability to mimic nature in smooth three-dimensions and rotations. I had never thought that way before. His goal was to create one new operation a year. Together we designed one a month or one a week, sitting for hours, visualizing new shapes that never had existed before. After we had developed a new flap reconstruction, we had plenty of chances to replicate it with the huge surgical volume at Wilford Hall.

In 1977 I organized the first Flap Symposium for the Plastic Surgery Educational Foundation (PSEF) in Norfolk. It was unbelievably successful, at least to all the planners. With 500 participants, a faculty of 69, and a microsurgery laboratory, it was the most financially successful PSEF symposium up to that time. The next year P.G. Arnold joined us for the First Norfolk Flap Workshop, extending annually to 1995. More than one third of the U.S. plastic surgeons came to Norfolk for this experience.

By 1980 reports of new flaps crowded the *Plastic and Reconstructive Surgery* journal. P.G. Arnold, Dave Dibbell, Luis Vasconez, Leonard Furlow, John Bostwick, Steve Mathes, Foad Nahai, Jim May, Pat Maxwell, Ian Jackson, Ian McGregor, Bill Futrell, Dennis Hurwitz, and others, including myself, were swept up in a frenzy of radical change in plastic surgery. Some became international stars of distant meetings. We shared willingly because we each learned more than we taught at every meeting. In a matter of months, the random flap, tube flap, delayed flap, and length-width ratio disappeared from plastic surgery consciousness. They were antiques of a distant past. It all started with these two 1977 papers on myocutaneous flaps.

CHAPTER 5

Classification of the Vascular Anatomy of Muscles: Experimental and Clinical Correlation

Mathes SJ, Nahai F. Plast Reconstr Surg 67:177-187, 1981

Reviewed by Ida Janelle Wagner, MD

Five patterns of muscle circulation, based on studies of the vascular anatomy of muscle, are described. Clinical and experimental correlation of this classification is determined by the predictive value of the vascular pattern of each muscle currently useful in reconstructive surgery in regard to the following parameters: arc of rotation, skin territory, distally based flaps, microvascular composite tissue transplantation, and design of muscle-delay experimental models. This classification is designed to assist the surgeon both in choice and design of the muscle and musculocutaneous flap for its use in reconstructive surgery. [1]

Research Question   What are the defined vascular pedicles of superficial muscles, and how can these be classified into a simple, consistent mechanism that can be used both to promote flap planning and communicate flap planning among surgeons?

Funding   Unknown

Study Dates   Based on anatomic studies performed by the authors in the late 1970s to early 1980s

Publishing Date   February 1981

Locations   San Francisco, CA, and Atlanta, GA

Subjects   Not applicable

Exclusion Criteria   Not applicable

Sample Size   Not applicable

Overview of Design   The paper describes a classification system based on previously existing anatomic studies of the vascular anatomy of superficial muscles.

Intervention   Not applicable

Follow-up   Not applicable

Endpoints   Not applicable

Results   All muscles can be classified into one of five categories based on the vascular pedicle blood supply to the muscle.

Criticisms/Limitations   The studies are based on the examinations of cadaver muscle; thus the observations are made in an "adynamic state" and require clinical correlation. A possible alternative would be to perform them by means of computed tomographic angiography or traditional angiography in a live patient.

Summary   Mathes and Nahai make two initial points: (1) Muscle flap success is based on reliable blood supply. (2) All muscles can be categorized into a type of vascular pedicle supply.

The paper then describes five patterns of muscle circulation based on extensive anatomic studies performed by the authors. The methods of studying the muscle vasculature include colored latex vascular injections, latex-barium vessel injections, anatomic dissections, and muscle angiograms. The patterns of circulation are determined by the following five variables: (1) regional source of the arterial pedicles, (2) size, (3) number, (4) location in relation to origin and insertion, and (5) angiographic patterns of internal muscle vessels.

The five patterns of muscle circulation are as follows: type I, one vascular pedicle; type II, dominant vascular pedicle plus minor pedicles; type III, two dominant pedicles; type IV, segmental vascular pedicles; and type V, one dominant vascular pedicle and secondary segmental pedicles.

These classifications have important clinical applications. They help predict muscle arc of rotation for pedicled flaps. Muscles categorized as types I, II, III, and V are able to survive solely on their dominant pedicle and thus are more amenable to rotation or transposition than a type IV flap. In addition, type III muscles have two potential arcs of rotation, given the two dominant pedicles. (They do not comment on the ability of type V flaps to also do this.) Flap classification also aids in the prediction of viable skin territories. Types II, III, and IV muscles are at risk of skin necrosis if distal segmental or minor pedicles are divided, whereas skin survival in type V flaps is robust.

Finally, the classification system aids in the design of flaps. Types II and IV flaps will be poor choices for distally based flaps because not all of the muscle may survive. These flaps may benefit from delay techniques or simply transposing a portion of the muscle closest to the pedicle. Types I, II, and V are recommended for free flap muscle transplantation.

Implications   Open any comprehensive plastic surgery text to the microsurgery section, and one will find the ubiquitous illustration from this landmark paper (Fig. 5-1).

The 1970s and early 1980s saw the emergence of microsurgery as a new discipline. It was a time of rapid discovery and investigation into the multitude of flap options available to reconstruct defects throughout the body. No longer limited by the reach of a local pedicle flap to cover a defect, plastic surgeons now had the entire musculature of the body at their disposal.[1] Lamberty and Cormack[2] describe this "revival in the anatomical basis of flaps, whether they be skin based, muscle based, or fascia based, [as] . . . one of the most significant factors in the huge advance we have seen in reconstructive techniques in the last decade." They proceed to define the 1970s as a critical time in the history of flap design and outlined the history of flaps as follows[2]:

- Distant origins from ancient Egypt through Tagliacozzi to Dieffenbach
- The birth of modern reconstructive surgery, 1900 to 1930
- Skin flaps and the age of the tube, 1930 to 1960
- An anatomical renaissance; the axial skin flap and microsurgery
- The 1970s, decade of the muscle and musculocutaneous flap
- The 1980s, decade of the fasciocutaneous flap

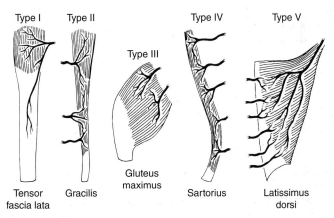

Fig. 5-1   Patterns of vascular anatomy of muscle: type I, one vascular pedicle; type II, dominant pedicle(s) plus minor pedicles; type III, two dominant pedicles; type IV, segmental vascular pedicles; type V, dominant pedicle plus secondary segmental pedicles. (From Mathes SJ, Nahai F. Classification of the vascular anatomy of muscles: experimental and clinical correlation. Plast Reconstr Surg 67:177-187, 1981.)

Stephen Mathes began his research career in the laboratory as an anatomist, investigating muscular vascular anatomy and applying this knowledge clinically as a reconstructive surgeon. Together with Foad Nahai, he completed hours of tedious dissection and anatomic research after operating all day, sometimes working late into the night only to return to the operating room early the next morning.[3] The two surgeon-scientists coauthored a book, *Clinical Atlas of Muscle and Musculocutaneous Flaps,* in 1979, based on this work. It was perfect timing for such a text, given the exploding climate of microsurgery. Mathes and Nahai published a second text, *Reconstructive Surgery: Principles, Anatomy & Technique,* in 1997, which became the seminal work on free flaps known colloquially as "Mathes and Nahai."

The identification of muscular vascular anatomy began in the late 1800s with the work of Carl Manchot, a German anatomist who used cutaneous injection studies to define cutaneous circulation. His work was expanded on by Michel Salmon in the 1930s, whose experimentation included both muscular and cutaneous circulation. Because these texts were published in German and French, respectively, they were largely ignored by the English-speaking world until the 1980s when they were translated into English. In 1919 Campbell and Pennefather[4] published "An Investigation Into the Blood Supply of Muscles With Special Reference to War Surgery," a paper that was meant to aid World War I trauma surgeons in the management of injured soldiers. In 1977 McCraw and Dibbell[5] published dissection and injection studies in cadavers and animated experiments in dogs to determine whether island myocutaneous flaps could be based on individual muscles. Building on the success of this work, McCraw et al[6] went on to define the cutaneous territories of muscles useful in reconstructive surgery. McGregor and Morgan[7] defined axial versus random pattern flaps in 1973. This paper builds on prior anatomic work and precedes the work of Lamberty and Cormack, who defined fasciocutaneous perforator flaps.

In 1982 Mathes et al[8] published a paper detailing the use of myocutaneous flaps in chronic osteomyelitis; they argued that the provision of a robust vascular supply to a wound affected by osteomyelitis is beneficial to wound healing. This concept was a direct clinical application of the outlined classification system of this paper and was used to change the dogma of flap reconstruction in the setting of chronic infection, suggesting that muscle flap reconstruction not only healed the chronic wound but also helped heal the infection that plagued such a wound.

In a letter to *The New England Journal of Medicine* in 1982, which commented on a study published in that edition by May et al, Mathes posed the question—"Does an operation to close an infected wound seem the worst kind of surgical heresy?" Because chronic wounds with osteomyelitis are often hypoxic, he suggested that bringing well-vascularized, axial, musculocutaneous flaps to cover the area helps not only with oxygenation of the skin (flap skin is well perfused by a rich capillary bed) but also to clear a bacterial load. He observed that musculocutaneous flaps "demonstrate superior resistance to necrosis after bacterial inoculation," whereas random pattern flaps undergo skin necrosis after such an inoculation.[9] He spent much of the rest of his career in the laboratory investigating the physiologic mechanisms underlying the superiority of musculocutaneous flaps for use in infected wounds.

This classification of muscle vascular anatomy is pragmatically designed for use in muscle transposition and microvascular transfer for reconstructive purposes. The findings presently indicate that there are five categories of vascular pedicle distribution in superficial musculature, which can be used to devise reconstructive muscle-based flap planning.

REFERENCES

1. Mathes SJ, Nahai F. Classification of the vascular anatomy of muscles: experimental and clinical correlation. Plast Reconstr Surg 67:177-187, 1981.
2. Lamberty BG, Cormack CG. Fasciocutaneous flaps. Clin Plast Surg 17:713-726, 1990.
3. Khan FN, Spiegel AJ. The evolution of perforator flaps. Semin Plast Surg 20:53-55, 2006.
4. Campbell J, Pennefather C. An investigation into the blood-supply of muscles, with special reference to war surgery. Lancet 1:294, 1919.
5. McCraw JB, Dibbell DG. Experimental definition of independent myocutaneous vascular territories. Plast Reconstr Surg 60:212-220, 1977.
6. McCraw JB, Dibbell DG, Carraway JH. Clinical definition of independent myocutaneous vascular territories. Plast Reconstr Surg 60:341-352, 1977.
7. McGregor IA, Morgan G. Axial and random pattern flaps. Br J Plast Surg 26:202-213, 1973.
8. Mathes SJ, Alpert BS, Chang N. Use of the muscle flap in chronic osteomyelitis: experimental and clinical correlation. Plast Reconstr Surg 69:815-828, 1982.
9. Mathes SJ. The muscle flap for management of osteomyelitis. N Engl J Med 306:294-295, 1982.

STUDY AUTHOR REFLECTIONS

Foad Nahai, MD, FACS

In the mid-1970s as a general surgery resident, Stephen Mathes investigated the blood supply of lower extremity muscles. He did this by injecting amputated specimens with latex and then dissecting the muscles. As interest in muscle and musculocutaneous flaps extended beyond the lower limb, Steve and I, as residents, began a search for other possible muscle flaps. This took us first to the anatomy dissection laboratory at Emory in Atlanta, later the anatomy laboratories at Washington University in St. Louis, and finally the morgue at Moffitt Hospital in San Francisco. Steve's preliminary work on the amputated specimens and my own background with a BSc in anatomy had prepared us well for this work. Initially, the dissections were performed on preserved cadavers and concluded with fresh specimens, which were injected with a latex-barium mixture. The fresh injected specimens allowed radiography and intramuscular dissections to further define the vascular supply of muscles.

The dissections led to the realization that there were five typical patterns of vascular supply to the muscles, which were emerging as the most clinically useful for flap transposition. The five types were described and our findings published in *Plastic and Reconstructive Surgery* in 1981. Steve and I were thrilled that at such an early stage in our academic careers our paper won the prestigious James Barrett Brown Award of the American Association of Plastic Surgeons for the best paper published in *Plastic and Reconstructive Surgery* in 1981. We did not realize that the paper and findings would have such a significant impact and that 33 years later would still be relevant and even end up in this book as one of the 50 most important papers in plastic surgery.

Although Steve and I collaborated for years dissecting more specimens, describing the "reconstructive ladder," and writing several more papers and three books, nothing ever matched our excitement over the publication of this paper, its reception, and long-lived relevance. I know Steve would be pleased and honored, as I am, to know that the work is still recognized as a significant contribution to the specialty.

CHAPTER 6

The Carpal-Tunnel Syndrome. Seventeen Years' Experience in Diagnosis and Treatment of Six Hundred Fifty-Four Hands

Phalen GS. J Bone Joint Surg Am 48:211-228, 1966

Reviewed by Ryan M. Garcia, MD, and David S. Ruch, MD

An accurate diagnosis of carpal tunnel syndrome can be made if the wrist-flexion test is positive, Tinel's sign is present over the median nerve at the wrist, and all objective sensory findings are strictly limited to the distribution of the median nerve distal to the wrist. These are the three most reliable clinical findings, and in almost every patient found to have the syndrome at least two of the three findings are present.[1]

Research Question   Phalen reviews the diagnosis and treatment of a large series of patients with carpal tunnel syndrome treated at The Cleveland Clinic. This is a single surgeon's experience (over a 17-year period) treating a large number of patients for a diagnosis that we now see as commonplace.

Funding   Not described

Study Dates   All patients seen and treated for carpal tunnel syndrome before August 1964; this is a report of the author's 17-year experience.

Publishing Date   March 1966

Subjects   All patients were seen and treated for carpal tunnel syndrome before August 1964. Patient ages ranged from 20 to 87 years. The duration of symptoms was less than 6 months in 32% of patients; 41% of patients in this series underwent a cortisone injection, and 40% (177 patients, 212 hands) underwent surgical release of the carpal tunnel.

Exclusion Criteria   Not described

Sample Size   654 hands in 439 patients

Overview of Design   A retrospective case series of patient evaluations and treatment for carpal tunnel syndrome at The Cleveland Clinic over a 17-year period

Intervention   The author first describes that all patients underwent a thorough history regarding their hand. He describes that patients usually present with progressive weakness and clumsiness in the hands, along with an associated hypesthesia and tingling in the median nerve distribution. Hypesthesia was noted in 79% of patients, and 32% reported symptoms for less than 6 months. The author notes that nocturnal symptoms are a frequent complaint, with patients awakened at night by burning pain in the thumb, index, and middle digits. During the physical examination, thenar atrophy was present in 41% of the hands. The wrist-flexion test, which was later called the *Phalen test,* is performed by asking the patient to hold the forearms vertical while allowing both hands to drop into complete flexion at the wrist (Fig. 6-1).[1] This position is held, thus squeezing the median nerve between the proximal edge of the transverse carpal ligament and the contents of the carpal canal. The results of this test were positive in 74% of patients.

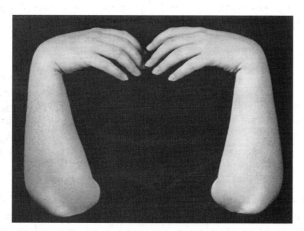

Fig. 6-1   The wrist-flexion test is positive when numbness and paresthesia in the median-nerve distribution in the hand are reproduced or exaggerated by holding the wrists in complete flexion from thirty to sixty seconds. (From Phalen GS. The carpal-tunnel syndrome. Seventeen years' experience in diagnosis and treatment of six hundred fifty-four hands. J Bone Joint Surg Am 48:211-228, 1966.)

The author describes the technique for the injection of steroids into the carpal tunnel, which was performed in 41% of patients (270 wrists). A local anesthetic is mixed with 25 mg of hydrocortisone or a similar amount of triamcinolone or methylprednisolone and then injected medial to the palmaris longus tendon into the carpal tunnel. Prompt and immediate relief of symptoms further supports the diagnosis of carpal tunnel syndrome.

All patients treated surgically (177 patients, 212 hands) underwent an extended open approach to the carpal tunnel. A pneumatic tourniquet is used and local or regional anesthesia is supplied. The author recommends the complete release of the entire transverse carpal ligament and further recommends transaction only under direct vision. The surgical incision is planned with an oblique incision extending from the hypothenar eminence laterally across the base of the palm to the distal flexion crease at the wrist. Exposure allows synovectomy when necessary. The author discourages routine median nerve neurolysis.

Follow-up   Only 12 patients (13 hands) in the surgical group (177 patients, 212 hands) were followed for less than 5 months, which was considered inadequate to determine treatment efficacy. Many patients were reported to have been followed for more than 10 years.

Endpoints   Complication rates, rate of thenar atrophy improvement, rate of hypesthesia improvement, and reoperation rate

Results   The author reported no major complications. Only one patient developed a superficial infection, and one patient developed complex regional pain syndrome, both of which resolved. Two patients underwent a reoperation. One hand had an incomplete release of the transverse carpal ligament, and the other hand required extensive neurolysis and tenolysis. Overall the author noted quicker patient recovery with a shorter initial duration of symptoms; 78% of patients without thenar atrophy and 76% of patients with thenar atrophy before surgery had an excellent result with the return of sensation and function.

Criticisms/Limitations   The article presented is a retrospective study of a nonrandomized patient population of a single surgeon's experience. The article is limited in patient demographics outside of age, occupation, and injury (if present). The outcomes are descriptive with very limited details on functional outcomes outside of sensory or thenar atrophy improvements. The article lacks further details of pain-related and hand-related functional disabilities and capabilities.

Relevant Studies   The article presented was the first to describe the clinical evaluation, diagnosis, and treatment options (surgical and nonsurgical) in a large number of patients with carpal tunnel syndrome. The article highlights a number of possible pathogeneses to explain the development of the condition. Possible etiologies include flexor tenosynovitis, ischemic events, a thickening of the transverse carpal ligament, increased content volume within the carpal canal, traumatic events, and hormonal or congenital causes. Phalen argued that the most likely etiology was a vasodilation and venous-stasis event that occurred at night, which resulted in an engorgement of the flexor synovialis, thus leading to an increased volume in the carpal canal contents. Gelberman et al[2] later scientifically studied the pressures exerted in the carpal canal with a wick catheter in patients with carpal tunnel syndrome and normal control subjects. They demonstrated significantly higher pressure readings in patients with carpal tunnel (32 mm Hg versus 2.5 mm Hg) particularly with wrist flexion (90 mm Hg versus 31 mm Hg) and extension (110 mm Hg versus 30 mm Hg) that was then relieved by carpal tunnel release. The authors from the same group later induced carpal tunnel syndrome in healthy volunteers by increasing tissue fluid pressure while monitoring neurophysiologic changes.[3] They again demonstrated an alteration in nerve viability with pressures between 30 and 60 mm Hg.

Phalen used steroid injections in 41% of patients presented in this article. In a prospective trial, Gelberman et al[4] followed patients for a mean of 18 months to demonstrate the use of a steroid injection for carpal tunnel. Overall they showed that 76% of patients were symptom free at 6 weeks, but this rate fell to 22% at 12 months. Furthermore, they concluded that patients were likely to respond favorably with less relapse to steroid injection if they had mild symptoms, symptoms of less than 1 year duration, normal sensibility, normal thenar strength and mass, and 1 or 2 millisecond prolongations of distal median motor or sensory latencies.

The surgical approach presented by Phalen would currently be considered an extended open approach. With improved surgical equipment and technique, progressively smaller incisions have been used. With this, multiple well-designed clinical trials have been performed to delineate the optimal treatment strategy for patients with carpal tunnel syndrome. An ulnar-based open approach to the carpal tunnel is still commonly used to avoid injury to the recurrent branch of the median nerve. In a classic anatomic description by Lanz,[5] the recurrent branch of the median nerve emerges from the carpal tunnel in an extraligamentous (46%), subligamentous (31%), or transligamentous (23%) fashion. More recent advancements include the minimally invasive endoscopic carpal tunnel release. In a prospective, randomized trial, Agee et al[6] were the first to demonstrate a quicker recovery and an earlier return to work but equal overall outcomes in patients treated by endoscopic release. The following year Brown et al[7] compared the endoscopic two-portal technique with the conventional open approach; they also demonstrated equal outcomes at final follow-up but a quicker recovery, an earlier return to work, and a lower rate of incisional pain in those patients treated with endoscopic release. Finally, Trumble et al[8] confirmed the findings of previous authors in a multicenter, prospective, randomized trial.

Summary   This classic article by Phalen on the diagnosis and treatment of carpal tunnel syndrome continues to have current applications. The wrist-flexion test (Phalen test) is used routinely in the evaluation of patients with median nerve symptoms. The release of the transverse carpal ligament remains one of the most common hand surgery procedures, and patients can routinely expect excellent outcomes.

Implications   The diagnosis and treatment of carpal tunnel syndrome are commonplace in hand surgery. This large series of patients treated both nonoperatively and operatively continues to give insight into the most common hand pathology seen by surgeons.

REFERENCES

1. Phalen GS. The carpal-tunnel syndrome. Seventeen years' experience in diagnosis and treatment of six hundred fifty-four hands. J Bone Joint Surg Am 48:211-228, 1966.

2. Gelberman RH, Hergenroeder PT, Hargens AR, et al. The carpal tunnel syndrome. A study of carpal canal pressures. J Bone Joint Surg Am 63:380-383, 1981.

3. Lundborg G, Gelberman RH, Minteer-Convery M, et al. Median nerve compression in the carpal tunnel—functional response to experimentally induced controlled pressure. J Hand Surg Am 7:252-259, 1982.

4. Gelberman RH, Aronson D, Weisman MH. Carpal-tunnel syndrome. Results of a prospective trial of steroid injection and splinting. J Bone Joint Surg Am 62:1181-1184, 1980.

5. Lanz U. Anatomical variations of the median nerve in the carpal tunnel. J Hand Surg Am 2:44-53, 1977.

6. Agee JM, McCarroll HR Jr, Tortosa RD, et al. Endoscopic release of the carpal tunnel: a randomized prospective multicenter study. J Hand Surg Am 17:987-995, 1992.

7. Brown RA, Gelberman RH, Seiler JG III, et al. Carpal tunnel release. A prospective, randomized assessment of open and endoscopic methods. J Bone Joint Surg Am 75:1265-1275, 1993.

8. Trumble TE, Diao E, Abrams RA, et al. Single-portal endoscopic carpal tunnel release compared with open release: a prospective, randomized trial. J Bone Joint Surg Am 84-A:1107-1115, 2002.

9. Bland JD. Do nerve conduction studies predict the outcome of carpal tunnel decompression? Muscle Nerve 24:935-940, 2001.

10. Katz JN, Losina E, Amick BC III, et al. Predictors of outcomes of carpal tunnel release. Arthritis Rheum 44:1184-1193, 2001.

11. Finson V, Russwurm H. Neurophysiology not required before surgery for typical carpal tunnel syndrome. J Hand Surg Br 26:61-64, 2001.

12. Redmond MD, Rivner MH. False positive electrodiagnostic tests in carpal tunnel syndrome. Muscle Nerve 11:511-517, 1988.

13. Edgell SE, McCabe SJ, Breidenbach WC, et al. Predicting the outcome of carpal tunnel release. J Hand Surg Am 28:255-261, 2003.

14. Melvin JL, Johnson EW, Duran R. Electrodiagnosis after surgery for the carpal tunnel syndrome. Arch Phys Med Rehabil 49:502-507, 1968.

15. Akman S, Erturer E, Celik M, et al. [The results of open surgical release in carpal tunnel syndrome and evaluation of follow-up criteria. Acta Orthop Traumatol Turc 36:259-264, 2002.

16. Palumbo CF, Szabo RM. Examination of patients for carpal tunnel syndrome sensibility, provocative and motor testing. Hand Clin 18:269-277, 2002.

EXPERT COMMENTARY

Wyndell H. Merritt, MD, FACS

There is a lesson to be learned when one rereads Phalen's clinical experience and conclusions—from his evaluations for carpal tunnel syndrome that were altogether clinical, with no use of electrodiagnostic studies unless he thought cervical compression possible, and no benefit from Semmes-Weinstein monofilament or two-point discrimination preoperative sensory measurements. His success rate is as good or better (more than 75% were excellent!) than cases reported today (currently with a 25% to 35% failure rate[9,10]). This may well be from our loss of respect for the clinical history and physical examination in favor of electrodiagnostic study as the best criterion for the diagnosis of and surgery for carpal tunnel syndrome.

In an interesting Canadian study, the electromyographers did not share the electrodiagnostic results with their two hand surgeons, who relied completely on the clinical examination and history for a diagnosis. Their surgical results were excellent; they had a 93% success rate but without correlation with the EMG nerve conduction study. Twenty percent of patients with a negative electrodiagnostic study had an excellent result, and 60% of their failures had a positive electrodiagnostic study for carpal tunnel syndrome. The authors concluded that the electrodiagnostic study was "of no value in carpal tunnel syndrome."[11] I would disagree; an electrodiagnostic study is just one piece of the diagnostic puzzle and can be very helpful as the only fully objective test available. However, it should never be regarded as having greater value than the history and physical evaluation. Off the street, as many as 46% of healthy volunteers have one or more positive electrodiagnostic signs of carpal tunnel syndrome, although they are asymptomatic and surely should not consider surgery.[12]

When in doubt Phalen used steroid injections, which remains a valuable diagnostic tool as long as the patient does not know exactly what to expect (especially when determining if a malingerer is seeking surgery). When the patient redevelops carpal tunnel syndrome (often 3 months or more after an injection), one can operate with greater confidence of success. Edgell et al[13] demonstrated that a steroid injection could be more accurate than an electrodiagnostic study or a two-point discrimination study, Phalen test, or survey instruments in predicting the outcome of surgery.

We need to revisit Phalen's dedication to an accurate clinical history and physical examination by now adding preoperative Semmes-Weinstein monofilament measurements, two-point discrimination sensory studies, and an electrodiagnostic study. We need to recognize that if there is postoperative confusion, the sensory measurements will more accurately reflect a change than the electrodiagnostic study, which remains abnormal for at least 2 years.[14,15]

We prefer to time (0 to 60 seconds) our provocative tests: median nerve compression, Phalen's wrist flexion, and fist testing as a rough measure of severity. However, when all the results are negative, the median Tinel sign is positive, and the Semmes-Weinstein monofilament measurements and two-point discrimination tests are severely altered in the median distribution, along with a weak or atrophic abductor pollicis brevis muscle, a severe median nerve compression is likely, and the patient's complaint is no longer pain or awakening at night but a loss of dexterity. Each of these factors, along with the history and measurements, must be weighed, and the final golden criterion for a diagnosis remains the clinician's opinion, just as it was in Phalen's day.[16]

CHAPTER 7

Primary Repair of Lacerated Flexor Tendons in "No Man's Land"

Kleinert HE, Kutz JE, Ashbell TS, Martinez E. J Bone Joint Surg Am 49A:577, 1967

Reviewed by Ryan M. Garcia, MD, and David S. Ruch, MD

Primary repair in no man's land is not recommended by the authors for the occasional operator in hand surgery. However, the authors concluded that the results obtainable by the experienced surgeon in selected patients support their contention that no man's land is some man's land.[1]

Research Question   The repair of flexor tendons has traditionally been fraught with complications and poor patient outcomes. This article presents the first large series that demonstrated good to excellent outcomes.

Funding   Not applicable

Study Dates   Not described; authors' 10-year experience

Publishing Date   April 1967; this was an abstract for the Proceedings of the 22nd Annual Meeting of the American Society for Surgery of the Hand, San Francisco, CA, January 13-14, 1967.

Subjects   Patients sustaining a laceration to the finger in zone II of the volar surface previously described by Bunnell[2,3] as "no man's land"

Exclusion Criteria   Lacerations involving open fractures, contaminated lacerations

Sample Size   Not described

Overview of Design   Retrospective case series of patients undergoing the repair of a flexor tendon laceration in zone II

Intervention   All patients who sustained a laceration to the flexor tendon in zone II were evaluated and treated with flexor tendon repair. Repairs were performed by a "skilled surgeon," and the surgical intervention was followed by a specific "postoperative rehabilitation" protocol. The exact details of the technique were not published in the 1967 abstract. However, expanded details can be found in a follow-up article published in 1973 in *Orthopedic Clinics of North America* entitled "Primary Repair of Flexor Tendons" by the same authors.[4] The described technique of flexor tendon repair involves the following:

- General or regional anesthesia (axillary block preferred) of the injured extremity
- Careful and thorough wound cleaning (delayed repair or secondary repair if there is evidence of infection)
- Use of a pneumatic tourniquet to create a bloodless field
- Surgical exposure with midlateral or zigzag extensions from the laceration
- Minimal surgical trauma (no-touch technique) in handling the tendon or peritendinous tissue (the use of fine delicate instruments designed specifically for hand surgery)
- Tendon repair that produces a firm and accurate juncture without bulging (a 5-0 crisscross primary suture followed by a 6-0 or 7-0 running paratenon suture)
- Use of a small-caliber, nonreactive suture material
- Hemostasis before wound closure
- Postoperative splint/cast for 3 to 3½ weeks with the wrist, hand, and finger held in partial flexion to prevent tension on the repair site
- Cast removal and initiation of a graded postoperative exercise program
- Dynamic splinting to minimize contractures and joint stiffness

Follow-up   Not described

Endpoints   A combination of patient outcomes as previously published (Table 7-1)[4]

Results   Good to excellent results were obtained in 87% of patients treated on the "private service" by a skilled hand surgeon. Good to excellent results were obtained in most patients regardless of which tendons necessitated repair. That is, the authors demonstrated good to excellent results in 86% of the repairs of both the flexor digitorum profundus and superficialis, 88% of isolated flexor digitorum profundus repairs, and 91% of isolated superficialis repairs. A "teaching service" group of patients was presented as having overall inferior results (76% had poor results).

Table 7-1   Patient Outcomes as Previously Published

	Flexion	Loss of Extension
Excellent	<1 cm to the distal palmar crease	<15 degrees of extension loss
Good	<1.5 cm to the distal palmar crease	<30 degrees of extension loss
Fair	2-3 cm to the distal palmar crease	30-50 degrees of extension loss
Poor	>3 cm to the distal palmar crease	>50 degrees of extension loss

From Kleinert HE, Kutz JE, Atasoy E, et al. Primary repair of flexor tendons. Orthop Clin North Am 4:865-876, 1973.

Criticisms/Limitations The article presented is a retrospective study of a nonrandomized patient population of a single surgeon's experience. A "private service" group of patients are compared with a "teaching service" group of patients and had markedly better results. These two groups are likely confounded by economics, mechanism of injury, support, and rehabilitation access, all of which contributed to patient outcomes. The article as an abstract is limited in the details on patient demographics, the extent of injury, and the degree of follow-up. The results presented as excellent, good, fair, or poor are determined on only two variables, namely, flexion and extension. The article lacks further details of pain-related and hand-related functional disabilities and capabilities.

Relevant Studies Early descriptions of flexor tendon repairs in zone II were fraught with complications and poor patient outcomes. Sterling Bunnell understood the importance of early tendon motion to prevent adhesions; however, the lack of adequate suture material and proper technique led to early tendon repair failure when early motion was started. This ultimately led Bunnell[2,3] to recommend wound debridement, resection of the tendon, and delayed tendon grafting. Bunnell[2,3] is also credited with labeling injuries in zone II of the flexor surface as "no man's land."

A meticulous flexor tendon repair, in addition to a progressive early motion rehabilitation protocol, resulted in the outstanding outcomes presented by Kleinert et al[4] and Lister et al.[5] The "Kleinert protocol" allows active extension with passive flexion of the digit through a series of rubber bands and pulleys (Fig. 7-1). Duran and Houser[6] developed a similar but unique early motion protocol that uses active participation by the patient to perform passive motion of the digit. Allowing early motion across a flexor tendon repair site improves healing[7] and reduces adhesion formation but relies heavily on the suture, suture technique,[8] the number of crossing suture strands,[9] and the elimination of gap formation.[10] In the original description by Kleinert et al,[4] a two-strand, grasping, nonlocking technique with a running epitendinous repair was advocated.

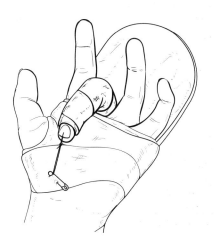

Fig. 7-1 The repaired digit is immobilized in a dorsal plaster splint to maintain the finger and wrist in moderate flexion. If there is no fracture, elastic dynamic traction is added. This permits some extension without stress on the site of repair and may prevent adhesions at the suture line. (Adapted from Kleinert HE, Kutz JE, Atasoy E, et al. Primary repair of flexor tendons. Orthop Clin North Am 4:865-876, 1973.)

Biomechanical studies followed, demonstrating that a greater number of core sutures crossing the repair site resulted in greater tensile strength.[9,11] Intrinsic tendon healing (primary tendon healing without ingrowth from the surrounding tendon sheath) was discovered to occur with early motion protocols if primary tendon failure was avoided and ultimately resulted in a reduction of adhesion formation and improved patient outcomes.[12] Preservation of the flexor tendon synovial sheath and its gliding surface was originally investigated in the 1960s by Hunter and Salisbury[13] with the development of the artificial gliding implant ("Hunter rod") for delayed tendon grafting and has recently been a focus of investigation after flexor tendon injury and repair.

Summary   Harold Kleinert's meticulous surgical technique and early passive motion protocol was a landmark advancement in the treatment of flexor tendon lacerations in zone II. Flexor tendon repair in "no man's land" can be performed routinely with good to excellent outcomes, making this area of concern "some man's land."

Implications   Flexor tendon repair in zone II of the flexor surface remains a challenge to the best of hand surgeons. Advancements in meticulous surgical technique, suture choice, and configuration followed by an early motion protocol have promoted our understanding of intrinsic tendon healing, gliding, and improved patient outcomes.

REFERENCES

1. Kleinert HE, Kutz JE, Ashbell TS, et al. Primary repair of lacerated flexor tendons in "no man's land." J Bone Joint Surg Am 49A:577, 1967.
2. Bunnell S. Surgery of the Hand. Philadelphia: JB Lippincott, 1944.
3. Bunnell S. Repair of nerves and tendons of the hands. J Bone Joint Surgery10:1-26, 1928.
4. Kleinert HE, Kutz JE, Atasoy E, et al. Primary repair of flexor tendons. Orthop Clin North Am 4:865-876, 1973.
5. Lister GD, Kleinert HE, Kutz JE, et al. Primary flexor tendon repair followed by immediate controlled mobilization. J Hand Surg Am 2:441-451, 1977.
6. Duran R, Houser R. Controlled passive motion following flexor tendon repair in zone 2 and 3. In Hunter J, Schneider L, Mackin E, et al, eds. Rehabilitation of the Hand, 3rd ed. St Louis: CV Mosby, 1975.
7. Woo SL, Gelberman RH, Cobb NG, et al. The importance of controlled passive mobilization on flexor tendon healing. A biomechanical study. Acta Orthop Scand 52:615-622, 1981.
8. Noguchi M, Seiler JG III, Gelberman RH, et al. In vitro biomechanical analysis of suture methods for flexor tendon repair. J Orthop Res 11:603-611, 1993.
9. Winters SC, Gelberman RH, Woo SL, et al. The effects of multiple-strand suture methods on the strength and excursion of repaired intrasynovial flexor tendons: a biomechanical study in dogs. J Hand Surg Am 23:97-104, 1998.
10. Gelberman RH, Boyer MI, Brodt MD, et al. The effect of gap formation at the repair site on the strength and excursion of intrasynovial flexor tendons. An experimental study on the early stages of tendon-healing in dogs. J Bone Joint Surg Am 81:975-982, 1999.

11. Winters SC, Seiler JG III, Woo SL, et al. Suture methods for flexor tendon repair. A biome-chanical analysis during the first six weeks following repair. Ann Chir Main Memb Super 16:229-234, 1997.
12. Manske PR, Gelberman RH, Vande Berg JS, et al. Intrinsic flexor-tendon repair. A morpho-logical study in vitro. J Bone Joint Am 66:385-396, 1984.
13. Hunter JM, Salisbury RE. Use of gliding artificial implants to produce tendon sheaths. Techniques and results in children. Plastic Reconstr Surg 45:564-572, 1970.
14. Thompson CJ, Lalonde DH, Denkler KA, et al. A critical look at the evidence for and against elective epinephrine use in the finger. Plast Reconstr Surg 119:260-266, 2007.
15. Howell JW, Merritt WH, Robinson SJ. Immediate controlled active motion following zone 4-7 extensor tendon repair. J Hand Ther18:182-190, 2005.
16. Merritt WH, Howell J, Tune R, et al. Achieving immediate active motion by using relative motion splinting after long extensor tendon repair and sagittal band ruptures with tendon subluxation. Operat Tech Plast Reconstr Surg 7:31-37, 2000.
17. Burns M, Derby B, Neumeister M. Wyndell Merritt immediate controlled active motion (ICAM) protocol following extensor tendon repairs in zone IV-VII: review of literature, or-thosis design, and case study—a multimedia article. Hand (NY) 8:17-22, 2013.
18. Hirth MJ, Bennet K, Mah E, et al. Early return to work and improved range of motion with modified relative motion splinting: a retrospective comparison with immobilization splint-ing for zones V and VI extensor tendon repairs. Hand Ther 16:86-94, 2011.

EXPERT COMMENTARY

Wyndell H. Merritt, MD, FACS

It is no accident that the 1967 abstract of Kleinert et al,[1] published in the *Journal of Bone and Joint Surgery*, did not result in the publication of a paper until 6 years later. His novel ideas were not easily accepted after the long-held dogma of "no man's land" and the new concept of early protected passive motion by dynamic splinting. Indeed, Kleinert told me he was severely criticized for such heresy!

Now that Kleinert's concept is an accepted standard, there is resistance to other well-established new ideas, such as the use of epinephrine and local anesthesia to obviate the need for a tourniquet and allow immediate assessment of the repair[14] and relative motion splinting that will permit immediate active motion and hand function after vari-ous extensor tendon injuries, which may also possibly afford protection for repaired flexor tendons.[15-18]

Kleinert et al introduced the concept of early motion reducing tendon adhesions that Furlow, Lineaweaver, Gelberman, Feehan, and many others later confirmed experi-mentally. The future strategy for better results in tendon surgery seems secure if we can just do away with the reluctance to question dogmas!

CHAPTER 8

Reconstruction of the Thumb by Transposition of an Adjacent Digit

Tanzer RC, Littler JW. Plast Reconstr Surg (1946) 3:533-547, 1948

Reviewed by Ryan M. Garcia, MD, and David S. Ruch, MD

> *The third method (adjacent digit pollicization) employs the transposition of an adjacent digit into the thumb position. We consider this procedure definitely superior to the preceding one (toe to thumb transfer) inasmuch as the continuity of vessels, nerves and tendons is preserved and the operative procedure simplified considerably.[1]*

Research Question   The thumb has long been paramount in the overall functional capabilities of the hand. The authors highlight three possible thumb reconstruction methods and further recommend pollicization as their preferred treatment method. This article attempts to standardize the operative preparation, plan, and execution of adjacent digit pollicization.

Funding   Not applicable

Study Dates   Not described; the authors present a 4-year military experience of severe hand injuries and ultimately derive seven cases of adjacent digit transposition to the thumb.

Publishing Date   September 1948

Subjects   Seven patients are presented as case examples for the procedure technique and execution.

Exclusion Criteria   The authors highlight that the only absolute contraindication to adjacent digit transfer for thumb reconstruction is inadequate circulation to the hand

and/or a transposed digit. The authors further recommend the following four criteria for a satisfactory reconstruction of the thumb:

1. There is an adjacent digit with sufficient and forceful flexion and extension allowing functional grasping.
2. The reconstructed thumb tip should be opposable to the pulp of at least one but preferably two adjacent digits.
3. The reconstructed thumb tip should have tactile sensibility.
4. Although less important, there should be an aesthetic, inconspicuous appearance and reasonable thumb contour.

Sample Size   7 cases

Overview of Design   A retrospective case series of patients undergoing adjacent digit pollicization after severe hand trauma and injury

Intervention   Tanzer and Littler[1] describe the procedure of transposing an adjacent digit to the thumb position, which is performed to allow thumb opposition and improved hand function. In the description they highlight that there may be local soft tissue deficiency for digit resurfacing. In their series of seven patients, five patients needed a pedicle abdominal flap for soft tissue coverage.

During the preparation phase, the authors first recommend the excision of any previous scar to improve circulation and soft tissue pliability. In many instances an abdominal pedicled flap may be necessary to fill a soft tissue defect. The laceration or loss of the digital nerves should also be repaired or grafted. The extensor tendon of the planned digit transposition should be transferred during the scar reconstruction/preparation phase.

The classic description is an index finger transposition for thumb reconstruction (Fig. 8-1). A longitudinal incision is made starting on the dorsal surface between the second and third metacarpals and extending to the midpalmar crease. The second dorsal interosseous muscle and intermetacarpal ligament are released. The first volar interosseous muscle and associated digital nerves and vessels are exposed and carried with the transposing digit. Ligation of the branching vessels to the middle digit at the bifurcation is necessary to allow the transposition of the index finger. The midshaft of the metacarpal is transected, and the digit is transposed to the thumb position and secured to the remaining metacarpal stump. A large wedge-shaped defect remains between the transposed digit and adjacent metacarpal. This is filled with a pedicled abdominal flap.

In a separate operative procedure, the digit is positioned. This often requires digit shortening in which the proximal phalanx of the transposed digit is either fused to the remaining metacarpal or the carpus. Maintaining the metacarpophalangeal joint of the

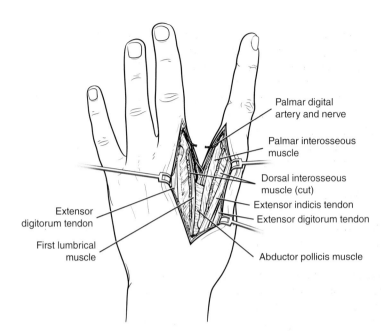

Palmar digital
artery and nerve

Palmar interosseous
muscle

Dorsal interosseous
muscle (cut)

Extensor indicis tendon

Extensor digitorum tendon

Abductor pollicis muscle

Extensor
digitorum tendon

First lumbrical
muscle

Fig. 8-1 Usual operative approach for mobilization of an index finger to replace the thumb. Following this step, the extensor tendons of the index finger are drawn under the skin flap and anchored with a removable wire suture. The second metacarpal, if not already fractured at the time of injury, is transected and the index finger moved into thumb position. (Adapted from Tanzer RC, Littler JW. Reconstruction of the thumb by transposition of an adjacent digit. Plast Reconstr Surg [1946] 3:533-547, 1948.)

transposed digit may lead to hyperextension and a compensatory flexion of the interphalangeal joints. This is corrected by metacarpophalangeal joint fusion in an ideal position or a tendon transfer. In patients in whom the flexor tendon is lost, a free graft or transfer of the flexor digitorum superficialis tendon can be used. The loss of the extensor tendon requires a free graft and should be oriented to provide some adductor function and lateral digit stability. Thumb opposition is ultimately gained by transferring the superficialis tendon of the ring finger around the flexor carpi ulnaris to the proximal phalanx of the transposed digit.

Follow-up Not routinely described

Endpoints Not described

Results The authors do not clearly detail their results. Each case report is given, and the ultimate outcomes are presented with variable flexion, extension, abduction, and opposition measurements. Occasional grip functions are given. The authors describe multiple revision procedures on each hand to refine and enhance its function.

Criticisms/Limitations   The article presented is a retrospective review of seven patients treated by a single surgeon over a 4-year period. All patients sustained severe hand injuries and the loss of their thumb. The article is limited in its details of patient demographics and the degree of follow-up. The article also lacks consistent and routine postoperative follow-up functional evaluations. It is difficult for the reader to grasp the ultimate outcomes of these procedures.

Relevant Studies   Tanzer and Littler[1] describe a method of thumb reconstruction by the transposition of an adjacent digit, the so-called, pollicization procedure. They describe this procedure in detail with limited drawings. Littler[2] expanded on his original technical description with a follow-up article in *Plastic and Reconstructive Surgery* in 1953. In this article Littler demonstrates that the use of a single neurovascular pedicle to the transposed digit is a sufficient arterial supply and allows the appropriate venous regression but requires careful dissection. This article also provides improved and extensive step-by-step illustrations of the pollicization procedure of the index finger. In 1952 Littler[3] described an alternate use of the pollicization procedure to reconstruct a "subtotal thumb." In some circumstances the entire index finger is unavailable for use, or the thumb may be shortened at the level of the metacarpophalangeal joint or distal metacarpal. Because a short thumb has limited functional value, Littler describes transferring a smaller portion of the adjacent digit to provide additional thumb length.

Although Tanzer and Littler[1,2] advocate the use of a single digital artery and accompanying venous system, others have argued that improved venous regression should be considered by retaining either a dorsal vein or a larger portion of dorsal skin with the accompanying venous system. Aston and Lankford[4] describe 20 pollicization procedures in which thin skin flaps were designed around the transposed index finger and argued for improved venous drainage. In a series of recent articles, Taghinia et al [5] and Taghinia and Upton[6] describe the refinements they have developed for the pollicization procedure of the index finger over a 30-year experience in 313 operations performed for either thumb aplasia or hypoplasia. In collaboration with Littler, these recent refinements include:
  • The avoidance of an unnatural deep web space by using improved and modified incisions that avoid the originally described Y-to-V component and V-shaped thenar skin flap
  • An improved understanding and positioning of the metacarpal head[7]
  • A rebalancing of the extrinsic and intrinsic tendons
  • The use of an adipofascial flap for thenar augmentation, cosmesis, and appearance

Buck-Gramcko[7] has made numerous advancements and contributions to the treatment of congenital differences of the hand. The approach and refinements in pollicization, including the proper positioning of the metacarpal head, are detailed in the first 100 cases performed.

Summary   J. William Littler's original article on adjacent digit pollicization was a landmark for both hand surgeons and plastic surgeons. By adhering to a number of surgical principles, he was able to provide a highly functional thumb in a series of seven severely mangled and injured hands. Over the years, his original description has undergone modifications and refinements, but the major components of the procedure still remain.

Implications   The thumb contributes to more than 50% of hand function, and its loss leads to severe functional limitations and life-altering events. Adjacent digit pollicization should be considered in cases of severe thumb trauma, thumb amputation, or developmental thumb aplasia or hypoplasia.

REFERENCES

1. Tanzer RC, Littler JW. Reconstruction of the thumb by transposition of an adjacent digit. Plast Reconstr Surg (1946) 3:533-547, 1948.
2. Littler JW. The neurovascular pedicle method of digital transposition for reconstruction of the thumb. Plast Reconstr Surg (1946) 12:303-319, 1953.
3. Littler JW. Subtotal reconstruction of the thumb. Plast Reconstr Surg (1946) 10:215-226, 1952.
4. Aston JW Jr, Lankford LL. Use of thin, mobile skin flaps in pollicization of the index finger. Plast Reconstr Surg 62:870-872, 1978.
5. Taghinia AH, Littler JW, Upton J. Refinements in pollicization: a 30-year experience. Plast Reconstr Surg 13:423e-433e, 2012.
6. Taghinia AH, Upton J. Index finger pollicization. J Hand Surg Am 36:333-339, 2011.
7. Buck-Gramcko D. Pollicization of the index finger. Method and results in aplasia and hypoplasia of the thumb. J Bone Joint Surg Am 53:1605-1617, 1971.
8. Bayot J. J. William Littler, 89, Specialist in Hand Surgery, Dies. New York Times, March 4, 2005.

EDITORIAL PERSPECTIVE

C. Scott Hultman, MD, MBA, FACS

William Littler's contributions to the field of hand surgery are staggering. A review of his work indexed on PubMed reveals "only" 58 publications, but most of these papers document landmark achievements in hand surgery, including pollicization, scaphoid arthroplasty, compartment reconstruction for de Quervain's tenosynovitis, repair of the thumb ulnar collateral ligament, management of trapeziometacarpal injuries, treatment of paronychial infections, tendon interposition arthroplasty in carpometacarpal reconstruction, flexor tendon transfer for proximal interphalangeal instability, treatment of mallet finger and boutonnière deformities, surgical management of neuroma, and of course neurovascular island and advancement flaps.

Dr. Littler's obituary, which was published in March 2005 in *The New York Times*, identified his early devotion to hand surgery as a major factor to the emergence of this field as a separate discipline. During World War II, while serving as a young Army surgeon first at Cushing General Hospital near Boston and later at Valley Forge Army Hospital in Pennsylvania, "he began shaping and refining surgical techniques still in use today. He worked on new ways to reconstruct missing thumbs, including replacing them with parts of forefingers, and he transplanted healthy bundles of nerves and arteries to areas that had lost feeling, a procedure known as a sensory neurovascular island transfer. To revive arms and hands paralyzed by nerve damage, he transferred tendons from areas that were unharmed."[8]

William Littler is the giant whose shoulders other giants stand on.

CHAPTER 9

Immediate Thumb Extension Following Extensor Indicis Proprius-to-Extensor Pollicis Longus Tendon Transfer Using the Wide-Awake Approach

Bezuhly M, Sparkes GL, Higgins A, Neumeister MW, Lalonde DH. Plast Reconstr Surg 119:1507-1512, 2007

Reviewed by Ryan M. Garcia, MD, and David S. Ruch, MD

In this article, we examine how the wide-awake approach to hand surgery has allowed us to perform simple tendon transfers with pure local anesthetic and without a tourniquet. The wide-awake approach (also) allows us to adjust tendon transfer tension with active movement to make sure the transfer is not too tight or too loose before the skin is closed.[1]

Research Question   The wide-awake approach to hand surgery consists of a local anesthetic injection with epinephrine to perform the procedure without general anesthesia or regional nerve block anesthesia and without a tourniquet. Historically, the use of epinephrine in the digits and hands has been forbidden. In this article Lalonde has challenged this concept. Additional supporting evidence has further suggested that it is safe to inject epinephrine in the hand and finger without evidence of distal ischemia or tissue loss. By performing a wide-awake tendon transfer, the surgeon is able to adjust the tension on the repair before the skin is closed. In addition, Lalonde made some interesting observations regarding cortical adaptation to the new tendon transfer.

Funding   None

Study Dates   February 2002 to May 2005

Publishing Date   April 2007

Subjects   Seven patients are presented after undergoing wide-awake hand surgery. Each patient underwent a tendon transfer of the extensor indicis proprius (EIP) to the extensor pollicis longus (EPL) tendon. Each patient sustained a prior EPL tendon rupture that was detected on physical examination and confirmed intraoperatively. One patient had a rerupture of the EIP-to-EPL transfer and was treated with an extensor carpi radialis longus to EPL transfer also under the wide-awake approach.

Exclusion Criteria   None described; inclusion criteria were patients with chronic, isolated ruptures of their EPL tendon.

Sample Size   7 cases

Overview of Design   A retrospective case series of seven consecutive patients who had prior ruptures of their EPL tendon

Intervention   The operative intervention begins with adequate anesthesia and vasoconstriction. Each patient was injected with 20 ml of 1% lidocaine and epinephrine (1:200,000) in the planned operative field (Fig. 9-1)[1] and allowed a minimum of 30 minutes to take effect. No tourniquet is used. A standard technique of EIP-to-EPL tendon transfer was then performed. After a temporary suture was placed, each patient was asked to actively extend the thumb. Patients were either allowed to look at the thumb while attempting to move it, were blocked from proprioception, or had a screen that blocked their direct vision of the thumb. Final sutures were then placed if the tension on the tendon transfer was appropriate. The authors note that in the absence of a tourniquet, all patients were comfortable, and the operative site had appropriate anesthesia and hemostasis. No additional anesthetic was required in any patient.

Follow-up   Mean follow-up of 16 months (range 6 to 36 months)

Endpoints   Follow-up measurements of the first five patients included range of motion, pinch strength, and grip strength.

Results   The authors describe a technique for wide-awake EIP-to-EPL tendon transfer with 1% lidocaine and epinephrine (1:200,000). They report that even in the absence of a tourniquet, all patients had appropriate hemostasis and an excellent surgical

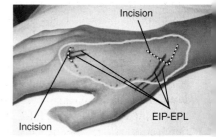

Fig. 9-1   The circled area was injected with 20 cc of 1% lidocaine with 1:200,000 epinephrine 30 minutes before the operative procedure. *Dashed lines* indicate incisions. *Black lines* outline the extensor indicis proprius and extensor pollicis longus tendons. *EIP,* Extensor indicis proprius; *EPL,* extensor pollicis longus. (From Bezuhly M, Sparkes GL, Higgins A, et al. Immediate thumb extension following extensor indicis proprius-to-extensor pollicis longus tendon transfer using the wide-awake approach. Plast Reconstr Surg 119:1507-1512, 2007.)

Table 9-1   Reported Outcomes for the First Five Patients Who Underwent Wide-Awake EIP-to-EPL Tendon Transfer

	Operative Thumb	Unoperated, Contralateral Thumb
Average thumb interphalangeal motion (degrees)		
Flexion	63	64
Extension	−4	−3
Average thumb metacarpophalangeal motion (degrees)		
Flexion	58	59
Extension	−7	−6
Average tripod pinch (kg)	5.8	4.9
Average lateral pinch (kg)	6.6	6
Average thumb grip (kg)	24	24

Data from Bezuhly M, Sparkes GL, Higgins A, et al. Immediate thumb extension following extensor indicis proprius-to-extensor pollicis longus tendon transfer using the wide-awake approach. Plast Reconstr Surg 119:1507-1512, 2007.

field. In addition, all patients reported to be comfortable throughout the procedure and were able to perform the necessary thumb motions when asked. Follow-up functional outcomes for the first five patients are represented (Table 9-1).[1] The authors comment and suggest that immediate cortical adaptation may occur after this tendon transfer because all patients were able to actively extend the thumb and index fingers independently without any hesitation on their first attempt (regardless if they were observing the thumb or blocked from viewing).

Criticisms/Limitations   This article represents a retrospective review of a nonrandomized patient population who underwent wide-awake tendon transfer. The article is limited in its small patient sample size and lack of a comparison group. The authors note that all patients were "comfortable" but give no objective measure of pain control. The authors comment and highlight that cortical adaptation may be immediate after tendon transfer. The concept of immediate cortical adaptation was later challenged[2]; an alternative explanation for this finding was shared innervation to the two muscles from the posterior interosseous nerve.

Relevant Studies   The primary goals of wide-awake tendon transfer surgery are to provide adequate anesthesia, a bloodless and hemostatic operative environment, and a comfortable patient who can actively participate in hand motion and function. This can allow the tendon transfer to be critically assessed and adjusted before closure of the skin. The classic and historic teaching is that epinephrine should be avoided in the distal extremity for fear of inducing an ischemic event. Lalonde has challenged this concept with the wide-awake approach to hand surgery. Further studies have also supported the use of epinephrine in hand surgery without any additional ischemia risks.[3-5] A single institution's prospective, randomized, clinical trial demonstrated increased durations of analgesia and no undesired ischemic complications associated with the use of epinephrine within digital nerve blocks.[3] This study was followed by a large, multicenter trial of 3110 patients, who were prospectively followed after an injection of low-dose epinephrine (1:100,000 or less) to the fingers or hand without a single case of distal digital tissue loss.[5] These findings were further substantiated in a large retrospective review of 1111 cases in which epinephrine was used in digital nerve blocks.[4] In the rare event that digital ischemia occurs after the use of epinephrine, phentolamine can be used as an antidote. A prospective, randomized trial was conducted on 22 healthy volunteers (18 of whom were hand surgeons) to investigate the effects of phentolamine on epinephrine reversal.[6] The 22 subjects underwent bilateral middle digit nerve block with 2% lidocaine and epinephrine (1:100,000), which was then followed by a randomized injection of either phentolamine or normal saline solution. The reversal of vasoconstriction was 85 minutes in the phentolamine group versus 320 minutes in the control group. No harmful vasoconstriction events occurred in any digit.

Lalonde[7] has further advocated the use of wide-awake surgery for flexor tendon repairs, Dupuytren's contracture,[8] wrist arthroscopy, and open triangular fibrocartilage complex repairs.[9] Lalonde advocates that a wide-awake approach to flexor tendon repair allows patients to actively participate in flexion and extension of the digit and may ultimately improve the outcome and success of repair.[7] Digital motion and observation allow the surgeon an opportunity to trim the flexor tendon repair, detect tendon bunching or gap formation, or open the pulley system as needed.[10] Cost savings are also implicated when wide-awake hand surgery can be performed in minor procedure rooms.[11]

Summary   Lalonde originally described wide-awake hand surgery in seven patients undergoing EIP-to-EPL tendon transfer. This approach can only be performed if adequate analgesia can be achieved, tourniquet use avoided, and a clear operative field attained with appropriate hemostasis. Multiple studies support the use and safety of epinephrine in the hand and finger, which challenges earlier teaching and dogma. The wide-awake approach allows surgeons to verify their work and make any necessary adjustments before skin closure. Wide-awake hand surgery appears to be safe and efficacious when EIP-to-EPL tendon transfers are performed.

Implications   Wide-awake hand surgery has multiple implications and potential uses throughout the field of hand surgery. Patient participation with finger and hand motion may have an added benefit because surgical adjustments can be made before the procedure is completed. The use of epinephrine as a vasoconstricting agent is paramount in wide-awake hand surgery and should be considered safe for the practicing physician.

REFERENCES

1. Bezuhly M, Sparkes GL, Higgins A, et al. Immediate thumb extension following extensor indicis proprius-to-extensor pollicis longus tendon transfer using the wide-awake approach. Plast Reconstr Surg 119:1507-1512, 2007.

2. Malaviya GN. Wide-awake approach. Plast Reconstr Surg 121:688; author reply 688-689, 2008.

3. Wilhelmi BJ, Blackwell SJ, Miller JH, et al. Do not use epinephrine in digital blocks: myth or truth? Plast Reconstr Surg 107:393-397, 2001.

4. Chowdhry S, Seidenstricker L, Cooney DS, et al. Do not use epinephrine in digital blocks: myth or truth? Part II. A retrospective review of 1111 cases. Plast Reconstr Surg 126:2031-2034, 2010.

5. Lalonde D, Bell M, Benoit P, et al. A multicenter prospective study of 3,110 consecutive cases of elective epinephrine use in the fingers and hand: the Dalhousie Project clinical phase. J Hand Surg Am 30:1061-1067, 2005.

6. Nodwell T, Lalonde D. How long does it take phentolamine to reverse adrenaline-induced vasoconstriction in the finger and hand? A prospective, randomized, blinded study: The Dalhousie project experimental phase. Can J Plast Surg 11:187-190, 2003.

7. Lalonde DH. Wide-awake flexor tendon repair. Plast Reconstr Surg 123:623-625, 2009.

8. Nelson R, Higgins A, Conrad J, et al. The wide-awake approach to Dupuytren's disease: fasciectomy under local anesthetic with epinephrine. Hand (NY) 5:117-124, 2010.

9. Hagert E, Lalonde DH. Wide-awake wrist arthroscopy and open TFCC repair. J Wrist Surg 1:55-60, 2012.

10. Higgins A, Lalonde DH, Bell M, et al. Avoiding flexor tendon repair rupture with intraoperative total active movement examination. Plast Reconstr Surg 126:941-945, 2010.

11. Leblanc MR, Lalonde J, Lalonde DH. A detailed cost and efficiency analysis of performing carpal tunnel surgery in the main operating room versus the ambulatory setting in Canada. Hand (NY) 2:173-178, 2007.

12. Lalonde DH, Kozin S. Tendon disorders of the hand. Plast Reconstr Surg 128:1e-14e, 2011.

13. Lalonde DH. How the wide awake approach is changing hand surgery and hand therapy: inaugural AAHS sponsored lecture at the ASHT meeting, San Diego, 2012. J Hand Ther 26:175-178, 2013.

STUDY AUTHOR REFLECTIONS

Donald H. Lalonde, MD, Hons BSc, MSc, FRCSC

This paper is important for two reasons:

1. It is the first description of wide-awake local anesthesia no tourniquet (WALANT) tendon transfers. WALANT has greatly improved the result of tendon transfers because the surgeon can adjust the tension of the transfer after watching the patient take the transfer through an active range of motion before the skin is closed. Before WALANT was used, some of my transfers were too tight and some were too loose. We also now know that WALANT has greatly improved the result of flexor tendon repairs with fewer ruptures, less need for tenolysis, and the progression to postoperative true active protected movement as opposed to place and hold.[9,12,13]

2. This is the first publication in which it was shown that some tendon transfers do not need to be "learned" by the patient after surgery. They can do it right on the operating table.

CHAPTER 10

Nerve Transfers for the Restoration of Hand Function After Spinal Cord Injury

Mackinnon SE, Yee A, Ray WZ. J Neurosurg 117:176-185, 2012

Reviewed by Brandon S. Smetana, MD, and J. Megan M. Patterson, MD

Nerve transfers using an expendable nearby motor nerve to reinnervate a denervated nerve have resulted in more rapid and improved recovery than traditional nerve graft reconstructions [and can restore] some hand function following a complete cervical spinal cord injury.[1]

Summary   Nerve transfers are used to restore function after peripheral nerve and brachial plexus injury.[2] These techniques have recently been applied to spinal cord injuries (SCIs).[3,4] Mackinnon et al[1] presented a case of improved finger flexion and hand function after transfer of the nerve to the brachialis to the anterior interosseous nerve (AIN) in a patient with a C7 American Spinal Injury Association (ASIA)-A SCI performed 23 months after the initial injury.

Research Question   Can bypassing a C7 level SCI with a brachialis nerve to AIN transfer restore volitional functional hand motion?

Funding   Departmental

Study Dates   The patient sustained his injury in June 2008. The initial evaluation by the study authors was in April 2010, and surgery was performed in May 2010. Follow-up was reported through August 2011 (15 months after surgery).

Publishing Date   July 2012

Location   Washington University School of Medicine, St. Louis, MO

Introduction   Spinal cord injuries (SCIs) occur with an incidence of 40 cases per million persons each year in the United States and involve young patients with an average age of less than 40 years. Recovery is unpredictable, and a growing number of young patients are left with significant disability, often requiring an advanced level of care.[1] Although data exist that investigate the role of neuroprotective and therapeutic agents after a SCI, there is a paucity of information regarding potential therapeutic interventions that result in reproducible improvements to functional status after injury. Currently nerve transfers are used to restore function in cases of both peripheral nerve and brachial plexus injuries; however, their use in the setting of SCIs has yet to be elucidated.

Study Goals   The aim of this study was to describe an intervention (brachialis nerve to AIN transfer in a patient with a C7 ASIA-A SCI), which resulted in improved hand function and patient independence. It also affirmed that unlike peripheral nerve injuries, the window of treatment for SCIs is much wider because of the preservation of the neuromuscular junction.

Patient   The patient was a 71-year-old man with a ASIA-A C7 level SCI who presented 22 months after the initial injury sustained in a motor vehicle accident in June 2008; he had no other reported extremity injury and underwent posterior and anterior cervical stabilization without complication soon after his injury. He was an International Classification for Surgery of the Hand in Tetraplegia grade 5 on the left and slightly less on the right, with the lowest active motor function during examination corresponding to wrist flexion (flexor carpi radialis) (Table 10-1).[1] There was no evidence of pinch, grip, finger flexion, or extension in either hand. He had intact static and moving two-point discrimination of 5 to 6 mm bilaterally in the median and ulnar nerves. There was significant intrinsic muscle atrophy and joint stiffness throughout all of his fingers with fixed contractures. Preoperative EMG and nerve conduction study demonstrated small motor unit potentials to the right flexor pollicis longus (FPL) and left flexor digitorum profundus (FDP) to the index and long fingers.

Procedure   Bilateral staged brachialis nerve to AIN transfers were performed 23 months after the initial injury. The patient was in the supine position under general anesthesia without muscle relaxants or paralytics to allow for intraoperative nerve stimu-

Table 10-1   Medical Research Council Motor Function of Bilateral Upper Extremities Before Operative Intervention

Motor Function	Wrist Extension	FCR	Pronation	BR	Shoulder Function	Elbow Flexion
Left (MRC)	5	5	4	5	5	5
Right (MRC)	4	3	4	4	5	5

Data from Mackinnon SE, Yee A, Ray WZ. Nerve transfers for the restoration of hand function after spinal cord injury. J Neurosurg 117:176-185, 2012.
BR, Brachioradialis; FCR, flexor carpi radialis; MRC, Medical Research Council.

lation. Medially based incisions were made in the brachium and carried down to the median nerve. Motor mapping of the median nerve with a nerve stimulator was performed to separate and protect the nerve fascicles innervating muscles above the level of the SCI (Fig. 10-1).[1] The AIN fascicle was identified in the medial and posterior portion of the median nerve and separated from the surrounding fascicles. Confirmation of endplate motor function was then performed with nerve stimulation. The AIN fascicle was then divided from the median nerve proximally. The brachialis nerve was identified and divided distally to ensure a tension free transfer. The repair was performed with 9.0 nylon and fibrin glue.

Outcome   The patient had voluntary movement in the FPL and FDP at 8 and 10 months after surgery in his left and right hands, respectively. At his final reported follow-up at 15 months after surgery, he had Medical Research Council grade 3 FPL and FDP strength bilaterally. He could perform simple hand-to-mouth movements with his right hand and was able to feed himself and perform rudimentary writing activities with his left.

Significance   This study provides the first description of the restoration of thumb and finger flexion after a SCI and confirms prior reports of reinnervation of muscle groups below the SCI level with nerve transfers. In conjunction with previously described nerve transfers for the treatment of SCIs,[3,4] it may fundamentally change the treatment of SCIs in select patients and allow improved function and independence in this growing patient population.

Criticisms/Limitations   Inherent in the study design as a case study, the project lacks the power to draw significant conclusions of treatment efficacy or comparison of functional outcome with alternative procedures such as tendon transfers. The study authors also note that the patient's preoperative joint contractures likely resulted in a less optimal outcome.

Relevant Studies   Nerve transfers have been reported in the literature since the early twentieth century. Tuttle in 1912 and Chiasserini in 1934 described the first reports, and early work done by Seddon, Kotani, and Gu in the decades to come provided the foundation for the use of nerve transfers in the setting of brachial plexus injury.[5] In 1994 Oberlin et al first reported on the transfer of ulnar motor fascicles of the flexor carpi ulnaris to the biceps branch of the musculocutaneous nerve to restore elbow flexion in the setting of upper brachial plexus injury.[6] Tung et al[6] and Ray et al[7] built on Oberlin's work by proposing a double fascicular nerve transfer to further improve elbow flexion in brachial plexus injury by adding a transfer of an expendable redundant branch of the median nerve to the brachialis branch of the musculocutaneous nerve. This additional transfer allowed improved elbow flexion and avoidance of salvage Steindler flexorplasties when compared with Oberlin's originally proposed transfer.[6,7]

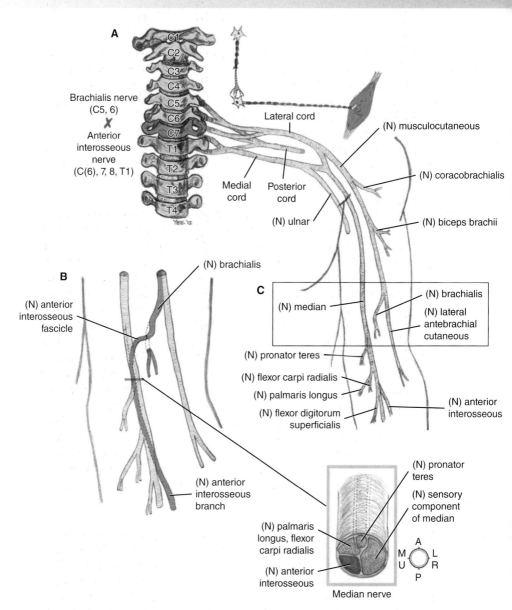

Fig. 10-1 Musculocutaneous and median nerve anatomy relevant to the brachialis nerve to AIN transfer in C-7 SCI. **A,** The donor brachialis branch divides from the musculocutaneous nerve on its medial aspect. After this branch point, the musculocutaneous nerve becomes the lateral antebrachial cutaneous nerve. **B,** The recipient AIN branches from the median nerve in the forearm on its lateral aspect, but courses proximally into the arm on its posterior/medial aspect. The donor brachialis nerve is transferred into the anterior interosseous fascicle in the arm. **C,** The AIN fascicle in the arm is located on the posterior/medial aspect of the median nerve, between the palmaris longus/flexor digitorum superficialis/flexor carpi radialis fascicle and the sensory component of the median nerve. The fascicular group to the pronator teres is located in the anterior portion of the median nerve, while the sensory fibers are lateral and the motor fibers medial. *A,* Anterior; *L,* lateral; *M,* medial; *N,* nerve; *P,* posterior; *R,* radial; *U,* ulnar. (From Mackinnon SE, Yee A, Ray WZ. Nerve transfers for the restoration of hand function after spinal cord injury. J Neurosurg 117:176-185, 2012.)

Nerve transfers have since become a common reconstructive technique used in many clinical situations.[2] The expanding indications are a direct result of the advantages nerve transfers impart over proximal nerve repair or grafting by decreasing the necessary length of regeneration, converting a proximal lesion into a more distal one, and thereby avoiding the detrimental effects of prolonged muscular denervation. These early successes and growing fund of knowledge contributed to the emergence of nerve transfers as a potential adjunct or initial alternative to traditional reconstructive methods of nerve grafting, tendon transfers, and joint fusions in the setting of peripheral nerve compression and/or traumatic peripheral nerve and brachial plexus injury.[8-10]

Although reports of nerve transfers for peripheral nerve and plexus injuries are published regularly in the literature, there remains a paucity of data surrounding the use of nerve transfers in the setting of central pathology within the spinal cord. This particular pathology poses a conundrum, and nerve transfers may afford a significant advantage over traditional treatment methodologies. In peripheral nerve injuries "time is muscle" and functional outcomes decrease with increased time from the initial injury because there is rapid atrophy and disintegration of muscle fibers after a period of a few months and apoptosis of distal Schwann cells leading to very poor if not irrecoverable function after 1 year.[2] As demonstrated in the presented study, in a SCI, continuity remains between anterior horn cells and motor endplates below the level of the injury with the preservation of muscle fibers over time. Thus timing is not as crucial in a SCI as it is in peripheral nerve injury, and the potential impact that nerve transfer may afford this patient population persists over a prolonged period of time. Moreover, in contrast to the clinical scenarios encountered with peripheral lacerations or brachial plexopathy, in a SCI postoperative mobilization is of paramount importance. The traditional surgical approaches to SCIs in the form of tendon transfers require prolonged immobilization to protect the integrity of the transfer. However, nerve transfers allow early mobilization after surgery, which avoids worsening stiffness in a patient population at risk of a contracture.

Because of the central and more profound nature of this pathologic process, the determination of an appropriate donor nerve in a SCI presents a significant challenge, because there are fewer available functional and expendable motor nerves in proximity to the recipient motor endplates. Dr. Mackinnon's creative adaptation of her early work with the brachialis nerve in double fascicular transfer for the restoration of elbow function as mentioned previously led to its application in SCIs. Both the expendability of the brachialis nerve and its proximity to the AIN make it a worthy candidate for transfer in the setting of SCIs as used in this landmark article.

Bertelli et al[3,4] have recently published two similar case reports detailing the use of nerve transfers in SCIs. In a similar manner in which Dr. Mackinnon's idea for the presented donor motor nerve came to fruition, Bertelli[3] transferred the teres minor motor branch of the axillary nerve, one of the nerves used in the common nerve transfers for the restoration of shoulder function, to the triceps nerve 9 months after injury to provide elbow extension. He also performed a transfer of the supinator motor branch to the posterior interosseous nerve to restore thumb and finger extension 7 months after the initial injury.[4] Both patients demonstrated functional improvements after surgery.

Conclusion   SCIs present a particularly interesting injury pattern, distinct from peripheral injury, because the damage affects one or a few levels but carries the potential for reinnervation below the level of the injury with preservation of the motor endplates. The highlighted study presents a patient who demonstrated the potential impact nerve transfers may carry in this neurologically devastated population. As a sole case study, further investigation is indicated to elucidate the reproducibility of the procedures and the significance of subsequent functional outcomes both within patient cohorts and in comparison with historical standards such as tendon transfers; however, the potential for significant functional impact of nerve transfers remains high.

Summary   There has been a recent paradigm shift in the treatment of peripheral nerve injuries with the advent of nerve transfers pioneered by Dr. Mackinnon. Nerve transfers are becoming a first-line treatment for proximal nerve injury with a reliance on tendon transfers as a salvage procedure if the desired functional outcome is not achieved. This article highlights a novel application of nerve transfers and emphasizes their potential role in the spinal cord injury population.

REFERENCES

1. Mackinnon SE, Yee A, Ray WZ. Nerve transfers for the restoration of hand function after spinal cord injury. J Neurosurg 117:176-185, 2012.
2. Tung TH, Mackinnon SE. Nerve transfers: indications, techniques, and outcomes. J Hand Surg Am 35:332-341, 2010.
    This summary article presents the current approaches to nerve transfers.
3. Bertelli JA, Ghizoni MF, Tacca CP. Transfer of the teres minor motor branch for triceps reinnervation in tetraplegia. J Neurosurg 114:1457-1460, 2011.
    This is a case report of a novel nerve transfer used to restore function in a SCI.
4. Bertelli JA, Tacca CP, Ghizoni MF, et al. Transfer of supinator motor branches to the posterior interosseous nerve to reconstruct thumb and finger extension in tetraplegia: case report. J Hand Surg Am 35:1647-1651, 2010.
    This is a case report of a novel nerve transfer used to restore function in a SCI.
5. Oberlin C, Ameur NE, Teboul F, et al. Restoration of elbow flexion in brachial plexus injury by transfer of ulnar nerve fascicles to the nerve to the biceps muscle. Tech Hand Up Extrem Surg 6:86-90, 2002.
    This is one of Oberlin's first papers describing the Oberlin procedure and its outcomes in a case series of patients.
6. Tung TH, Novak CB, Mackinnon SE. Nerve transfers to the biceps and brachialis branches to improve elbow flexion strength after brachial plexus injuries. J Neurosurg 98:313-318, 2003.
    This landmark article presents a case series of patients who underwent a modification of the Oberlin procedure with a double fascicular transfer and the research that served as the foundation for the procedure.

7. Ray WZ, Pet MA, Yee A, et al. Double fascicular nerve transfer to the biceps and brachialis muscles after brachial plexus injury: clinical outcomes in a series of 29 cases. J Neurosurg 114:1520-1528, 2011.

8. Bertelli JA, Ghizoni MF. Transfer of the accessory nerve to the suprascapular nerve in brachial plexus reconstruction. J Hand Surg Am 32:989-998, 2007.

9. Bertelli JA, Kechele PR, Santos MA, et al. Axillary nerve repair by triceps motor branch through axillary access: anatomical basis and clinical results. J Neurosurg 107:370-377, 2007.

10. Haase SC, Chung KC. Anterior interosseous nerve transfer to the motor branch of the ulnar nerve for high ulnar nerve injuries. Ann Plast Surg 49:285-290, 2002.

11. Kuhn TS. The Structure of Scientific Revolutions, 3rd ed. Chicago: University of Chicago Press, 1996.

12. Logan D, King J, Fischer-Wright H. Tribal Leadership: Leveraging Natural Groups to Build a Thriving Organization. New York: Harper Collins, 2008.

13. Ericsson KA, Charnes N, Feltovich PJ, et al. The Cambridge Handbook of Expertise and Expert Performance. New York: Cambridge University Press, 2006.

14. Johnson S. Where Good Ideas Come From. The Natural History of Innovation. New York: Penguin Group (USA), 2010.

15. Kiwerski J. Recovery of the simple hand function in tetraplegia patients following transfer of the musculo-cutaneous nerve into the median nerve. Paraplegia 20:242-247, 1982.

16. Carlsen BT, Kircher MF, Spinner RJ, et al. Comparison of single versus double nerve transfers for elbow flexion after brachial plexus injury. Plast Reconstr Surg 127:269-276, 2011.

17. Ray WZ, Yarbrough CK, Yee A, et al. Clinical outcomes following brachialis to anterior interosseous nerve transfers. J Neurosurg 117:604-609, 2012.

STUDY AUTHOR REFLECTIONS

Susan E. Mackinnon, MD, FACS

I have been fortunate to have practiced during two major paradigm shifts in nerve surgery: nerve repair to nerve graft and nerve graft to nerve transfer. These radical changes in the management of nerve injuries illustrate Thomas Kuhn's concept[11] of scientific development "as a succession of tradition-bound periods punctuated by sudden breaks or paradigm shifts."

Trained in the era of nerve grafting and stimulated by the "average" results especially with long grafts, in April 1991 I expanded the use of nerve transfer for high ulnar nerve injuries and upper brachial plexus injuries with the anterior interosseous nerve to deep ulnar and medial pectoral to musculocutaneous nerve transfers. The academic environments at the University of Toronto and Washington University School of Medicine in St. Louis provided strong clinical and basic neuroscience research communities with outstanding colleagues and collaborators.[12]

Decades of hard work[13] and some moments of good luck and serendipity combined to provide the "adjacent possibilities"[14] that facilitated the micro-internal dissection of major nerves and an understanding of the complex but reproducible and reliable internal topography of the peripheral nerve. We recently became aware of a 1982 study in which the musculocutaneous nerve was divided in the midarm and transferred to the entire median nerve.[15] It was certainly a "good idea, but before its time."[14] A report, critical of the need to innervate the brachialis nerve with our double fascicular technique, freed us to use the brachialis nerve as an expendable nerve donor to provide hand function in patients with lower brachial plexus injuries.[16,17]

However, it was a truly serendipitous event that led to this case of restoration of hand closing function in a C7 quadriplegic patient. Dr. Martin C. Robson brought his life-long friend since their surgical internship to my clinic and requested a nerve transfer to restore hand function. Now 4 years after that procedure, this patient continues to have increased hand function, which is critical to his independence and enhancement of his quality of life. My associate, Dr. Ida K. Fox, is leading our effort in nerve transfers in the spinal cord–injured population and has replicated this result. Nerve transfer in the spinal cord–injured population is a field in its infancy. Specifically, this operation is challenging, because the success of the nerve transfer procedure for hand closure in the patient with a spinal cord injury requires experience and understanding of the very complex internal anatomy of the median nerve so that the portions of the median nerve under voluntary control above the spinal cord injury are protected (that is, wrist flexion and pronation) and the fascicles for thumb and finger flexion are specifically identified and reinnervated.

This single case report reflects decades of work and would not have occurred in my practice without that critical balance between the clinic and the bench and those key ingredients described by Ericsson et al,[13] Johnson,[14] and Logan et al[12]: persistence and effort spurred on by failure, outstanding collaborations, a dedicated team, and occasionally some very good fortune and good luck.

CHAPTER 11

Refinements in Rotation-Advancement Cleft Lip Technique

Millard DR Jr. Plast Reconstr Surg 33:26-38, 1964

Reviewed by Jeyhan S. Wood, MD

> *Genius is an infinite capacity for taking pains [attributed to Sir Arthur Conan Doyle]. This is true not only in the art of detection; but it should be an incentive for us to pay greater attention to detail, which in surgery is merely a striving for perfection by refinement of broader principles.*[1]

Research Question   How can the rotation-advancement cleft lip repair technique be improved to provide patients with better aesthetic outcomes?

Funding   Not applicable

Study Dates   8 years (1955 to 1963)

Publishing Date   January 1964

Location   University of Miami School of Medicine, Miami, FL

Subjects   Children with incomplete or complete unilateral cleft lip, who have undergone the rotation-advancement technique by Dr. Millard

Exclusion Criteria   Not applicable

Sample Size   Not applicable

Overview of Design   A retrospective review of healed results of patients undergoing Millard's rotation-advancement lip repair

Intervention   Not applicable

Follow-up   Not reported

Endpoints   Critical and detailed observation of healed results over 8 years

Results   Seven refinements of Millard's rotation-advancement technique are presented, which he noted after criticizing his own postoperative results over an 8-year period.

1. The first is lengthening of the unilateral short columella with the C flap. He suggests holding up the affected nostril arch to approximate the unaffected side in height. The resultant defect at the base of the cleft side columella indicates the amount of tissue deficiency that is needed. This defect may be filled with the C flap.

2. He suggests extending the incision of the lateral flap into the nasal vestibule to increase the length of the advancement flap, particularly for wide clefts. This decreases tension across the repair by recruiting the excess tissue within the vestibule that may otherwise be discarded.

3. Millard advocates maintaining the white roll across the cleft defect at the mucocutaneous junction line to provide a clear separation between the red vermilion and pink scar.

4. He recommends revising the alar web with a crescent excision. This not only thins the excess bulky tissue from within the cleft side ala but also lifts the nostril arch, which contributes to nostril symmetry.

5. He proposes the use of autogenous rib for alveolar bone grafting to provide a supportive base for the nose and lip. Millard describes supplementing the bony alveolar gap with rib after turning over the mucoperiosteal flaps to expose the cleft. The rib is covered with lip mucosa that has been freed from its adjacent maxillary attachments. This strut provides the needed support to the alar base, resulting in improved symmetry of the nose and vermilion.

6. He recommends correcting the often attenuated vermilion border through adjacent tissue rearrangement, specifically, V-Y advancements and Z-plasty of the posterior lip mucosa. Millard suggests adjusting the unaffected "normal" side when needed.

7. Although incomplete clefts have less missing tissue and baseline distortion, they often require just as much or even more rotation versus their complete cleft counterparts. Therefore most of these refinements also apply to the incomplete cleft. According to Millard, the principles of the rotation-advancement technique are "to save the most tissue, rearrange natural landmarks to the best advantage, place the scars in the least objectionable positions, and offer less difficulty for secondary corrections."

Criticisms/Limitations   This is a single author's observations of his own technique.

Relevant Studies   Unilateral cheiloplasty began as a simple straight-line repair. The recognition that Cupid's bow is present in a cleft lip was a major turning point, with subsequent techniques focusing on the preservation and proper alignment of this important anatomic structure. At the time of Millard's original[2] description of his rotation-advancement technique, many other methods were being implemented, such as the quadrangular flap, triangular flap, and straight-line repairs.[3] Numerous surgeons have offered their own refinements to improve the classically described rotation-advancement repair while preserving the fundamental goals, which include preserving Cupid's bow and the normal philtral column line and minimizing tension across the free border of the lip. These modifications have developed to address observed limitations of the repair, such as inadequate rotation of the medial lip segment, deficient vermilion at the cleft, and scarring along the philtral column.[3] Today 84% of cleft surgeons use the rotation-advancement technique with or without modification; the most popular variations are the Noordhoff vermilion flap, triangular advancement flap, and Mohler modification.[3] For those surgeons who prefer a triangular flap technique, the most common are the Randall-Tennison repair and Fisher anatomical subunit approach.[3]

Furthermore, the nasal component of primary lip repair has evolved over the years to become a major focus of correction, with over half of cleft surgeons performing some type of primary nasal correction in their patients with complete unilateral cleft lip.[3] Innumerable techniques have been described to address the cleft nasal deformity with the underlying principle that cartilage shape and position are the contributing factors behind surrounding soft tissue changes. Innovators in the field of cleft nasal deformity have emphasized the placement of the cleft-side alar cartilage into the proper alignment even before the repair of the nasal floor or lip.[4]

Although most of the technical refinements described in this paper have become common practice among cleft surgeons when rotation-advancement lip repair is performed, some have not. Primary alveolar bone grafting in the first year of life as described here by Millard continues to be an area of debate, because studies have shown both a negative impact on subsequent maxillary growth[5] and no midface growth restriction.[6] Secondary bone grafting with cancellous bone from the iliac crest at the time of mixed dentition has become the gold standard. Advocates claim predictability in graft take with reliable support for the alar base and the supportive role of the graft in the eruption of the cleft dentition.[5] Furthermore, most anterior maxillary growth has ceased by the age of 6 years, minimizing any potential growth impairments by the bone graft.[5]

Although Millard repaired most lips at the average age of 3 months, he recommended considering a delay in surgery in those children with exceptionally wide clefts. Today, nasoalveolar molding would be offered at many institutions to help narrow the cleft before surgical repair. Presurgical infant orthopedics has impacted the surgical repair of wide unilateral and bilateral cleft lips since its original introduction in the 1950s.[7]

Nasoalveolar molding has evolved through several modifications in device design and function. This has ranged from active molding to passive alignment of the cleft segments and from primarily addressing the lip deformity to comprehensive treatment of the lip, palate, and nasal deformity.[8,9] On completion of nasoalveolar molding, the medial and lateral lip segments may be in such close proximity to one another at the time of lip repair to allow primary gingivoperiosteoplasty, which has been reported to eliminate the need for future alveolar bone grafting in some instances.[10]

Summary   Millard may have said it best: "There cannot be enough emphasis placed on the value of modifying a flexible method to the individual differences of each case and later embellishing it rather than forcing a rigid method into the mouth of every cleft. Our end point is the ideal normal, an extremely limiting and inelastic goal."

Implications   The Millard rotation-advancement technique has become the standard for the repair of unilateral complete and incomplete cleft lips for most cleft surgeons. This technique is under continual evolution to make the repair of a cleft lip even less conspicuous. The presence of a multitude of techniques and modifications of the rotation-advancement repair is a testament to the fact that the ultimate goal of achieving reproducible, lasting symmetry for the lip and nose remains elusive.

REFERENCES

1. Millard DR Jr. Refinements in rotation-advancement cleft lip technique. Plast Reconstr Surg 33:26-38, 1964.
2. Millard DR Jr. A radical rotation in single harelip. Am J Surg 95:318-322, 1985.
3. Sitzman TJ, Girotto JA, Marcus JR. Current surgical practices in cleft care: unilateral cleft lip repair. Plast Reconstr Surg 121:261e-270e, 2008.
4. McComb HK, Coghlan BA. Primary repair of the unilateral cleft lip nose: completion of a longitudinal study. Cleft Palate Craniofac J 33:23-31; discussion 30-31, 1996.
5. Grisius TM, Spolyar J, Jackson IT, et al. Assessment of cleft lip and palate patients treated with presurgical orthopedic correction and either primary bone grafts, gingivoperiosteoplasty, or without alveolar grafting procedures. J Craniofac Surg 17:468-473, 2006.
6. Dado DV, Rosenstein SW, Alder ME, et al. Long-term assessment of early alveolar bone grafts using three-dimensional computer-assisted tomography: a pilot study. Plast Reconstr Surg 99:1840-1845, 1997.
7. McNeil C. Orthodontic procedures in the treatment of congenital cleft palate. Dent Rec (London) 70:126-132, 1950.
8. Grayson BH, Cutting C, Wood R. Preoperative columella lengthening in bilateral cleft lip and palate. Plast Reconstr Surg 92:1422-1423, 1993.
9. Grayson BH, Maull D. Nasoalveolar molding for infants born with clefts of the lip, alveolus, and palate. Semin Plast Surg 19:294-301, 2005.
10. Santiago PE, Grayson BH, Cutting CB, et al. Reduced need for alveolar bone grafting by presurgical orthopedics and primary gingivoperiosteoplasty. Cleft Palate Craniofac J 35:77-80, 1998.

EXPERT COMMENTARY

H. Wolfgang Losken, MD, MBChB, FCS(SA), FRCS(Ed)

Ralph Millard first performed the rotation-advancement cleft lip repair while in Vietnam during the war. This was an exceptional contribution to cleft surgery. This publication is the most significant one on cleft lip repair. As a Maytag-McCahill Fellow with Dr. Millard during 1972, I was impressed that he was a great teacher and a superb surgeon. His most significant quality was that every cleft lip repair was a challenge to achieve a better result. He would constantly try new ways that would result in a better outcome. In this article he identifies seven refinements to the repair. That was Millard at his best and this was plastic surgery at its best. His many residents and fellows benefited from this inquiring approach and were challenged to do the same in their future careers in plastic surgery. Their contributions to the field of plastic surgery attest to the influence Ralph Millard had on the field of plastic surgery.

I spent time with him in the last year before he passed away. He was proud of his wonderful contribution to cleft lip care, and he was delighted at the improvement that followed his rotation-advancement cleft lip repair. It is remarkable that 84% of all surgeons are still doing the Millard repair or a modification 50 years after it was first presented. Is there another operation that can achieve this degree of success?

CHAPTER 12

Cleft Palate Repair by Double Opposing Z-plasty

Furlow LT Jr. Plast Reconstr Surg 78:724-738, 1986

Reviewed by Daniel J. Krochmal, MD, FACS

> *It is hoped that double opposing Z-plasty palate repair will be another step toward the surgical goals of normal speech, growth, and hearing for the child with a cleft of the palate.[1]*

Research Question   Previous techniques of cleft palate repair have resulted in mid-facial growth retardation or required multiple stages that resulted in poor speech. Does a single-stage Z-plasty palate repair effectively close the cleft and result in adequate speech function?

Funding   None mentioned

Study Dates   November 1976 to the time of manuscript preparation in 1985

Publishing Date   December 1986

Location   Craniofacial Unit at the University of Florida, Gainesville, FL

Subjects   Twenty-two consecutive patients, ages 6.75 to 15 months at the time of palate repair; eight patients had unilateral cleft lip and palate, eight had bilateral cleft lip and palate, and six had postalveolar clefts.

Exclusion Criteria   None

Overview of Design   A case series; a retrospective review of 22 patients who underwent double opposing Z-plasty palatoplasty with routine postoperative monitoring and speech assessment

Intervention   A novel technique for cleft palatoplasty was performed. The repair involved a "mirror image" procedure on either side of the cleft. The central limb of the Z-plasty is the cleft. The anteriorly based flaps are composed of mucosa only (either palatal or nasal), whereas the posteriorly based flaps are composed of both palatal muscle and mucosa (either palatal or nasal) as a myomucosal flap. The lateral limbs of the Z-plasty end at the hamuli. Transposing the myomucosal flaps creates a muscle sling. For hard palate repair, mucoperiosteal flaps are elevated and sutured together in the midline. Often, relaxing incisions are not necessary because the tissue is taken from a curved arch of the palate and brought into a shorter horizontal plane.

Follow-up   Routine postoperative and speech follow-up was in an academic craniofacial center. Median follow-up was 3.75 years (range 0.33 to 8.33 years). Twenty patients underwent velopharyngeal assessment, and 16 patients underwent subsequent formal speech evaluation.

Endpoints   Velopharyngeal competence, secondary palatal surgery, presence of a crossbite, audiologic status, and postoperative complications

Results   The two patients with mild velopharyngeal insufficiency had unilateral cleft lip and palate repairs.

Regarding postoperative complications, one child had a fistula that was subsequently repaired, one child had a postoperative fever that delayed her hospital discharge, and one child had postoperative stridor that resolved with expectant management (Table 12-1).[1] In one patient with a wide bilateral cleft, buccal mucosal flaps were used to close the large back cuts.

Criticisms/Limitations   Taken on its own, the limitations of this study include a single surgeon's experience, limited case numbers, and descriptive statistics. Regarding the technique, it may be inadequate in very wide horseshoe-shaped clefts, leading to the inability to close the hard palate mucoperiosteal flaps in the midline even though the posterior soft palate myomucosal flaps may close easily. (Dr. Furlow cites this unique case in this paper.)

Table 12-1   Degree of Velopharyngeal Insufficiency in Treatment of Cleft Patients

Velopharyngeal Insufficiency	No. of Patients	Percentage
None	18/20	90
Mild	2/20	10
Moderate or severe	0/20	0
Pharyngeal flap	0/20	0

Data from Furlow LT Jr. Cleft palate repair by double opposing Z-plasty. Plast Reconstr Surg 78:724-736, 1986.

Relevant Studies   Leonard Furlow[2] presented his initial work at the Southeastern Society of Plastic and Reconstructive Surgeons in 1978. Other groups embraced the technique and have reported improved speech results compared with prior techniques.[3] A nonrandomized comparison between the double opposing Z-plasty and a two-flap palatoplasty has shown that the Furlow repair is associated with improved velopharyngeal closure.[4] A prospective, randomized study also showed improved velopharyngeal function compared with the von Langenbeck procedure, although in this study the fistula rate for the Furlow palatoplasty was higher.[5] At our institution, when limiting the Furlow palatoplasty to Veau type I or II repairs that are less than 8 mm wide, no postoperative fistulas were noted in 36 patients.[6] For children who develop velopharyngeal incompetence after palatoplasty, the Furlow double opposing Z-plasty technique can be an effective treatment.[7,8] Thus far, the Furlow double opposing Z-plasty palate repair has withstood the test of time and has become a standard procedure in the cleft surgeon's armamentarium.

Summary   Dr. Furlow's double opposing Z-plasty appears to be an effective method to close a primary cleft and lengthen the palate to provide velopharyngeal competence. It is also useful in secondary revision procedures to increase palatal length in an effort to forego pharyngeal flap surgeries.

Implications   The ability to simultaneously address the hard and soft palates while not significantly inhibiting maxillary growth has obviated the need for a two-stage approach to palatoplasty. Compared with earlier techniques, the double opposing Z-plasty has improved postoperative speech function and has a low fistula rate. After 40 years, it remains the procedure of choice for some cleft surgeons.

REFERENCES

1. Furlow LT Jr. Cleft palate repair by double opposing Z-plasty. Plast Reconstr Surg 78:724-738, 1986.
2. Furlow LT Jr. Cleft palate repair: preliminary report on lengthening and muscle transposition by Z-plasty. Presented at the Annual Meeting of the Southeastern Society of Plastic and Reconstructive Surgeons, Boca Raton, FL, May 16, 1978.
3. Kirschner RE, Wang P, Jawad AF, et al. Cleft-palate repair by modified Furlow double-opposing Z-plasty: the Children's Hospital of Philadelphia experience. Plast Reconstr Surg104:1998-2010; discussion 2011-2014, 1999.
4. Dong Y, Dong F, Zhang Z, et al. An effect comparison between Furlow double opposing Z-plasty and two-flap palatoplasty on velopharyngeal closure. Int J Oral Maxillofac Surg 41:604-611, 2012.
5. Williams WN, Seagle MB, Pegoraro-Krook MI, et al. Prospective clinical trial comparing outcome measure between Furlow and von Langenbeck palatoplasties for UCLP. Ann Plast Surg 66:154-163, 2011.
6. Losken HW, van Aalst JA, Teotia SS, et al. Achieving low cleft palate fistula rates: surgical results and techniques. Cleft Palate Craniofac J 48:312-320, 2011.

7. Chen PK, Wu JT, Chen YR, et al. Correction of secondary velopharyngeal insufficiency in cleft palate patients with the Furlow palatoplasty. Plast Reconstr Surg 94:933-941, 1994.
8. Hudson DA, Grobbelaar AO, Fernandes DB, et al. Treatment of velopharyngeal incompetence by the Furlow Z-plasty. Ann Plast Surg 34:23-26, 1995.
9. Furlow LT Jr. Double opposing Z-plasty palate repair. In Losee J, Kirchner R, eds. Comprehensive Cleft Care. New York: McGraw Hill, 2009.
10. LaRossa D, Kirschner RE, Low DW. The Children's Hospital modification of the Furlow double-opposing Z-plasty. In Losee J, Kirschner, R, eds. Comprehensive Cleft Care. New York: McGraw Hill, 2009.
11. McCraw JB, Furlow LT Jr. The dorsalis pedis arterialized flap. A clinical study. Plast Reconstr Surg 55:177-185, 1975.

STUDY AUTHOR REFLECTIONS

Leonard T. Furlow, Jr., MD, FACS

A far too high velopharyngeal insufficiency (VPI) rate (52%) in my von Langenbeck (VL) and VL + intravelar veloplasty repairs led me to search for a one-stage repair that would provide adequate velar length, good levator function, and minimal hard palate scarring to ensure good maxillary growth. From my familiarity with Z-plasties in other sites, I realized that two Z-plasties could realign the velar muscles and lengthen the velum without taking mucoperiosteum from the hard palate

In private practice I did 37 cases—33 infants and 4 older patients; 10 were syndromic. The VPI rate was 8%, down from 52%. I am sorry that space restraints require me to present my patients as data in a table.

The case results for the 33 infants are shown in Table 12-2.

After I retired, I performed some 300 double opposing Z-plasty palate repairs on volunteer surgery trips; it was a great operative experience marred by minimal follow-up.

Table 12-2 Private Practice Experience With Double Opposing Z-Plasty for Cleft Palate Repair

Type	No.	Postoperative VPI	Fistulas	LeFort I	Lateral Relaxing Incisions
UCLP	2	1/12	0	0	0
BCLP	10	1/10	0	2	0
CP	11	1/11	2	0	0
Total	33	3/33 (9%)	2/33 (6%)	2	0
9-34 y/o	4	0/4	0	0	0
Total	37	3/37 (8%)	2/37 (5%)	2	0

BCLP, Bilateral cleft lip palatoplasty; *CP,* cleft palatoplasty; *UCLP,* unilateral cleft lip palatoplasty; *VPI,* velopharyngeal insufficiency.

From these I learned:

1. The importance of the posteriorly based Z-plasty lateral limb incisions, which automatically divide the palatal aponeuroses, to free the muscles for rotation.
2. The importance of the anteriorly based Z-plasty lateral limb incisions, which determine the AP, lateral, and posterior pharyngeal wall distances of the tip of the levators and position the flap tips directly under/over the base of the contralateral levator where it enters the velum from behind the superior constrictor; this automatically produces a precisely transverse levator sling.
3. That closure of the hard palate depends not on cleft width but on the available mucoperiosteal flap width.
4. That hard palate mattress sutures avoid fistulas.
5. How to preplan the operation by measuring the available mucoperiosteal flap width before incision.
6. How to make accurate cleft margin incisions when the mucoperiosteal flap width is adequate.
7. What to do when there is insufficient mucoperiosteal flap width for closure without lateral relaxing incisions.

These and a number of other tips are in my last article in *Comprehensive Cleft Care*.[9]

Peter Randall of the University of Pennsylvania liked the description of my first four cases in 1978, and he has taught it worldwide. His modifications—the liberal use of relaxing incisions, space of Ernst dissection, smaller Z-plasties, and a less well-defined levator dissection and inset[10]—have probably become the most used version of the operation. Although I prefer my version, it is not clear which produces better results.

EDITORIAL PERSPECTIVE

C. Scott Hultman, MD, MBA, FACS

Dr. Maurice "Josh" John Jurkiewicz, Past President of the American College of Surgeons and former Chief of Plastic Surgery at Emory University, told me that that Leonard Furlow's double opposing Z-plasty was the most ingenious operation of the twentieth century. This opinion serves as the highest of endorsements for this procedure. Also of note, Dr. Furlow was one of the first residents to graduate from The University of North Carolina's plastic surgery residency program in 1965 under the leadership of Erle Peacock, Jr., MD, JD. After finishing his hand surgery training at The University of North Carolina, Dr. Furlow then completed his craniofacial training under Dr. J at the University of Florida. In 1975 Dr. Furlow, in conjunction with John McCraw, was also the first surgeon to describe the dorsalis pedis fasciocutaneous flap for the coverage of local defects of the foot, ankle, and lower leg.[11]

The birth of axial, pedicled, composite fasciocutaneous flaps had just occurred.

CHAPTER 13

Lengthening the Human Mandible by Gradual Distraction

McCarthy JG, Schreiber J, Karp N, Thorne CH, Grayson BH. Plast Reconstr Surg 89:1-8; discussion 9-10, 1992

Reviewed by Daniel J. Krochmal, MD, FACS

> *If a hypoplastic mandible can be increased in length and volume, one can speculate whether there is also the potential for improvement in neuromuscular function (functional matrix) and attendant growth and development of the affected jaw. The answer obviously awaits and the development of an internal expansion device and long-term observation of a larger number of patients.*[1]

Research Question Previous work had already demonstrated the efficacy and safety profile of the distraction technique on the extremities of humans to obviate the need for bone grafts and the mandible of canines. What is the effectiveness and morbidity profile of the distraction osteogenesis technique on the pediatric human mandible?

Funding None mentioned; after submission, the authors "entered into an agreement with the Howmedica Company to modify the expansion device."[1]

Study Dates May 1989 until manuscript submission in 1991

Publishing Date January 1992

Location New York University Medical Center Institute of Reconstructive Plastic Surgery, New York, NY

Subjects A case series of four pediatric subjects: a 23-month-old male with right-sided craniofacial microsomia, an 8-year-old male with Nager syndrome (bilateral distraction), a 5-year-old male with left-sided craniofacial microsomia, and a 10-year-old male with left-sided craniofacial microsomia

Exclusion Criteria   None

Overview of Design   A case series—a prospective pilot study that used an external distraction device for mandibular distraction; photographs, radiographs, and dental models were obtained preoperatively, postoperatively, at distractor removal, and every 6 months thereafter.

Intervention   An external mandibular distractor was placed. With the use of a modified Risdon incision, the mandible was exposed in a supraperiosteal plane. Four distractor holes were drilled bicortically at 10 and 14 mm away from the eventual corticotomy site. The pins were placed in the mandible, the site was closed, and the external lengthening device was attached to the pins. Expansion began at 7 days at a rate of 1 mm/day for 20 days, with a subsequent 9-week consolidation phase.

Follow-up   Patients were followed every 6 months until manuscript submission. Follow-up ranged from 11 to 20 months.

Endpoints   Chin position, subjective evidence of mandible lengthening on radiography, and surgical outcomes and complications

Results   The 23-month-old male patient underwent a successful unilateral expansion of 18 mm; at 17 months afterward, his chin remained deviated to the contralateral side, with considerable radiographic evidence of increased mandibular length. The 8-year-old male patient with Nager syndrome underwent a successful bilateral expansion, with 24 mm on the left side and 22 mm on the right side; on follow-up he had a 5 mm relapse and scars that were considered nonsatisfactory. The 5-year-old male patient underwent a successful unilateral expansion of 20 mm; "long-term" clinical and radiographic follow-up demonstrated a significant increase in mandibular dimensions. The 10-year-old male patient underwent a successful unilateral expansion of 20 mm; his chin position moved to a more midline position.

Criticisms/Limitations   The longest follow-up was 20 months. Therefore following bone length and mandible position with continued facial growth could not be assessed initially. This limitation has been subsequently addressed, and the surgical correction has been shown to be stable.[2]

Relevant Studies   Gavriil Abramovich Ilizarov,[3] a self-trained Russian internist, surgeon, obstetrician, pediatrician, and orthopedist, developed and popularized his technique for the gradual lengthening of bone in the 1960s and 1970s. Preliminary work on lengthening canine mandibles was successful and thus paved the way for study in humans.[4] Several authors published their thoughts on the technique a decade after the initial manuscript.[5] They noted that the treatment of micrognathia with sleep apnea and upper airway obstruction had been revolutionized: distraction of Pruzansky type II mandibles had replaced rib graft reconstruction, and distraction could lengthen a bone graft that had become insufficient in length; that the simultaneous lengthening of soft tissues limits relapse; and if needed secondary and tertiary distraction can be performed. Since this publication, distraction osteogenesis has become a very powerful, widespread tool for lengthening the pediatric mandible and has also found uses in other areas of craniomaxillofacial dysmorphology.[6-8] The distractor apparatus has evolved and now includes options for internal distractor and resorbable devices.

Summary   Distraction osteogenesis of the pediatric mandible with an external device achieves excellent mandibular lengthening and has a satisfactory morbidity profile. On short-term follow-up, bone resorption does not appear to be an issue

Implications   This technique allows lengthening the pediatric mandible without a need for a secondary surgical site for bone grafting or intermaxillary fixation. The efficacy and safety profile of mandibular distraction have allowed this procedure to expand beyond the mandible, and it is used in both midfacial and cranial vault expansion procedures. The ability to simultaneously lengthen soft tissues without muscle or nerve dysfunction makes distraction osteogenesis a very powerful tool.

REFERENCES

1. McCarthy JG, Schreiber J, Karp N, et al. Lengthening the human mandible by gradual distraction. Plast Reconstr Surg 89:1-8; discussion 9-10, 1992.
2. Shetye PR, Grayson BH, Mackool RJ, et al. Long-term stability and growth following unilateral mandibular distraction in growing children with craniofacial microsomia. Plast Reconstr Surg 118:985-995, 2006.
3. Ilizarov GA, Ledyaev VI. The replacement of long tubular bones defects by lengthening distraction osteotomy of one of the fragments. 1969. Clin Orthop Relat Res 280:7-10, 1992.
4. Karp NS, Thorne CH, McCarthy JG, et al. Bone lengthening in the craniofacial skeleton. Ann Plast Surg 24:231-237, 1990.
5. McCarthy JG, Katzen JT, Hopper R, et al. The first decade of mandibular distraction: lessons we have learned. Plast Reconstr Surg 110:1704-1713, 2002.
6. Shetye PR, Boutros S, Grayson BH, et al. Midterm follow-up of midface distraction for syndromic craniosynostosis: a clinical and cephalometric study. Plast Reconstr Surg 120:1621-1632, 2007.
7. Hopper RA. New trends in cranio-orbital and midface distraction for craniofacial dysostosis. Curr Opin Otolaryngol Head Neck Surg 20:298-303, 2012.
8. Saman M, Abramowitz JM, Buchbinder D. Mandibular osteotomies and distraction osteogenesis: evolution and current advances. JAMA Facial Plast Surg 15:167-173, 2013.
9. Caballero M, Pappa AK, Roden KS, et al. Osteoinduction of umbilical cord and palate periosteum-derived mesenchymal stem cells on poly (lactic-co-glycolic) acid nanomicrofibers. Ann Plast Surg 72(Suppl 2):S176-S183, 2014.
10. Deshpande S, James AW, Blough J, et al. Reconciling the effects of inflammatory cytokines on mesenchymal cell osteogenic differentiation. J Surg Res 185:278-285, 2013.

STUDY AUTHOR REFLECTIONS
Joseph McCarthy, MD, FACS

This paper was the first one published on the clinical application of the technique of distraction osteogenesis on the craniofacial skeleton. It followed two previous canine studies that were rejected by *Plastic and Reconstructive Surgery* as "irrelevant" and "of little clinical utility."

When our team at the Institute of Reconstructive Plastic Surgery performed the first and historic operation (a unilateral mandibular distraction) in May 1989 (a quarter of a century ago), we were confident that it would be successful because of the findings of our previous laboratory studies. The patient was just shy of 2 years of age and had unilateral craniofacial microsomia. Now a university graduate, he is on the executive staff of the New York Giants football team. We proceeded to continue distraction studies on the mandible, midface, zygoma, and cranium; all of these anatomic sites have undergone successful clinical distraction.

All of the above truly represent "translational research," a term that I prefer to modify as "bidirectional research": clinical to laboratory to clinical. Distraction osteogenesis is actually tissue engineering, or as Joseph Murray wrote, "inductive surgery." In the coming years, fewer interventive techniques will be found to apply distraction; the devices will be miniaturized, and laboratory research will result in a shortening of the consolidation phase. It will be exciting to see future research and developments.

EDITORIAL PERSPECTIVE
C. Scott Hultman, MD, MBA, FACS

The very first presentation I ever gave in plastic surgery was on distraction osteogenesis in 1989. As a fourth-year medical student at the University of Pittsburgh, Bill Futrell, then the Chief of Plastic Surgery, asked me to "look into some old Russian technique that lengthens bone, by an orthopod named Ilizarov [1921-1992]." With cardboard slides and pictures photocopied from Eastern European journals, I delivered a Grand Rounds that was both educational and provocative—and felt like science fiction! Dr. Futrell commented: "Someday we will lengthen mandibles, femurs, and thumbs with that device." Michael Bentz, future Chief of Plastic Surgery at the University of Wisconsin, Madison, was in the audience that day as Dr. Futrell's Chief Resident. Mike has been a mentor of mine for more than 20 years, and I cannot help but think that he tucked that idea away and was stimulated in some small part to pursue a career in pediatric plastic surgery.

One cannot overstate how all of the innovations and innovators in plastic surgery are interconnected. Dr. McCarthy's conceptualization that we can replace bone with new bone—tissue with new tissue—launched the true beginning of tissue engineering on a clinical level. Today discovering even newer ways to create, modulate, and manipulate bone[9,10] has reinvigorated plastic surgery as a field defined by "problem-solving." We are the innovators of surgery, the rightful guardians of tissue engineering, in our quest to restore and enhance both form and function.

CHAPTER 14

Technical Advances in Ear Reconstruction With Autogenous Rib Cartilage Grafts: Personal Experience With 1200 Cases

Brent B. Plast Reconstr Surg 104:319-334; discussion 335-338, 1999

Reviewed by Jeyhan S. Wood, MD, and H. Wolfgang Losken, MD, MBChB, FCS(SA), FRCS(Ed)

Surgically constructed ears remain durable, withstand trauma well, and provide consistent emotional relief and psychological benefits through the repair.[1]

Research Question To present the author's rationale for his current methods of managing total ear reconstruction

Funding None

Study Dates 25-year period

Publishing Date August 1999

Locations Woodside, CA, and Stanford University Medical Center, Palo Alto, CA

Subjects Both children and adults with microtia and traumatic auricular deformities

Exclusion Criteria Not reported

Sample Size There were 1094 completed ears in 1000 patients with microtia: 582 right, 324 left, and 94 bilateral. There were 125 cases of traumatic ear injuries.

Overview of Design This is a retrospective review of total ear reconstructions with autologous cartilage performed by Dr. Brent, with a discussion of the author's current techniques, the general guidelines for each stage of reconstruction, special considerations for different patient populations, and future directions of autologous ear reconstruction. A questionnaire survey on the long-term outcome of ear repair was conducted with patients with microtia.

Intervention   Not applicable

Follow-up   1 to 18 years, with an average of 7.7 years

Endpoints   Observation of healed results and outcomes of 1200 ear reconstructions over a 25-year period

Results   Brent followed Tanzer in perfecting the ear reconstruction. Brent was the pioneer of ear reconstruction. Brent reports that his favorite age to perform ear reconstruction is between 7 and 8 years old when the child is large enough for substantial rib cartilage graft harvest and is becoming aware of the deformity. In his experience Medpor (Porex Surgical Products Group, Newnan, GA) implants are not as resistant to trauma as autogenous grafts and are more prone to infectious complications with resultant draining sinus tracts. Brent reported that he had not lost an ear cartilage graft to trauma after 10 days of the operation. Although prefabrication was originally attempted in the 1940s,[2] the technique resulted in inconsistent results. Prefabrication has been revisited in recent years as tissue engineering has become more popular. This technique is still in the early stages of development, and sculpting autogenous rib cartilage currently remains the procedure of choice for ear reconstruction.

The first stage entails harvesting the rib cartilage from the contralateral chest with a cartilage-sparing technique to limit chest wall deformity. This is accomplished by leaving a small rim of the upper margin of the sixth rib cartilage. The creation of a sufficient ear with minimal cartilage requires the efficient use of the harvested cartilage and is based on Brent's original[3] principle of an expansile framework. In designing the framework, he emphasizes limiting unnecessary trauma by using scalpels and chisels rather than power tools and preserving the perichondrium to promote skin adherence. He advocates the use of 4-0 and 5-0 clear nylon for securing the framework together. Brent describes an advancement to create the tragus within the original framework by including a tragal strut (Fig. 14-1).[1]

Brent touches on several pearls throughout the stages of reconstruction. Regarding framework modifications in older patients, he recommends carving the ear as one piece because the cartilages are often fused into a solid block. He describes the sliding helical advancement technique to increase the projection of the framework if needed. When the cutaneous cover is designed, he marks the position of the ear with the previously made template and makes the incision along the backside of the ear vestige. He describes the careful removal of the deformed cartilage, then the creation of a thin skin pocket with a fine dissection scissors, and dissection beyond the marked ear margin. He uses two small drains. He inserts one drain from under the frame, through the conchal region, and then over the inferior helical crus. The second drain is placed beneath and behind the framework and drains into the vacuum tubes. After surgery he suggests

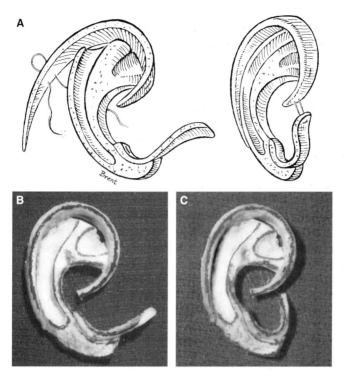

Fig. 14-1 Ear framework fabrication with integral tragal strut. **A,** Construction of the frame. The floating cartilage creates a helix, and second strut is arched around to form the antitragus, intertragal notch, and tragus. This arch is completed when the tip of the strut is affixed to the crus helix of the main frame with horizontal mattress suture of clear nylon. **B** and **C,** Actual framework fabrication with the patient's rib cartilage. (From Brent B. Technical advances in ear reconstruction with autogenous rib cartilage grafts: personal experience with 1200 cases. Plast Reconstr Surg 104:319-334; discussion 335-338, 1999.)

packing the convolutions of the constructed ear with Vaseline gauze and then covering the construct with a bulky noncompressive dressing. He suggests that the tubes should be changed regularly to ensure constant suction. He prefers to remove the drains on postoperative day 5. The sutures are removed at 1 week and then the dressing at day 12. Patients are released to return to school after 2 weeks and to participate in sports after 4 to 5 weeks for children and 6 weeks for teenagers and adults. Regarding sleep, Brent protects the construct for 1 month and then patients are released from the restrictions.

A low hairline at the site of the ear reconstruction is a major problem. He recommends the creation of a hairline before reconstruction is begun. He advises pretreatment of the area with serial laser treatments because this will make the skin softer and finer.

Subsequent stages include earlobe transposition, which Brent believes is safer and aesthetically better to perform as a separate stage as opposed to combining it with framework placement. The ear construct is then lifted with one of the two described methods. The auriculocephalic sulcus may be created by raising the framework with its connective tissue covering through an incision several millimeters remote from the framework and then applying a split-thickness skin graft. If greater projection is desired, the cartilage-wedging technique can be used, which involves placing a wedge of cartilage behind the ear and covering it with a turnover flap of occipitalis fascia, followed by a skin graft. This piece of cartilage is banked beneath the scalp during the first stage of rib cartilage harvest. Brent describes harvesting this piece of cartilage by splitting the outer cartilage from the rib, resulting in desirable warping of the cartilage wedge into an ideal shape to form the posterior conchal wall. Tragus construction can be accomplished through one of the two described methods. By using the tissue from the contralateral ear, adjustments may be made to ensure frontal symmetry. The tragus may be constructed at the first stage by the addition of an extra strut of cartilage (see Fig. 14-1). This technique is particularly helpful in bilateral microtia, in which there is no excess tissue available from which to construct a tragus. The creative use of remnant vestiges presents more of a surgical challenge when a more normal ear exists in conjunction with the remnants.

To determine the long-term results of his microtia repairs, a questionnaire survey was conducted with his patients with microtia; he had a 50.8% response rate. Brent found that reconstructed ears can withstand trauma remarkably well with more than 70 cases of major trauma reported, which resulted in no ear construct losses. The ears reportedly did not have any issues with shrinkage of the cartilage over time. He concluded that autogenous ear frameworks are likely to grow in younger patients and unrepaired microtia causes a significant impact as a child ages and enters school.

Criticisms/Limitations   A single surgeon's experience; it does not provide the questions asked in the survey.

Relevant Studies   The major turning point for modern ear reconstruction was Tanzer's introduction[4] of the use of autologous rib cartilage carved in a solid block. He identified four primary difficulties in ear reconstruction, which remain true today: obtaining an adequate skin envelope, utilizing a framework that is permanent and inert, achieving the delicacy and appropriate contour of a natural ear, and attaining symmetry with the contralateral auricle.[4] He addressed each of these issues with his described technique and achieved results that have lasted over the years.

Carving a delicate ear framework takes considerable time and skill. In an effort to try to simplify the operation, Peer[2] described a prefabricated ear composed of "diced" costal cartilage grafts buried within a Vitallium mold under an abdominal wall skin flap. Months later, the mold would be removed, and the new framework was inserted into a subcutaneous pocket. The main problem with this method was blunting of the desired fine detail of the construct.

Other alternatives to carving an ear framework were and continue to be investigated. In 1966 Cronin[5] introduced implantable silicone ear frameworks. Although the results were aesthetically promising, the Silastic prostheses ultimately had an unacceptably high incidence of extrusion. Despite efforts to cover the frameworks with living tissue, such as fascia lata, galeal, or fascial flaps, the implants still extruded. Although porous polyethylene implants historically have similar complications with extrusion, in recent years improved outcomes have been reported when the implants were covered with temporoparietal fascia flaps.[6]

Today the gold standard for ear reconstruction is with autologous costal cartilage. Several leaders in this field, including Brent,[1] Nagata,[7] and Firmin,[8] follow the same basic principles with slight variations in technique regarding the age at reconstruction, number of stages, and laterality of the donor site. Nagata[7] reduced the number of operations required for ear reconstruction from four (as suggested by Brent) to three by transposing the earlobe at the first operation and also reducing it to two operations by inserting the tragus cartilage graft to the reconstructed ear. For those patients who are not surgical candidates and for adult patients, prosthetic ears may be a practical option.

As alluded to in Brent's article, the future direction of ear reconstruction involves tissue engineering. Proponents of alternate methods of ear reconstruction cite potential downsides to the use of autologous cartilage, including the inconsistent, unreliable shape of the framework, an increase in operative time for harvesting and carving the cartilage, and donor site morbidity, including the risk of pneumothorax, bleeding, and chest wall deformity.[9] Previous attempts to create a tissue-engineered ear cartilage framework found that the neocartilage was not rigid enough to withstand the external deforming forces of the contracting skin envelope unless externally stented for a prolonged period.[9] Brent emphasizes the importance of developing a framework that is durable enough to withstand the deforming, flattening forces of the overlying tight skin envelope. Recent advances in tissue engineering include covering an alloplastic framework with tissue-engineered cartilage to improve the stability between the structure and surrounding tissue.[10] Although the early work is promising, staged autologous ear reconstruction remains the current standard of care for patients with microtia.

Summary   This article presents Brent's latest framework fabrication technique, including cartilage sparing, minimizing donor-site morbidity, tragus reconstruction as part of the original framework, achieving ear projection with a scalp-banked cartilage wedge, and addressing the low hairline with preoperative laser therapy. His survey of 1000 patients with microtia portends to the lasting physical stability of these constructs and the lasting emotional benefits these reconstructions have on this patient population.

Implications   Ear reconstruction is a surgical challenge, requiring considerable skill, meticulous technique, attention to detail, and ability to adapt to each patient because each patient varies in the deformity and the quantity and quality of available donor cartilage. By sharing the refinements of his technique, Brent has allowed quality ear reconstruction with an autologous framework to be widely practiced.

REFERENCES

1. Brent B. Technical advances in ear reconstruction with autogenous rib cartilage grafts: personal experience with 1200 cases. Plast Reconstr Surg 104:319-334; discussion 335-338, 1999.
2. Peer L. Reconstruction of the auricle with diced cartilage grafts in a Vitallium ear mold. Plast Reconstr Surg 3:653-666, 1948.
3. Brent B. Ear reconstruction with an expansile framework of autogenous rib cartilage. Plast Reconstr Surg 53:619-628, 1974.
4. Tanzer R. Total reconstruction of the external ear. Plast Reconstr Surg 23:1, 1959.
5. Cronin TD. Use of a Silastic frame for total and subtotal reconstruction of the external ear: preliminary report. Plast Reconstr Surg 37:399-405, 1966.
6. Reinisch JF, Lewin S. Ear reconstruction using a porous polyethylene framework and temporoparietal fascia flap. Facial Plast Surg 25:181-189, 2009.
7. Nagata S. A new method of total reconstruction of the auricle for microtia. Plast Reconstr Surg 92:187-201, 1993.
8. Firmin F. State-of-the-art autogenous ear reconstruction in cases of microtia. Adv Otorhinolaryngol 68:25-52, 2010.
9. Cao Y, Vacanti JP, Paige K, et al. Transplantation of chondrocytes utilizing a polymer-cell construct to produce tissue-engineered cartilage in the shape of a human ear. Plast Reconstr Surg 100:297-302; discussion 303-304, 1997.
10. Hwang C, Lee BK, Green D, et al. Auricular reconstruction using tissue-engineered alloplastic implants for improved clinical outcomes. Plast Reconstr Surg 133:360e-369e, 2014.

STUDY AUTHOR REFLECTIONS

Burt Brent, MD

I have now done 2000 autogenous rib cartilage grafts for patients with microtia or trauma. The former made up 90% of my experience. I have not really changed my technique in the past decade other than in the stage of separating the ear from the head with a skin graft. I have switched from using split-thickness skin grafts to full-thickness grafts because (1) there is less contraction and shrinkage and (2) the donor site is much more comfortable for the patient and the healing is less problematic.

EDITORIAL PERSPECTIVE

C. Scott Hultman, MD, MBA, FACS

What can you add to a paper that includes the world's largest series of procedures performed by a technical genius over the course of that surgeon's career? I first met Burt Brent as a Visiting Professor at Emory University in 1999 and was humbled, to say the least, to be in the presence of one of the greatest masters of our time. John Bostwick, as Chief of Plastic Surgery, had invited Dr. Brent to help us learn about his techniques for ear reconstruction. What impressed me the most, however, was Dr. Brent's commitment to the psychological, social, and emotional recovery of patients with congenital and traumatic deformities. Although I have never performed a total ear reconstruction, as a faculty member, Dr. Brent's philosophy about total patient care—including the longitudinal component—has deeply and profoundly affected my own practice in burn reconstruction. I am constantly reminded that as surgeons, we perform four-dimensional reconstruction, with the fourth element being time: how we manipulate the reconstruction over time, how the reconstruction matures over time, and how the patient's reconstructive needs may change over time.

CHAPTER 15

The Definitive Plastic Surgical Treatment of the Severe Facial Deformities of Craniofacial Dysostosis. Crouzon's and Apert's Diseases

Tessier P. Plast Reconstr Surg 48:419-442, 1971

Reviewed by H. Wolfgang Losken, MD, MBChB, FCS(SA), FRCS(Ed)

In this paper we shall suggest a surgical method of treatment of the facial deformities associated with certain types of craniostenosis, . . . craniofacial dysostosis, . . . and other facial dysmorphias.[1]

Subject The LeFort III osteotomy and advancement was described in detail by Paul Tessier. After Tessier published this paper, the procedure was performed by surgeons throughout the world. This article was the birth of craniofacial surgery, and Paul Tessier has been considered the father of craniofacial surgery.

Although the LeFort III osteotomy had previously been performed and published by Sir Harold Gillies and S.H. Harrison[2] and Obwegeser,[3] Paul Tessier[1] popularized it.

Crouzon's and Apert's syndromes have maxillary hypoplasia, and the LeFort III osteotomy and advancement will correct this deformity. These children also have craniosynostosis with a varying degree of recession of the forehead, but this operation does not correct this deformity. The LeFort III osteotomy and advancement corrects the flat zygomas and infraorbital border, correcting the appearance of exorbitism. It advances the nose and maxilla and also corrects the class III malocclusion and open bite.

Funding Unknown

Study Dates 1960s

Publishing Date 1971

Location Plastic-Surgical Service, Centre Médico-Chirurgical Foch, Paris, France

Clinical Material Tessier performed the first LeFort III osteotomy in 1958 and reported on three cases. The same procedure is performed in Crouzon's and Apert's syndromes. The exorbitism is corrected by the advancement of the infraorbital margin and the enlargement of the orbital volume. Sagittal and vertical correction is achieved to correct the malocclusion. In Crouzon's and Apert's syndromes there may be craniosynostosis and a receding forehead that may need correction. There may also be hypertelorism that may require a surgical procedure.

Craniofacial Development The growth of the cranium is influenced by the growth of the brain. The growth of the orbit is influenced by the growth of the eyeballs. The growth of the maxilla is directly related to the eruption of the teeth. Craniosynostosis of the skull and face interferes with growth.

Description of Crouzon's Disease There may be brachycephaly or oxycephaly and a bregmatic bump. There is a recession of the forehead, which is caused by coronal craniosynostosis. The maxillary hypoplasia causes the severe exorbitism of Crouzon's syndrome. The reduction in the orbital depth causes this. The shallow bony orbits and hypoplasia of the malar bone result in lateral canthal dystopia.

Difference Between Crouzon's and Apert's Syndromes In Apert's syndrome the supraorbital rim is recessed to a greater degree than in Crouzon's syndrome. In Apert's syndrome there is a cleft of the palate and the nose is always deviated. Apert's syndrome has an open bite. There may be mandibular hypoplasia in both Crouzon's and Apert's syndromes. Children with Apert's syndrome also have syndactylism.

Objective of Surgical Correction Crouzon's and Apert's syndromes have reduced projection of the face and a class III occlusion, which need correction. The vertical dimension of the face is reduced and this also needs correction. The goal is to correct the exorbitism, which is caused by a reduction in the size of the orbit. The vertical height of the orbit needs enlargement, and the advancement of the infraorbital border needs to be achieved.

Outline of Our Method The incisions are a coronal (bitemporal), infraorbital, and intraoral posterior vestibular. The coronal incision allows good exposure of the orbit and medial canthal ligaments and temporal fossa. In the temporal fossa an osteotomy is made in the lateral orbital wall and to the sphenomaxillary fissure (Fig. 15-1).[1] In the front nasal area the medial orbital wall osteotomy is made superior and posterior to the medial canthal ligament, and an osteotomy is then made above the front nasal suture, obliquely inferiorly for 10 to 15 mm. The osteotomy of the vomer is then performed.

The infraorbital incision exposes the floor of the orbit, infraorbital margin, and malar bone. Perform malar step osteotomies (Fig. 15-1)[1], plus those of the orbital floor and medial and lateral orbital walls.

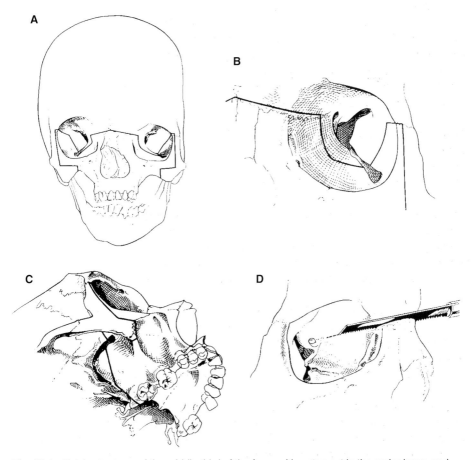

Fig. 15-1 Total osteotomy of the middle third of the face, *with* a step cut in the malar bone, and *with* sagittal splitting of the lateral orbital walls. **A,** The facial retrusion and exorbitism are noted, the keel-shaped osteotomy is outlined, and the step cut osteotomies in the zygomas are shown. **B,** Outline of the orbital osteotomies, through which one does a sagittal splitting of the lateral orbital walls with a chisel. **C,** The osteotomy between the maxilla and the pterygoid process is done bilaterally. **D,** The main basal osteotomy is done, either a straight horizontal one or a keel-shaped one.

Continued

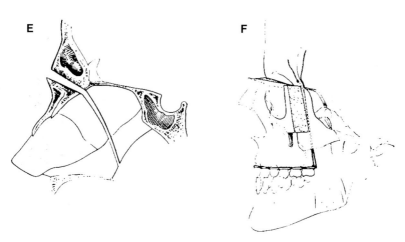

Fig. 15-1, cont'd   E, The oblique sectioning of the vomer. **F,** Bringing the facial mass forward, exposing the extent of the diastasis between the cranium and the face. Bone grafts are inserted into the step cuts in the zygomas. (From Tessier P. The definitive plastic surgical treatment of the severe facial deformities of craniofacial dysostosis. Crouzon's and Apert's diseases. Plast Reconstr Surg 48:419-442, 1971.)

The vestibular incisions expose the pterygomaxillary fissure for the osteotomy (Fig. 15-1).[1]

The LeFort III disjunction is then performed to correct the deformity and overcorrect it 10 mm. Interdental fixation is achieved to obtain a perfect occlusion. Bone grafts are then inserted in the front nasal area, lateral orbital wall, and pterygomaxillary osteotomy. All the osteotomies and grafts are fixed with stainless steel wires. The bone graft of the pterygomaxillary osteotomy is not fixed. Additional onlay bone grafts are applied to the zygoma and frontal bone. It is suggested that the use of a Diadem orthopedic frame will prevent interdental fixation after surgery.

An alternate osteotomy could be performed in which an osteotomy can be made through the anterior zygomatic arch and lateral orbital wall (Fig. 15-2).

Complications:
1. Fracture of the zygomatic arch.
2. CSF rhinorrhea; this is avoided by an accurate radiologic, preoperative evaluation of the anatomy of the front nasal area. The osteotomy is in an oblique inferior direction to ensure that the osteotomy does not go intracranial.
3. Trismus from the displacement of the bone graft in the pterygomaxillary osteotomy; a secondary procedure may need to be performed 6 months later. The operations were performed at 10 to 12 years of age.

Discussion   Paul Tessier described the LeFort III osteotomy and advancement of the face in Crouzon's and Apert's syndromes. He had a craniofacial fellowship and had

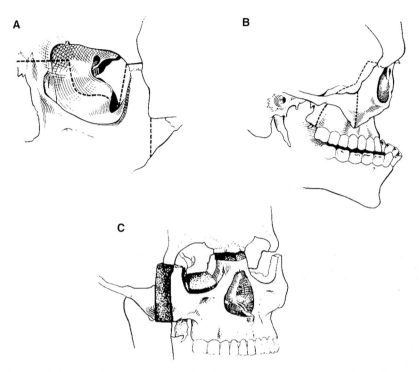

Fig. 15-2   Variation. **A-B,** Total osteotomy of the mid-face *without* the step cut in the malar and *without* sagittal splitting of the lateral orbital walls. Deep orbital osteotomies, plus a cut across the frontal process near the frontomalar surture, plus a cut across the junction of the zygomatic arch with the zygoma. The posterior face of the main cuts, and the cranial base. **C,** Bringing the facial mass forward. Inserting bone grafts into the main gaps. (From Tessier P. The definitive plastic surgical treatment of the severe facial deformities of craniofacial dysostosis. Crouzon's and Apert's diseases. Plast Reconstr Surg 48:419-442, 1971.)

surgeons from many countries around the world train under him. He also had visitors from many centers around the world spend time watching and learning from him. I visited Paul Tessier in 1975 after I had performed a few LeFort III osteotomies based on this article. Paul Tessier also presented his work in many centers and visited centers throughout the world. He visited us in South Africa and spent time in our Craniofacial Center in 1980 discussing craniofacial deformities and their treatment.

The LeFort III osteotomy and advancement was followed by more radical procedures. Ortiz Monasterio et al[4] expanded the procedure to do a fronto facial advancement, advancing the frontal bone and maxilla simultaneously. This procedure was performed by many surgeons.[5] The age at which the operation was performed became younger, and the procedure was performed at the age of 4 years.

Combining face advancement and correction of hypertelorism was presented by van der Meulen.[6]

Mühlbauer et al[7] used miniplates to fix the craniofacial skeleton in craniofacial surgery. Subsequently, biodegradable plates were used, and this avoided the additional procedure to remove the plates and screws.

Bone distraction made it possible to do the osteotomy, attach a distractor, advance the face, and overcorrect the deformity and thus possibly avoid a future operation.[8] This procedural advancement reduced the operating time because bone grafts did not have to be taken and fixed into position.

REFERENCES

1. Tessier P. The definitive plastic surgical treatment of the severe facial deformities of craniofacial dysostosis. Crouzon's and Apert's diseases. Plast Reconstr Surg 48:419-442, 1971.
2. Gillies H, Harrison SH. Operative correction by osteotomy of recessed malar maxillary compound in a case of oxycephaly. Br J Plast Surg 3:123-127, 1950.
3. Obwegeser H. Surgical correction of small or retrodisplaced maxillae. The "dish-face" deformity. Plast Reconstr Surg 43:351-365, 1969.
4. Ortiz Monasterio F, Del Campo AF, Carrillo A. Advancement of the orbits and midface in one piece, combined with frontal repositioning, for correction of Crouzon deformity. Plast Reconstr Surg 61:507-515, 1978.
5. Losken HW, MorrisWMM, Uys PB, et al. Crouzon's disease. Part 1. One-stage correction of combined face and forehead advancement. S Afr Med J 75:274-279.
6. van der Meulen JC. Median faciotomy. Br J Plast Surg 32:339-342, 1979.
7. Mühlbauer W, Anderl H, Ramatschi P, et al. Radical treatment of craniofacial anomalies in infancy and the use of miniplates in craniofacial surgery. Clin Plast Surg 14:101-111, 1987.
8. Polley JW, Figueroa AA. Management of severe maxillary deficiency in childhood and adolescence through distraction osteogenesis with an external adjustable, rigid distraction device. J Craniofac Surg 8:181-186, 1997.

EDITORIAL PERSPECTIVE

C. Scott Hultman, MD, MBA, FACS

I never had the privilege of meeting Dr. Tessier, but I have met scores of craniofacial surgeons who trained under him and worked with him directly, including Dr. Losken. In addition to creating the entire field of craniofacial surgery, Dr. Tessier really taught us that the only limitation to what we could accomplish was our imagination. Perhaps no other surgeon has radically transformed a field like Dr. Tessier—introducing novel techniques, combining standard and unorthodox principles, and resetting expectations—to transform the malformed face into one that is "normal." I maintain that Dr. Tessier is the most courageous surgeon our discipline has ever known. His greatest gift is to believe that the impossible may be achievable.

A Two-Stage Method for Pharyngoesophageal Reconstruction With a Primary Pectoral Skin Flap

Bakamjian VY. Plast Reconstr Surg 36:173-184, 1965

Reviewed by Shunsuke Yoshida, MD, MS

All of the existing methods for reconstruction of the pharynx and cervical esophagus following total laryngopharyngectomy for advanced cancer are short of ideal, some of them considerably so. A new pedicle flap technique that accomplishes the major part of the reconstruction at the time of the resection has been developed, and reduces some of the disadvantages to an acceptable minimum.[1]

Research Question   Is it possible to reconstruct a full-thickness, total laryngopharyngectomy defect with regional, vascularized, composite tissue? How does the deltopectoral flap compare with simpler methods involving skin grafts and bolsters and more complex methods such as stomach, jejunal, or colonic interposition?

Funding   Unknown

Study Dates   Early 1960s

Publishing Date   August 1965

Location   Roswell Park Memorial Institute, Buffalo, NY

Subjects   Patients with total laryngopharyngectomy defects after extirpation for advanced cancer

Exclusion Criteria   Not reported

Sample Size   Six patients are discussed; 10 patients are reported in the summary section.

Study Design   A case series, retrospective

Intervention   Reconstruction of 360-degree, full-thickness esophageal defects with a staged deltopectoral flap

Follow-up   All six patients had successful reconstruction of the cervical esophageal defects, with no reported cases of flap failure, proximal necrosis, or exposure of the carotid artery. Problems with minor distal flap necrosis and dehiscence, stricture, and temporary salivary fistula occurred but were successfully corrected at secondary flap division.

Endpoints   Restoration of continuity of the alimentary tract

Procedure   A tracheostomy is performed first. The procedure is executed through a parallel, transverse neck incision or a single collar incision with posterosuperior extension. After resection of the legion, an "oblong rectangular flap of skin from the pectoral region into the neck" is inverted to form a hollow epidermal tube. Perforators of the internal mammary vessels supply the medial skin flap while the lateral tip of the skin flap is placed over the acromial or subacromial region. This pectoral flap is passed underneath the bipedicled cervical skin flap, inverted to form a tube, and anastomosed end-to-end at the oropharyngeal opening. An end-to-side anastomosis is created between the esophageal stump and the unsutured opening in the seam in the lower part of the skin tube. The cervical skin is closed over the reconstructed pharynx, and the pectoral donor site is resurfaced with a split-thickness skin graft. The patient is given nutrition through a nasogastric tube introduced during this first stage of the operation. In 3 to 5 weeks, the base of the flap is divided and the flap is closed at the pectoral outlet. Dilation of any anastomotic strictures can be undertaken at that time.

Commentary   There are three possible explanations for the successful viability of an undelayed, horizontal upper chest flap:
1. The blood supply from the internal mammary branch perforators.
2. The dependent position of the flap base that reduces venous engorgement.
3. The typical anatomy of a total laryngopharyngectomy allowed flap creation to conform to the recommended safe ratio of 2:1. The author noted two distinct advantages of this method. First, the ability to create a pedicled tube graft without delay allowed the timely eradication of cancerous lesions and the option to immediately reconstruct the laryngopharynx after a significant excision. Second, the inferior and lateral positions of the open end of the epidermal tube allowed saliva to drain on to the chest wall without spillage into the tracheostoma.

Results   The results of six patients with undelayed pectoral flaps are discussed.[1] One patient had a subtotal pharyngectomy with laryngectomy and radical neck dissection.

A primary pectoral flap was used successfully to cover the anterior three fourths of the pharynx. Two patients had previously undergone laryngopharyngectomies with failed free-inlay graft reconstructions with marked scarring and contracture on the neck. Minor infection and external wound separation occurred, resulting in annular stricture at the superior anastomosis after repair with a pectoral flap. This was corrected at the second stage operation. Two patients with extensive tonsillar carcinoma underwent en bloc radical excision, resulting in the removal of the lateral half of the oropharyngeal circumference. Overambitious reach of the pectoral flap caused marginal necrosis and moderate suture line separation near the tip of the flap but without adverse effects except slow healing by secondary intention. One patient underwent a total glossectomy, laryngectomy, and radical neck dissection. Bilateral, medially based pectoral flaps were used in an attempt to reconstruct the entire oropharyngeal passage, reaching as high as the gingival border of the mandible. Flap tip necrosis led to anterior separation of the flaps from the mandible, creating a fistulous defect at the floor of the mouth. Distant flaps were later fashioned for closure.

Criticisms/Limitations   The main disadvantages of the deltopectoral flap are the multistaged nature of the reconstruction and the large, conspicuous, donor-site defect that requires skin grafting.[1,2] In addition, the wide base limits the arc of rotation.[3]

Relevant Studies   Dr. Vahram Bakamjian[4] was born in 1918 in Aleppo, Syria. He received his Bachelor of Science degree in 1940 and his Doctor of Medicine degree in 1945 from the American University of Beirut. He trained in an ear, nose, and throat residency at Columbia University and completed his plastic surgery residency under Dr. Webster. He was recruited to Roswell Park Memorial Institute and the Department of Head and Neck Surgery in 1965. His innovative spirit as a plastic surgeon was evident in the head and neck articles he published and the numerous trainees he attracted from around the world. His achievements earned him the Special Recognition Award of the Society of Head and Neck Surgeons, the Distinguished Fellow Award from the American Association of Plastic Surgeons, and an honorary fellow designation from the Japanese Society of Plastic and Reconstructive Surgery. He was known for his "deltopectoral flap design," but as a man with great vision, he quickly embraced the concept of musculocutaneous flaps and free flaps later in his career. Dr. Bakamjian retired from the Roswell Park Cancer Institute in 1996. Widely considered the "father of modern-day head and neck reconstruction," he passed away in 2010.

Dr. Bakamjian[5] first used the medially based deltopectoral flap in 1962. He was unsatisfied with the options for the reconstruction of the pharynx after total laryngopharyngectomy. He was also experimenting with a variety of L-shaped flaps to prefabricate a hollow tube with the short limb of the "L" when in 1959 he was faced with the reconstruction of a low and short laryngopharyngeal defect. It occurred to him that a hollow skin tube could be fashioned at the end of a laterally based pectoral flap. Then in 1962 faced with a similar problem, he modified his approach to a medially based pectoral flap supplied by internal mammary artery perforators. By 1964 he had used the flap nine times, and at the encouragement of his chairman, he submitted his work to *Plastic and Reconstructive Surgery.* The editor originally indicated that it seemed "foolhardy" to use a long, medially based flap. Dr. Bakamjian sent a resume with pictures and the article was published in 1965. Citing his dislike for public speaking, he did not present this work until 1968 at a symposium on cancer of the head and neck in Pittsburgh.

The 20-year experience of the use of the deltopectoral flap has been published from the Roswell Park Memorial Institute.[6] Six hundred four patients with a total of 678 delto-pectoral flaps were included. Five hundred thirty patients received a single deltopec-toral flap, 496 of which (82%) required no additional flaps. The indications for sur-gery varied. Most patients needed reconstruction after resection of a malignancy in the upper aerodigestive tract, salivary or thyroid glands, or skin. The overall complication rate was 51%, of which 22% were considered major. The risk factors for complications were multifactorial; however, the highest rate of flap necrosis occurred when the flap was tubulated, used in an irradiated bed, had a slit to receive a stoma or an esophageal anastomosis, or was used for major or total reconstructions of the pharynx. The rate of major necrosis was not statistically significant between delayed and nondelayed flaps. Therefore the authors stood against the routine use of a delayed flap. They also found that the complication rates were comparable with their experience with myocutaneous flap reconstructions.

Since the original description now a half a century ago, the use of myocutaneous flaps and free flaps have replaced the deltopectoral flap in head and neck reconstructions. Complications of adjuvant radiotherapy after a complex reconstruction of composite head and neck defects have limited management options. Pedicled fasciocutaneous, myocutaneous, or free flaps are considered the mainstays in secondary reconstruction. However, irradiated, fibrotic skin on the neck can preclude tunneling of flaps, and free flap reconstruction of an irradiated field can be challenging with high complication rates.[7] Furthermore, patients may object to the thought of another complex free flap re-construction.[7] The deltopectoral flap continues to be a viable option in these settings.

Summary   A new pedicle flap technique that allowed immediate and dependable reconstruction with improved postoperative salivary control after a partial or total pharyngectomy was described in 1965.

Implications   This paper was the first to describe a medially based axial skin flap for reconstruction after a major pharyngeal resection. Although myocutaneous flaps and free flaps have become the mainstay of reconstructive options after resection of head and neck cancer, the deltopectoral flap is still recognized as a viable option, especially in the setting of adjuvant radiotherapy.

REFERENCES

1. Bakamjian VY. A two-stage method for pharyngoesophageal reconstruction with a primary pectoral skin flap. Plast Reconstr Surg 36:173-184, 1965.
2. Mureau MAM, Hofer SO. Maximizing results in reconstruction of cheek defects. Clin Plast Surg 36:461-476, 2009.
3. Neligan PC, Gullane PJ, Vesely M, et al. The internal mammary perforator flap: new variation on an old theme. Plast Reconstr Surg 119:891-893, 2007.
4. Serletti JM, Cohen MN, Shedd DP. Vahram Y. Bakamjian, M.D., 1918 to 2010. Plast Reconstr Surg 129:1218-1220, 2012.
5. Bakamjian VY. An interview with Vahram Bakamjian, M.D.: conducted by William D. Morain, M.D. Ann Plast Surg 13:253-256, 1984.
6. Gilas T, Sako K, Razack MS, et al. Major head and neck reconstruction using the deltopectoral flap. A 20 year experience. Am J Surg 152:430-434, 1986.
7. Krijgh DD, Mureau MA. Reconstructive options in patients with late complications after surgery and radiotherapy for head and neck cancer: remember the deltopectoral flap. Ann Plast Surg 71:181-185, 2013.

EDITORIAL PERSPECTIVE

C. Scott Hultman, MD, MBA, FACS

The Spanish philosopher George Santayana warned, "Those who cannot remember the past are condemned to repeat it."

I first used the deltopectoral flap as a resident at Grady Memorial Hospital in Atlanta in 1999 to cover a previous free flap that had gone horribly, miserably wrong. A 30-year-old woman had attempted suicide and instead blew out her anterior mandible, including skin, bone, and mucosal lining, as well as the base of her tongue. After reviewing the case with our attending, Jack Culbertson (one of Emory's finest, most versatile surgeons, who died far too soon, at the age of 62 in 2013), we planned a scapular/parascapular free flap with a large, cruciate skin island, including the lateral portion of the scapula, to restore the missing bone. We even harvested this flap the night before as a dress rehearsal in the fresh tissue cadaver laboratory. On postoperative day 4, the patient developed a salivary fistula and quickly had a thrombosis of her venous outflow, rendering the flap unsalvageable. In the operating room, quite panicked, I called Jack to explain the situation, and after telling me to "put the flap in the bucket," he asked, "have you ever done a deltopectoral flap?" "No," I responded, "never heard of it." Jack replied, "It's one of the oldest flaps in the book. Just read the book. You residents jump all the way to the top of the reconstructive ladder, with complex free flaps that require microsurgery, but you need to learn the foundations first, so that you can salvage a failed reconstruction like this." So we got out the book, left her titanium bar in place, and covered the entire defect (floor of the mouth, gingival and buccal mucosa, and chin and neck skin) with a flap that had been described decades earlier by Vahram Bakamjian.

I have never used the deltopectoral flap as a primary method of reconstruction, but this flap has served as a lifeboat for me multiple times over the past 15 years. I am really glad I read the book. Thanks, Jack. I will see you someday in the skies over Shiprock, under a canopy of countless stars.

CHAPTER 17

The Pectoralis Major Myocutaneous Flap. A Versatile Flap for Reconstruction in the Head and Neck

Ariyan S. Plast Reconstr Surg 63:73-81, 1979

Reviewed by Saif Al-Bustani, MD, DMD

> [The pectoralis major myocutaneous flap] has enough bulk to fill cavities, to augment contour, and to provide structural support in one step.[1]

Research Question   As extensive head and neck resections become common and immediate reconstruction becomes more acceptable, what are the advantages of the newly introduced pectoralis major myocutaneous flap?

Funding   Not applicable

Study Date   1978

Publishing Date   January 1979

Location   Yale University School of Medicine, New Haven, CT

Subjects   Patients with extensive head and neck defects, including orbital and oropharyngeal

Exclusion Criteria   Not applicable

Sample Size   4 patients

Overview of Design   This is a retrospective case series of four patients requiring pedicled pectoralis major myocutaneous flaps for orbital or oropharyngeal defect coverage. Reconstruction was performed immediately in all patients. Fresh cadaver dissection was performed to delineate the anatomy and the operative technique was detailed.

Intervention   The pectoralis myocutaneous flap was used for orbital and oropharyngeal defects. Flap design and skin island placement were dependent on defect requirements. All donor sites were closed primarily. In two of the patients undergoing orbital reconstruction, flap division was required at a second stage. In the other two patients undergoing oropharyngeal reconstruction, the flap was tunneled over the clavicle in a single stage. When needed, a portion of the skin paddle was deepithelialized and buried for dead space obliteration and coverage of duraplasty fascial grafts.

Follow-up   Not mentioned

Endpoints   Successful flap transfer and flap division when indicated

Results   All flaps were transferred successfully with defect coverage, obliteration of dead space, restoration of contour and symmetry, and coverage of duraplasty fascial grafts.

Criticisms/Limitations   This is a small case series meant to introduce this pedicled myocutaneous flap to the readership and its potential indications for head and neck reconstruction in the immediate setting with inherent limitations as such. There was no mention of follow-up or specific endpoints.

Relevant Studies   Since its inception in 1979 with this landmark study, the pectoralis major myocutaneous flap became the workhorse flap for reliable reconstruction of defects in the head and neck until the widespread use of microvascular surgery techniques in the 1980s. Since then, the role of this flap has evolved to that of salvage in patients with failed microvascular reconstruction. It is also often considered the pedicled flap of choice in patients too compromised to tolerate the lengthy nature of microsurgery. In addition, it is not uncommon for this flap to be an adjunct to microsurgery for extensive defects requiring multiple flaps. In their experience detailing their current indications, Schneider et al[2] performed 53 pectoralis major flaps over a 10-year period from 2002 to 2012. Thirty-eight percent of the flaps were used after a free flap complication such as flap failure, fistula, or great vessel exposure; 33% were performed concurrently with a free flap for dead space obliteration or neck/great vessel coverage; and 29% were indicated for primary reconstruction in comorbid patients or in patients in whom neck coverage was required in a tenuous wound bed.

In a subsequent study from the same year as his original account, Ariyan[3] detailed his experience with a larger case series of 14 patients. He described outlining the skin paddle directly over the vascular pedicle of the muscle. He reported no total or partial flap loss or fistulas and only partial dehiscence at the skin level in three patients. Ariyan cited a number of advantages to this flap, including a large area of available skin for coverage, a large amount of muscle for bulk and carotid coverage, incorporating rib for bone grafting, and enough length for frontoorbital and temporoparietal coverage.

Baek et al[4] described their experience with 133 pectoralis major flaps for various head and neck defects and reported a low complication rate. Of importance they detailed a variation on the operative technique with placement of the skin paddle outside the vascular pedicle of the muscle relying on perforators for skin perfusion. Since then various modifications and applications have been introduced in the literature. Dennis and Kashima[5] introduced the Janus flap; a prefabricated pectoralis major flap with a split-thickness skin graft on the muscle surface for two back-to-back skin surfaces used in the staged reconstruction of the pharyngoesophagus and cervical esophagus. Meyer et al[6] described a bilobed flap that incorporates both the pectoralis myocutaneous flap and the ipsilateral medially based deltopectoral flap for the reconstruction of the cervical esophagus. The pectoralis major limb is used for pharyngoesophageal/esophageal reconstruction, whereas the deltopectoral limb is used for coverage of the exposed undersurface of the myocutaneous flap. Lee and Loré[7] reported partially tubing the pectoralis myocutaneous flap for the reconstruction of the anterior and lateral walls of total laryngectomy or total pharyngectomy defects, whereas a dermal graft is used for the posterior wall to allow better deglutition. Sharzer et al[8] outlined the parasternal and inframammary paddles to reduce bulk and minimize distortion, especially of the breast in the female patient. This modification in paddle placement represents the most popular design for this flap when it is currently used for oropharyngeal reconstruction.

Although Ariyan[3] and Baek et al[4] reported low complication rates, Shah et al[9] relayed a different experience with 211 flaps at Memorial Sloan Kettering. Their overall complication rate was 63%. These included flap necrosis, suture line dehiscence, fistula, infection, and hematoma. Significant global risk factors for the development of complications included age over 70 years, female gender, obesity, hypoalbuminemia, and the presence of other systemic diseases. The only local significant risk factor identified was reconstruction in the oral cavity after major glossectomy. That said, most of these complications (74%) were minor, managed conservatively, and did not require a reoperation. Total flap necrosis occurred in only 3%, whereas a fistula occurred in 26%. More recently, however, McLean et al[10] conveyed favorable outcomes in their review of 136 patients from 1998 to 2008. The overall complication rate was 13%, including total flap necrosis (0.8%), partial flap necrosis (3%), fistula (3%), hematoma (3%), and neck contracture (5%). Flap revision was required in 3.5% of the patients. Radiation was a significant risk factor for developing complications. It is interesting to note that Schneider et al[2] also reported neck contractures in their complication profile but at a higher rate (26%). They attributed that to muscle atrophy related to their initial practice of routinely dividing the pectoral nerves to limit muscle contraction.

Summary   The pectoralis major myocutaneous flap is reliable and versatile, with many applications in head and neck reconstruction. The anatomy is consistent, the dissection is relatively straightforward, the arc of rotation is adequate for most head and neck defects, and the amount of muscle and surface area of skin is abundant.

Implications   This landmark study introduces the pectoralis major myocutaneous flap for head and neck reconstruction to the readership. It is time-tested and continues to play a major role with real indications.

REFERENCES

1. Ariyan S. The pectoralis major myocutaneous flap. A versatile flap for reconstruction in the head and neck. Plast Reconstr Surg 63:73-81, 1979.
2. Schneider DS, Wu V, Wax MK. Indications for pedicled pectoralis major flap in a free tissue transfer practice. Head Neck 34:1106-1110, 2012.
3. Ariyan S. Further experiences with the pectoralis major myocutaneous flap for the immediate repair of defects from excisions of head and neck cancers. Plast Reconstr Surg 64:605-612, 1979.
4. Baek SM, Lawson W, Biller HF. An analysis of 133 pectoralis major myocutaneous flaps. Plast Reconstr Surg 69:460-469, 1982.
5. Dennis D, Kashima H. Introduction of the Janus flap. A modified pectoralis major myocutaneous flap for cervical esophageal and pharyngeal reconstruction. Arch Otolaryngol 107:431-435, 1981.
6. Meyer R, Kelly TP, Abul Failat AS. Single bilobed flap for use in head and neck reconstruction. Ann Plast Surg 6:203-206, 1981.
7. Lee KY, Loré JM Jr. Two modifications of pectoralis major myocutaneous flap (PMMF). Laryngoscope 96:363-367, 1986.
8. Sharzer LA, Kalisman M, Silver CE, et al. The parasternal paddle: a modification of the pectoralis major myocutaneous flap. Plast Reconstr Surg 67:753-762, 1981.
9. Shah JP, Haribhakti V, Loree TR, et al. Complications of the pectoralis major myocutaneous flap in head and neck reconstruction. Am J Surg 160:352-355, 1990.
10. McLean JN, Carlson GW, Losken A. The pectoralis major myocutaneous flap revisited: a reliable technique for head and neck reconstruction. Ann Plast Surg 64:570-573, 2010.

STUDY AUTHOR REFLECTIONS

Stephan Ariyan, MD, MBA, FACS

The pectoralis major myocutaneous flap was developed out of necessity for a patient who presented in 1977 with a recurrent squamous cell carcinoma of the ethmoid sinuses after working many years painting watch dials with radium paint. She had been treated elsewhere with full-course radiation therapy to the orbit and forehead. She had already lost her vision in that eye but still refused surgery.

I knew she would return soon with pain, bleeding, or both and require radical resection of the anterior cranial fossa and orbital region with exposure of the dura. The most reliable flap at the time was the deltopectoral flap of Bakamjian, but I would not be able to bring enough bulk to the reconstruction site. I therefore dissected fresh cadavers to see if I could bring a portion of the pectoralis major under the deltopectoral flap to fill in the large empty resection site. As the original paper shows, I found that the thoracoacromial artery and accompanying veins were the blood supply. She came in for the surgery and we were prepared for the reconstruction. In fact, this very first case was filmed by the American College of Surgeons (ACS) for the Cine Clinics session of the fall 1977 meeting and is available in the ACS Film Library.

We soon established the versatility of this flap. Indeed, the film and first paper show that only a narrow segment of the muscle overlying the vessels is all that is necessary for its vascular pedicle.

We also found this flap very versatile for major skull base resections, pharyngoesophageal reconstructions, and major defects of the floor of the mouth after glossectomy.

Subsequently, we demonstrated that if we can move any segment of vascularized muscle, we can transfer any skin overlying that muscle and any bone attached under the muscle. We verified with fluorescent microscopy the viable transfer of the pectoralis major muscle and segments of attached rib.

Despite those successful flaps, I believe that the microvascular transfer of the fibula is still the most appropriate choice.

Finally, it should be noted that the use of the pectoralis major flap for pharyngeal reconstruction will most often demonstrate a salivary or pharyngocutaneous fistula. That is because the flap is sutured to the pharyngeal tissue that has no strength to hold the suture line. This fistula almost always closes and heals without requiring any additional surgical intervention.

Moreover, any loss of the skin paddle is either because of an extension too far beyond the muscle itself or because the weight of the muscle pulls away from under the surface of the skin paddle, which is sutured to the periphery of the wound. Indeed, the muscle needs to be securely anchored to the periosteum or nearby fascia before the skin paddle is repaired to avoid this mechanical separation of fine vessels from the muscle to the skin.

EDITORIAL PERSPECTIVE

C. Scott Hultman, MD, MBA, FACS

Many people claim to have "invented" the pectoralis flap for head and neck reconstruction, but only one person really did: Stephan Ariyan. Riding an unprecedented wave of innovation sparked by John McCraw in the 1970s, Dr. Ariyan, Chief of Plastic Surgery at Yale, was the first to report the use of this pedicled flap for multiple, different complex defects (cephalad to the clavicle) when these wounds required lining, bulk, obliteration of dead space, revascularization, coverage of hardware, and replacement of irradiated skin. Although the pectoralis muscle flap had been used for years as an advancement or turnover flap in the chest wall and mediastinal reconstruction, Dr. Ariyan quickly refined and modified this flap, which became the gold standard for reliable, nonmicrosurgical reconstruction of the head and neck.

So successful was Dr. Ariyan in demonstrating the efficacy and safety of the pectoralis muscle and myocutaneous flap that other specialties appropriated this flap for their own use. But then again, this is the story of plastic surgery: we develop new techniques and technologies, apply these innovations to clinical care, and move on to the next surgical problem. Plastic surgery is not just general surgery done well as some have championed, but rather plastic surgery may be the surgery of applied innovation in which creativity and discipline merge to yield better ways to achieve form and function. In many ways the "success" of the pectoralis flap represents both the climax of the myocutanous flap revolution but also the transition to the modern era, in which plastic surgery could be pursued by nonplastic surgeons, sometimes for the better, often for the worse.

CHAPTER 18

A 10-Year Experience in Nasal Reconstruction With the Three-Stage Forehead Flap

Menick FJ. Plast Reconstr Surg 109:1839-1855; discussion 1856-1861, 2002

Reviewed by Saif Al-Bustani, MD, DMD

> *The technique ensures a maximal blood supply, a thin covering flap, unimpeded surgical exposure, controlled shaping, and the maximal use of all lining options. The aesthetic results are improved, and the need for later revisions is minimized.*[1]

Research Question   What are the advantages of the three-stage forehead flap?

Funding   Not applicable

Study Dates   1991 to 2001

Publishing Date   May 2002

Location   Tucson, AZ

Subjects   Patients with partial-thickness and full-thickness nasal defects

Exclusion Criteria   None

Sample Size   90 patients with nasal defects

Overview of Design   This is a retrospective review of 90 patients undergoing the three-stage forehead flap technique for reconstruction; both partial-thickness and full-thickness defects were reconstructed with the same approach. After surgery, patients were evaluated subjectively by the surgeon for general aesthetic assessment.

Intervention   Nasal reconstruction is achieved in three stages. In the first stage, a full-thickness forehead flap is elevated without thinning except for the columellar inset. If a vascularized intranasal lining is present, primary cartilage grafts are placed. If it is absent, the forehead flap may be folded to create the missing intranasal lining, or it may be lined with a skin graft. In either case, primary cartilage grafts are not placed. When folding is planned, the flap is extended distally on the forehead with an additional 2 to 3 mm for rolling over the margin, or it may be lined with a skin graft. The donor site is closed primarily or allowed to heal with secondary intention. In the second intermediate stage 3 weeks later, the physiologically delayed forehead flap is elevated with 3 to 4 mm of subcutaneous fat except for the columella, which remains attached. If the forehead flap was folded for intranasal lining in the first stage, it is elevated at the rim, separating the lining from the cover. Once the flap is elevated, the underlying construct (made of subcutaneous fat and frontalis muscle) is thinned and sculpted in the subunit principle if primary cartilage grafts were initially placed over the intact lining. Delayed primary cartilage grafting is performed during this intermediate second stage to support the newly reconstructed lining, which is created from a skin graft or folded forehead flap. The cover skin is then replaced. In the third stage 3 weeks later, the pedicle is divided. The distal flap is again elevated with 3 to 4 mm of subcutaneous fat, and the underling construct is thinned and sculpted as needed to create the expected subunit contours, defining the dorsal lines, alar crease, and sidewall junction. If the initial skin graft placed for lining does not "take," it is debrided and a second skin graft is reapplied.

Follow-up   Not mentioned

Endpoints   Postoperative complications, requirements for subsequent minor and major revisions, and overall aesthetic outcomes

Results   Intranasal lining flaps were used in 15 patients, prelaminated forehead flaps with full-thickness skin grafts for lining in 11, folded forehead flaps for lining in 3, turnover flaps in 5, prefabricated flaps in 4, and free flaps for lining in 2. No flap necrosis was observed. One infection observed was related to lining loss. In partial-thickness defects reconstructed with this technique, only minor revisions were required. In full-thickness defects, one major revision or more than two minor revisions were required in less than 5% of patients. Overall aesthetic results approached normal.

Criticisms/Limitations   This is primarily a technique paper with little emphasis on objective results. There is no mention of follow-up intervals or duration. There is no direct comparison with a two-stage forehead flap group. The rate of minor revisions is not mentioned.

Relevant Studies   The history of nasal reconstruction dates back to 3000 BC, as evidenced in the *Edwin Smith Surgical Papyrus.* This impressive Egyptian surgical treatise detailed 48 case reports for the treatment of mostly traumatic injuries. Four of those cases dealt with nasal injuries, including two nasal bone fractures, a nasal cartilage fracture, and an open nasal wound. The cases emphasized the removal of blood clots from the nasal cavity. For an open wound, the dressings consisted of fresh meat applied directly to the wound for the first day and then daily dressing changes with oil and honey until the patient recovered. Nasal fracture repair was achieved with simple manipulation. Internal nasal splints were fashioned from two plugs of cloth soaked in oil. External splints were fabricated from thin wood padded with linen.[2,3] Arguably, the next major contribution to nasal reconstruction came from Sushruta's work, the *Samhita,* from approximately 600 BC. Here he described a staged pedicled cheek or forehead flap for nasal reconstruction. The wound edges are freshened, the flap is transferred, and the pedicle is divided once it is healed.[2] In fifteenth century Europe, the Italian Branca family and the German wound specialist and Bavarian army surgeon Heinrich von Pfalzpaint guarded their nasal reconstruction techniques for a staged arm flap to the nose. This was a two-stage flap from the biceps region, in which the arm was bandaged to the head and the flap was divided 8 to10 days later. During the second stage, inset and sculpting were performed. In his text *Wundarznei,* Pfalzpaint says to his pupil: "If one comes to you with a cut off nose, let no one watch and make him swear to tell nobody how you cured him."[2] Gasparo Tagliacozzi's delayed upper arm flap to the nose, which was described 100 years later, required six stages and 4 months to exact the repair.[2]

In the modern era, McCarthy et al[4] performed the first anatomic study to delineate the redundancy in blood supply to the forehead flap, building on Kazanjian's popularized median forehead flap and Millard's paramedian forehead flap. They found that the terminal branch of the facial artery, the angular artery, provided enough vascularity to support the forehead flap independent of the supraorbital and supratrochlear arteries, allowing extensive mobilization of the flap.[4]

The three-stage forehead flap, however, may be attributed to Millard.[5] He introduced an intermediate stage, designed to thin and tailor the distal most portion of the flap, covering the nasal tip, safely, while the pedicle was still intact. He wanted to avoid the nasal reconstruction that tended to "blob up." He then proceeded to say that "only a slob is satisfied with a blob."

Expanding on this concept, Burget and Menick published their landmark work on defining the topographic subunits of the nose. Although the nose was designated a unit of the face by González-Ulloa, Burget and Menick[6] described the dorsum, tip, alae, sidewalls, and soft triangles as subunits separated by shallow valleys and ridges. To maximize the aesthetics, they advocated excising and resurfacing an entire subunit if more than 50% is involved in a defect.

Emphasizing the need to functionally and aesthetically reconstruct the basic three layers of the nose (cover, framework, and lining), Burget and Menick[7] take it a step further with refinements to achieve the fourth dimension in repair—normalcy. Although the cover and lining provide length and width, the nasal cartilages provide projection, airway patency, and the subtle shape that give a nose its distinction. The latter is only true if the cover is thin to allow it. Their techniques of using thin, well-vascularized vestibular membrane and septal chondromucosal flaps for lining, primary cartilage grafts, and a forehead flap for cover in the subunit principle promoted normalcy in function and aesthetics. In the current study, Menick uses the prelaminated or folded forehead flap for lining, accomplishing great results.

Menick[8] provides further practical details in a more recent article. The timing of reconstruction must ensure control of contamination or infection, demarcation of tissues, clear margins in tumor cases, resolution of edema, stability of tissue tension, and stability of scar contraction. Using quarter-inch paper tape and foil, the surgeon fabricates an exact template for each planned subunit reconstruction, based on the contralateral, normal subunit. As a general guide, large, deep nasal defects require regional flaps. Those include defects >1.5 cm in diameter, those requiring cartilage replacement, full-thickness defects, and infratip or columellar defects. The two-stage nasolabial flap is best reserved for isolated superficial alar defects. Otherwise the three-stage forehead flap is the regional flap of choice. Significant reconstructions often require a revision for refinement. This includes the donor site.

Moreover, Menick[9] described his approach to the late revision of a failed reconstruction in a methodical way. He classifies the deformities into minor and major. If the overall dimension, volume, and position are acceptable, nasal landmarks are lacking, and the nostrils are small or asymmetrical, then the deformity is minor. Major deformities diverge from normal in a fundamental way and are often shapeless, bulky, stenotic, and without landmarks. Revisions of minor defects are accomplished in one stage and usually involve direct incisions in subunit borders, disregarding old scars to correct local problems. Revisions of major defects will require staging. Gross debulking is achieved with incisions along flap borders, whereas finesse revisions are approached by direct incisions to improve landmarks. In severe cases the entire reconstruction must be redone with the use of a second regional flap, usually a forehead flap.

In pediatric nasal reconstruction, Burget[10] detailed his successful experience with the forehead flap. It has acceptable donor site morbidity, especially because it is nonsebaceous and grows with the patient. Reconstruction may start as soon as 3½ years of age in the hope of completion by 5 years of age, before the child begins school. A diagnosis of nasal defects in children may be more difficult than in adults. It is prudent to visualize or recreate the defect to formulate the appropriate plan. For the most part, a three-stage forehead flap is used with similar principles in mind. In large defects two layers of framework are reconstructed. This requires grafts for nasal dimension and grafts for nasal contour. With the exception of projection, the reconstructed nose will grow with the patient. Augmentation may be required at 8 to 12 years.

Summary   The three-stage forehead flap is superior to its two-stage counterpart. It allows the creation of a thin and supple nasal cover. It allows delayed primary cartilage grafting or revision of primary cartilage grafts during the intermediate stage. It creates an ideal rigid substructure reflected through thin overlying skin. It expands the options for intranasal lining with skin grafts or folded forehead flaps. It preserves the option of salvaging the forehead flap in cases of infection by raising a well-vascularized, full-thickness flap during the first stage. It ensures maximal blood supply to all nasal layers. It decreases the number of revisions and the degree of difficulty of subsequent revisions. Finally, it improves the aesthetic results.

Implications   The three-stage forehead flap refined by Dr. Menick represents the gold standard in aesthetic nasal reconstruction of both partial-thickness and full-thickness defects. It achieves superb results while minimizing the number and complexity of required revisions.

REFERENCES

1. Menick FJ. A 10-year experience in nasal reconstruction with the three-stage forehead flap. Plast Reconstr Surg 109:1839-1855; discussion 1856-1861, 2002.
2. Whitaker IS, Karoo RO, Spyrou G, et al. The birth of plastic surgery: the story of nasal reconstruction from the Edwin Smith Papyrus to the twenty-first century. Plast Reconstr Surg 120:327-336, 2007.
3. The Edwin Smith Surgical Papyrus. Turning the Pages Online. National Library of Medicine. Available at *http://archive.nlm.nih.gov/proj/ttp/flash/smith/smith.html.*
4. McCarthy JG, Lorenc ZP, Cutting C, et al. The median forehead flap revisited: the blood supply. Plast Reconstr Surg 76:866-869, 1985.
5. Millard DR Jr. Reconstructive rhinoplasty for the lower half of a nose. Plast Reconstr Surg 53:133-139, 1974.
6. Burget GC, Menick FJ. The subunit principle in nasal reconstruction. Plast Reconstr Surg 76:239-247, 1985.
7. Burget GC, Menick FJ. Nasal reconstruction: seeking a fourth dimension. Plast Reconstr Surg 78:145-157, 1986.
8. Menick FJ. Practical details of nasal reconstruction. Plast Reconstr Surg 131:613e-630e, 2013.
9. Menick FJ. An approach to the late revision of a failed nasal reconstruction. Plast Reconstr Surg 129:92e-103e, 2012.
10. Burget GC. Preliminary review of pediatric nasal reconstruction with detailed report of one case. Plast Reconstr Surg 124:907-918, 2009.

STUDY AUTHOR REFLECTIONS

Frederick J. Menick, MD

The transfer of a forehead flap in three stages should become the workhorse of nasal reconstruction for large and deep nasal defects. It maximizes the blood supply during transfer and the intermediate operation. It permits the surgeon to modify a flap from the thick and stiff forehead to create a uniformly thin skin cover. It permits widespread soft tissue scoping and the opportunity to reposition, recontour, or add cartilage grafts before pedicle division. It permits the aesthetic use of a forehead flap or skin graft as a thin supple lining that is useful for unilateral or bilateral lining defects.

Presently, I completely elevate the forehead flap during the intermediate operation to allow complete exposure, soft tissue sculpting, and delayed primary grafting. The flap is not left connected to the columella as a bipedicled flap. Because of the applicability and effectiveness of the folded forehead flap for lining, it is the primary method to restore the nasal lining. When a lining deficiency is apparent during surgery, additional skin is added to the distal end of a forehead flap in the area of the normal dog-ear excision to supply a lining without an additional intranasal lining injury or significant additional morbidity to the forehead donor. The skin graft lining technique is used only in salvage situation areas.

EDITORIAL PERSPECTIVE

C. Scott Hultman, MD, MBA, FACS

Nasal reconstruction with the forehead flap remains my favorite procedure to perform, well into my third decade of clinical practice as a surgeon. Perhaps this is because of the intricate balance of aesthetics and function, or because the reconstruction requires four-dimensional planning, with meticulous consideration of lining, support, and coverage. Maybe my fascination with this set of operations can be explained by realizing that thousands of years of evolution went into the creation and refinement of this procedure. Plastic surgery is as old as all of medicine, which hopefully means that plastic surgery will thrive well into the future. Until we solve the problems of immunosuppression and can justify the transplantation of composite nasal allografts, forehead flaps will remain at the top of the algorithm for nasal reconstruction, the apogee of our accomplishments, until someday another innovation may make them obsolete.

CHAPTER 19

A Review of 60 Consecutive Fibula Free Flap Mandible Reconstructions

Hidalgo DA, Rekow A. Plast Reconstr Surg 96:585-596; discussion 597-602, 1995

Reviewed by Saif Al-Bustani, MD, DMD

> *The fibula is an ideal donor site for mandible reconstruction because of its length, uniform shape, blood supply anatomy, adjacent soft tissue availability, and convenient location.*[1]

Research Question   With a narrow recommended list of free flaps used for mandibular reconstruction, when is the free fibular flap indicated?

Funding   Not applicable

Study Dates   October 1986 to February 1992

Publishing Date   September 1995

Location   Memorial Sloan Kettering Cancer Center and Cornell University Medical College, New York, NY

Subjects   Patients with oncologic defects of the mandible, both composite and osseous only; primary and secondary cases were included.

Exclusion Criteria   Not applicable

Sample Size   60 patients; 81% had primary reconstructions, and 62% of the patients were men.

Overview of Design   A retrospective review of 60 consecutive patients requiring free fibular flaps for mandibular reconstruction after oncologic resections; reconstruction was performed primarily when possible. Oropharyngeal function was evaluated by a physical examination and questionnaire. Static and dynamic donor-site functions were evaluated by a physical examination. Aesthetic outcomes were evaluated by a subjective examination and photography.

Intervention   The fibula was used in all anterior mandibular defects and most lateral defects. A skin island was planned when mucosal and/or skin defects were anticipated. Donor sites with skin islands exceeding 4 cm were closed with skin grafting. Preoperative templates and intraoperative specimens were used to shape the bone and perform the appropriate fibular osteotomies. The primary method of bone fixation was miniplates. In the disease-free and nonradiated patient, osseointegrated dental implants were subsequently indicated for placement.

Follow-up   In 38 patients the average follow-up was 39.2 months. Death and recurrence of disease precluded long-term follow-up in the remainder of patients.

Endpoints   Overall successful flap transfer, bony healing between the osteotomized fibular segments and to the remaining mandible, skin island viability, donor-site morbidity (both early and late), oropharyngeal function, and aesthetic outcomes

Results   Ninety-eight percent of the flaps were transferred successfully. There was one fibrous union and one nonunion. Ninety percent of the skin islands raised remained viable. Donor-site cellulitis occurred in two patients. On long-term follow-up, all patients ambulated independently, whereas two patients had difficulty running. Fifteen patients experienced persistent pain, hypoesthesia, edema, and/or ankle weakness. Almost all patients had limitation on flexion of the hallux. Fifty-one percent of the patients evaluated tolerated a regular diet, whereas 42% tolerated a soft diet. Thirty-nine percent of the patients evaluated had normal speech, 32% had mild impairment, 19% were hard to understand, and 10% were unintelligible. The average maximal incisal opening was 35.2 mm. Only 18 patients were candidates for osseointegrated implants, and 56% of those had them placed. Forty-eight percent of the patients had a good aesthetic result, 30% were fair, and 22% were poor.

Criticisms/Limitations   This is a retrospective case series, with inherent limitations as such. Long-term follow-up was limited to a subset of the patients. Aesthetic outcomes were not measured by independent evaluators.

Relevant Studies   The free fibula flap was first introduced by Ian Taylor[2] in 1975. However, Hidalgo[3] first applied its use to mandibular reconstruction in 1989. Cadaver studies by Wei et al[4] established the anatomic basis for harvesting the fibula flap as an osteoseptocutaneous flap with a reliable blood supply to the skin on the lateral aspect of the lower leg by means of the septocutaneous perforators of the peroneal artery. Since then, the technique for raising the fibula flap with or without a skin paddle has been refined, and it has become the mainstay flap for the reconstruction of composite segmental mandibulectomy and osseous-only defects in the patient after ablation and trauma.

The fibula is ideal for several reasons. It provides sufficient bony length to reconstruct the entire mandible,[5] and it offers an adequate shape for osseointegrated dental implant placement to improve masticatory function. The segmental blood supply allows multiple osteotomies, accommodating most mandibular defects. In addition, the adjacent lateral skin paddle can be reliably harvested for composite oromandibular defects. The axial blood supply is predictable and the harvest is relatively straightforward. Finally, donor-site morbidity is minimal.[1]

To optimize the functional and aesthetic outcome of the fibular flap, Hidalgo[6] emphasized the importance of preoperative planning with CT images to construct mandibular templates to aid in shaping the bone and deciding on osteotomy sites. Intraoperatively, the resected specimen is also used to that end. Today it is possible to prebend the fixation plates with a stereolithographic model. Also, one can plan the mandibular and fibular osteotomies with prefabricated cutting guides based on three-dimensional CT images of the mandible and donor leg, all of which use virtual surgical planning.[7] The use of the "double barrel" fibula flap may also contribute to improving function and aesthetics by achieving more bone height to match the native mandible, especially in the nonatrophic or dentate mandible.[8]

Although radiated fibulas were excluded from osseointegrated dental implant placement in this paper, in a more recent paper Salinas et al[9] reported a success rate of 82.4% for implants placed in radiated fibulas compared with 88% in the radiated native mandibles. The difference was not significant. All patients received hyperbaric oxygen therapy according to a standard protocol.[9]

One of the limitations of this study was the lack of independent evaluators of aesthetic outcomes. Interestingly, in a subsequent follow-up study, Hidalgo and Pusic[10] established the long-term results of their mandibular reconstructions, and functional and aesthetic outcomes were again measured. This time aesthetic measures were assessed by independent evaluators. Remarkably, over a 10-year-period, both functional and aesthetic outcomes were favorable and stable. Bone resorption was minimal, even in the face of adjuvant radiation.[10]

In another subsequent paper, Cordeiro et al[11] established an algorithm (Fig. 19-1) that expanded the indications for the use of the fibula flap in mandibular reconstructions. They assert that the fibula should be the first choice in most patients, especially those with anterior and large defects. They put forth an algorithm for mandibular reconstruction that accounts for the bony and skin/soft tissue defects. They also confirm their long-term experience with good functional and aesthetic outcomes.[11]

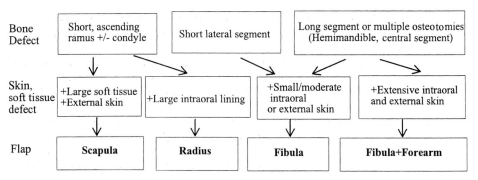

Fig. 19-1 Algorithm for mandible reconstruction with osseous free flaps. Donor-site selection is based primarily on the location and extent of the bony defect and the associated soft-tissue requirements. (From Cordeiro PG, Disa JJ, Hidalgo DA, et al. Reconstruction of the mandible with osseous free flaps: a 10-year experience with 150 consecutive patients. Plast Reconstr Surg 104:1314-1320, 1999.)

Summary   The free fibula flap, whether osseous or osseocutaneous, is indicated for most mandibular or oromandibular reconstructions with excellent functional and aesthetic outcomes.

Implications   This study solidified the role of the free fibula flap in mandibular reconstruction. It presents the readership with a refined approach to the harvest that also incorporates a reliable skin paddle. Hidalgo communicates his extensive favorable experience with this workhorse flap

REFERENCES

1. Hidalgo DA, Rekow A. A review of 60 consecutive fibula free flap mandible reconstructions. Plast Reconstr Surg 96:585-596; discussion 597-602, 1995.
2. Taylor GI, Miller GD, Ham FJ. The free vascularized bone graft. A clinical extension of microvascular techniques. Plast Reconstr Surg 55:533-544, 1975.
3. Hidalgo DA. Fibula free flap: a new method of mandible reconstruction. Plast Reconstr Surg 84:71-79, 1989.
4. Wei FC, Chen HC, Chuang CC, et al. Fibular osteoseptocutaneous flap: anatomic study and clinical application. Plast Reconstr Surg 78:191-200, 1986.
5. Wei FC, Seah CS, Tsai YC, et al. Fibula osteoseptocutaneous flap for reconstruction of composite mandibular defects. Plast Reconstr Surg 93:294-304; discussion 305-306, 1994.
6. Hidalgo DA. Aesthetic improvements in free-flap mandible reconstruction. Plast Reconstr Surg 88:574-585; discussion 586-587, 1991.

7. Antony AK, Chen WF, Kolokythas A, et al. Use of virtual surgery and stereolithography-guided osteotomy for mandibular reconstruction with the free fibula. Plast Reconstr Surg 128:1080-1084, 2011.
8. He Y, Zhang ZY, Zhu HG, et al. Double-barrel fibula vascularized free flap with dental rehabilitation for mandibular reconstruction. J Oral Maxillofac Surg 69:2663-2669, 2011.
9. Salinas TJ, Desa VP, Katsnelson A, et al. Clinical evaluation of implants in radiated fibula flaps. J Oral Maxillofac Surg 68:524-529, 2010.
10. Hidalgo DA, Pusic AL. Free-flap mandibular reconstruction: a 10-year follow-up study. Plast Reconstr Surg 110:438-449; discussion 450-451, 2002.
11. Cordeiro PG, Disa JJ, Hidalgo DA, et al. Reconstruction of the mandible with osseous free flaps: a 10-year experience with 150 consecutive patients. Plast Reconstr Surg 104:1314-1320, 1999.

EDITORIAL PERSPECTIVE

C. Scott Hultman, MD, MBA, FACS

Very often a complex defect requires a complex flap. Although the free fibula osseoseptocutaneous flap is a technically challenging and exciting flap to harvest and shape into a mandible—while it is still attached to the leg!—insetting of the actual flap remains even more difficult. What is remarkable about this operation is the level of success that Hidalgo achieved in a very short period of time in terms of aesthetic and functional outcomes. I have reconstructed many mandibles to date with this flap (and lost a lot of skin paddles), but none have achieved the artistic and mechanical success as those shown by Dr. Hidalgo. In fact early in my career, I would watch a battered VHS tape over and over again, gleaning new insights on every viewing, picking up pearls or even crumbs of wisdom, about the harvest, shaping, and insetting of the free fibula flap. I sat in awe each time, marveling at his speed and precision, always aware of the next step (him, not me). In that process, I became a little better each time, but I never felt that I had mastered the operation. In fact that is probably true for most plastic surgeons. And that is why we love plastic surgery.

CHAPTER 20

Comprehensive Management of Pan-facial Fractures

Manson PN, Clark N, Robertson B, Crawley WA. J Craniomaxillofac Trauma 1:43-56, 1995

Reviewed by H. Wolfgang Losken, MD, MBChB, FCS(SA), FRCS(Ed)

> *The last 20 years have seen considerable advances in facial injury management, . . . (through) . . . improved use of craniofacial exposures, development of techniques that rigidly stabilize remaining bone and allow for replacement of bone that has been destroyed, . . . and a better understanding of soft tissue changes following fracture.[1]*

Research Question   What is the most effective algorithm for the treatment of pan-facial fractures? In what order and how should the fractures be reduced and stabilized to optimize form and function?

Funding   Not applicable

Study Dates   1980s and 1990s

Publishing Date   September 1995

Location   Johns Hopkins Medical Institution, Baltimore, MD

Overview of Design   A review article of the primary surgeon's practice; a monograph

Subjects   The publication by Paul Manson et al[1] deals with a very difficult aspect of reconstructive surgery. All face and skull fractures are difficult to correct perfectly so that the patient regains the shape that it was before the injury. In the pan-facial fracture, the fractures are extensive, and the challenge is that much more difficult. The operating time can be long. The patient may have additional injuries that make it unadvisable to correct the displaced fractures immediately. The delay in treatment makes the reduction more difficult and because of scar tissue more likely that a perfect result has not been achieved. Manson advises that the fractures should be treated immediately and not to wait for the reduction in swelling. Undoubtedly, the immediate reduction in the face fractures results in the fractures clicking back into place, and thus a perfect reduction is more likely to be achieved.

This article is the result of 20 years of experience in the treatment of face and skull fractures and covers every fracture of the face and skull exceptionally well. Those 20 years saw the advances in craniofacial surgery by Paul Tessier[2] and the principle of adequate exposure of the craniofacial skeleton. The correct surgical treatment of face fractures was influenced by the experience of treating secondary face deformities resulting from trauma and the problem that a perfect result was not always possible. Bone grafts were required to correct gross deformities of the bony skeleton. When there were severe fractures with bones fractured into multiple small fragments that could not be corrected with reduction and fixation alone, bone grafts were required as described by Gruss and MacKinnon.[3]

In pan-facial fractures the standard approach is to correct the occlusion and then work from bottom to top. Because the treatment of fractures of the skull had improved so much since the advent of craniofacial surgery and the fixation of the midface to the skull had been perfected, the top-to-bottom approach was an alternative in some fractures. The fractures of the cranium involve the supraorbital border and frontal sinuses; the midface may be LeFort I, II, or III; and the mandible may be fractured in the horizontal of vertical ramus.

Investigations   CT scans were invaluable to identify all of the fractures, and more important, to identify the direction in which the bones were displaced so that we can work out the directional reduction of the bones. It was essential to evaluate the correction of the pan-facial fracture deformity in craniofacial height, face width, and most important the projection of the face (Fig. 20-1). If it is possible to obtain photographs of the patient before the injury, this will be of assistance in achieving a perfect facial profile and shape. These are essential in the reduction of the fractures to achieve projection of the face, width correction, and height. When we review our long-term results after pan-facial fractures, we unfortunately see some faces that we made too long. This must be corrected accurately at surgery to avoid exophthalmia or enophthalmia of an orbit that has been made too big with increased vertical height or an inadequate correction of the displaced orbital wall, most commonly the floor of the orbit.

Incisions   Craniofacial surgery had introduced the more radical incisions for the exposure of the skull and face.[4,5] The coronal incision allowed the exposure of the forehead, lateral and medial walls of the orbit, zygoma, and nose. The great exposure resulted in more accurate reduction and fixation of the fractured and displaced bones. The change from eyelid incisions to conjunctival incisions and extension laterally to the lateral canthotomy made it possible to expose the orbital floor perfectly and ensure a perfect reduction of the bony orbit. Intraoral incisions made the exposure of the maxilla and mandible without outside scars. Exposure and a perfect reduction of the subcondylar mandibular fractures with preauricular-retromandibular incisions made it

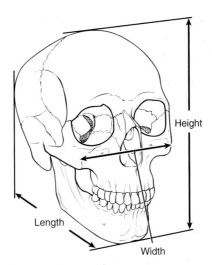

Fig. 20-1 In the repair of the pan-facial fractures it is essential to correct the displaced projection, facial height, and facial width.

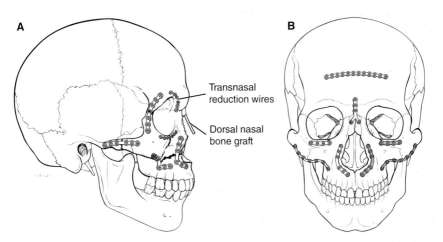

Fig. 20-2 **A,** Fixation of the face fractures with plates and screws to achieve stability of the face. **B,** Biodegradable plates on the right of the skull and miniplates on the left.

necessary to do skin incisions. If there were lacerations, this made it possible to repair the fractures through the incisions. This was another good reason for doing the fracture reduction immediately after the injury.

The change from wire fixation to plate and screw fixation by Luhr[6] (Fig. 20-2, *A*) has resulted in better reduction and fixation of the bones (Fig. 20-2, *B*). Many of the bones may be displaced in any of three directions.

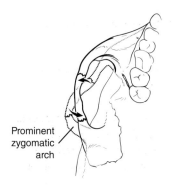

Prominent
zygomatic
arch

Fig. 20-3   Fracture of the zygoma results in a flat cheek bone and excess prominence of the zygomatic arch. This must be corrected with adequate and appropriate reduction and plate and screw fixation.

Zygoma Fractures   In the zygoma fracture the bone may be displaced medially, down and inferiorly, and it is essential that all must be corrected before the plates are applied. The zygomatic arch may become more prominent with the fracture, and the reduction must correct this excess projection and allow the zygomatic bone to be reduced adequately to achieve adequate prominence of the cheek bones (Fig. 20-3). This will require adequate reduction with a bone hook or an appropriate instrument when the bone plates are fixed. If the zygomatic arch needs to be plated, this can only be achieved through a coronal incision.

Cranial Fractures   A craniotomy may be required to operate on any intracranial injury. If only the anterior wall of the frontal sinus is fractured, this can be reduced and fixed. If the posterior wall of the frontal sinus is fractured, a craniotomy is required. The posterior wall of the frontal sinus is removed, the mucosa of the frontal sinus is stripped, and the nasofrontal duct bone is grafted. It is essential to remove all of the mucosa from the sinus. It may even be necessary to bur the sinus wall to ensure that the mucosa has been removed. If there is comminution of the frontal bone bar resulting in an inadequate projection of the forehead, a bone graft may be indicated.

Nasoethmoid and Orbital Fractures   The nasoethmoid fracture may be comminuted and result in telecanthus or a flat nose. If the canthi are wider than they should be, this must be corrected with a transnasal wire.[7] The wires are placed superiorly to the medial canthal ligament. This will correct the medial orbital wall. If there is also a laceration and the medial canthal ligament is displaced, a transnasal wire correction of the medial canthal ligament attachment is essential. The front nasal bones are then fixed to the frontal bone.[8] The nose must be reduced; one must correct the displacement to one side and ensure that the bones of the nose are adequately projected. If this is inadequate, a bone graft may be necessary on the nose. Hopefully, this will rarely be necessary if an adequate reduction of the medial canthi is achieved. Every effort should be made to reduce the deformed nasal septum.

After the zygoma and nasoethmoid fractures are reduced correctly, the floor of the orbit is explored, and a split calvarial bone graft with the periosteum attached is taken and molded into the floor of the orbit to prevent enophthalmos.[9] Metal in the mesh in the floor of the orbit is not advised because of the danger of blindness if a second major face injury occurs. A silicone sheet is also not advised because it commonly extrudes and must be removed.

Palate Fractures   A fracture of the palate and an expansion of the maxillary dental arch must be reduced, and it may be necessary to fix this with a metal plate.

Mandibular Fractures   Open reduction and plate fixation are essential in all mandibular fractures of the horizontal ramus and the angle of the mandible. Subcondylar fractures may need to be exposed and fixed with a plate. Arch bars and interdental wires ensure that a perfect occlusion is achieved. Patients with pan-facial fractures may require a tracheotomy.

Order of Treatment of Pan-facial Fractures   Paul Manson outlines his preference for the order of treatment of pan-facial fractures. He applies arch bars and achieves correct occlusion. Plating of the palate may need to be done first. The mandible fractures would then be stabilized. The supraorbital border is fixed and the nasoethmoid fractures are reduced. The zygoma is then reduced and the floor of the orbit is corrected. The LeFort I fracture is then reduced and fixed. If there is significant bone loss over the maxillary sinus, a bone graft may be necessary.

Discussion   This article by Paul Manson deals with fractures of every area of the craniofacial skeleton. His recommendations for treatment could be applied to any of the areas of the face or skull. The difficulty arises when multiple areas are fractured, and the goal is to obtain a perfect correction of the projection of that area and the width and height of the face. When it is a pan-facial fracture, the problems become compounded. If each of the reductions is only a millimeter from perfect, this could result in a significant and unacceptable deformity. Our goal should be to never need to operate on this skeletal deformity again. Every bone reduction must be perfect.

This raises the controversial issue regarding the statement that a bony gap of more than 4 to 5 mm should be corrected with a bone graft. If there is so much comminution of the bone that there is a bone gap, then a bone graft is indicated. However, more important a gap of 4 to 5 mm may be an indication that we have not adequately and perfectly reduced the fracture. We should not accept that. If we identify that a site we have reduced and fixed is not perfect, we should remove the plates and screws and fix it in the correct position.

One of the next advances that influenced our treatment of pan-facial fractures is the introduction of biodegradable plates[5,10] (see Fig. 20-2, *B*). In Europe it is common to remove all metal plates, and this requires a second operation later. The use of biodegradable plates avoids this additional operation. One of the problems of biodegradable plates is that the plates are not as stable as metal plates. Miniplates have had the advantage of containing less metal than standard metal plates. Miniplates are not as stable as standard metal plates. We must identify when it is safe to use biodegradable plates instead of metal plates.

The treatment of pan-facial fractures is not easy. It is very time-consuming. To achieve a good functional and cosmetic result, it is essential to correct every fractured face bone accurately to achieve correct projection of the face and facial height. It must be the same as the patient had before the injury.

REFERENCES

1. Manson PN, Clark N, Robertson B, et al. Comprehensive management of pan-facial fractures. J Craniomaxillofac Trauma 1:43-56, 1995.
2. Tessier P. Complications of facial trauma. Principles of later reconstruction. Ann Plast Surg 17:411-420, 1986.
3. Gruss JS, Mackinnon SE. Complex maxillary fractures: role of buttress reconstruction and immediate bone grafts. Plast Reconstr Surg 78:9-22, 1986.
4. Wolf SA. Application of craniofacial surgical precepts in orbital reconstruction following trauma and tumor removal. J Maxillofac Surg 10:212-223, 1982.
5. Losken HW, van Aalst JA, Mooney MP, et al. Biodegradation of Inion fast-absorbing biodegradable plates and screws. J Craniofac Surg 19:748-756, 2008.
6. Luhr HG. Indications for use of a microsystem for internal fixation in craniofacial surgery. J Craniofac Surg 1:35-46, 1990.
7. Markowitz BL, Manson PN, Sargent L, et al. Management of the medial canthal tendon in nasoethmoid orbital fractures: the importance of the central fragment in classification and treatment. Plast Reconstr Surg 87:843-853, 1991.
8. Jackson IT. Classification and treatment of orbitozygomatic and orbitoethmoid fractures. The place of bone grafting and plate fixation. Clin Plast Surg 16:77-91, 1989.
9. Kawamoto HK Jr. Late posttraumatic enophthalmos: a correctable deformity? Plast Reconstr Surg 69:423-432, 1982.
10. Losken HW. Rigid fixation of the craniofacial skeleton. Probl Plast Reconstr Surg 3:172-181, 1994.
11. Manley G. Precision medicine approach for neurotrauma [abstract]. Presented at the 32nd Annual Symposium of the National Neurotrauma Society, San Francisco, CA, June 29–July 2, 2014.
12. Manson P, Clark N, Robertson B, et al. Subunit principles in midface fractures: the importance of sagittal buttresses, soft-tissue reductions, and sequencing treatment of segmental fractures. Plast Reconstr Surg 103:1287-1306, 1999.
13. Manson P, Markowitz B, Mirvis S, et al. Toward CT-based facial fracture treatment. Plast Reconstr Surg 85:202-212; discussion 213-214, 1990.
14. Manson P, Iliff N. Management of blow-out fractures of the orbital floor. II. Early repair for selected injuries. Surv Ophthalmol 35:280-292, 1991.
15. Markowitz B, Manson P, Sargent L, et al. Management of the medial canthal tendon in nasoethmoid orbital fractures: the importance of the central fragment in treatment and classification. Plast Reconstr Surg 87:843-853, 1991.
16. Hendrickson M, Clark N, Manson P. Sagittal fractures of the maxilla: classification and treatment. Plast Reconstr Surg 101:319-332, 1998.
17. Crawley W, Azman P, Clark N, et al. The edentulous LeFort fracture. J Craniofacial Surg 8:298-308, 1997.
18. Rodriguez ED, Stanwix MG, Nam AJ, et al. Twenty-six-year experience treating frontal sinus fractures: a novel algorithm based on anatomical fracture pattern and failure of conventional techniques. Plast Reconstr Surg 122:1850-1856, 2008.

19. Manson PN, Stanwix M, Yaremchuk M, et al. Frontobasilar fractures: anatomy, classification and clinical significance. Plast Reconstr Surg 124:2096-2106, 2009.

20. Lee RH, Gamble WB, Robertson B, et al. The MCFONTZL classification system for soft-tissue injuries to the face. Plast Reconstr Surg 103:1150-1157, 1999.

21. Lee RH, Gamble B, Mayer MH, et al. Patterns of facial lacerations from blunt trauma. Plast Reconstr Surg 99:1544-1554, 1997.

22. Clark N, Birely B, Manson PN, et al. High-energy ballistic and avulsive facial injuries: classification, patterns, and an algorithm for primary reconstruction. Plast Reconstr Surg 98:583-601, 1996.

23. Robertson B, Manson P. The importance of serial debridement and "a second look" procedures in high-energy ballistic and avulsive facial injuries. Operat Tech Plast Reconstr Surg 5:236-246, 1998.

24. Rodriguez ED, Martin M, Bluebond-Langner R, et al. Microsurgical reconstruction of post-traumatic high-energy maxillary defects: establishing the effectiveness of early reconstruction. Plast Reconstr Surg 120(7 Suppl 2):103S-117S, 2007.

25. Rodriguez E, Bluebond-Langner R, Park J, et al. Preservation of contour in periorbital and midfacial craniofacial microsurgery: reconstruction of the soft tissue elements and skeletal buttresses. Plast Reconstr Surg 121:1738-1747, 2008.

26. Fisher M, Dorafshar A, Bojovic B, et al. The evolution of critical concepts in aesthetic craniofacial microsurgical reconstruction. Plast Reconstr Surg 130:389-398, 2012.

STUDY AUTHOR REFLECTIONS

Paul Manson, MD, FACS, and Eduardo D. Rodriguez, MD, DDS

In the past 30 years, much progress has been made regarding classification, treatment options, timing, and technique of reductions of both the bone and soft tissue in the treatment of facial injuries.

In particular, clinicians have recently benefited from refined classifications for many diseases, which have yielded outcome data that have produced noticeable treatment improvements. Because all disease occur in patterns, the recognition of those patterns permits a better understanding of how to manage disease. The continuing process of diagnosis, treatment, and outcome analysis yields consistent changes and improvements to both the taxonomy and thereby future treatment, perpetuating the cycle of improvement.[11]

The most challenging facial injuries to treat are pan-facial fractures,[12] which by definition must include at least two of the three major areas of the facial skeleton: frontal bone, midface, and mandible. Practically, further division of the facial skeleton into functional and anatomic parts creates a treatment algorithm organized by the concept of "CT-based facial fracture treatment"[13] determined by (1) the anatomic area and

(2) the energy or "comminution and displacement" of the particular anatomic part of the skeleton injured.

The 1999 paper[12] proposed a comprehensive treatment organization for both the bone and soft tissue; it covered exposure, reduction, and fixation for each degree of bone injury in each anatomic area and then dealt with how to improve the quality of the soft tissue in the original injury, the timing of fracture repair, and the closure and replacement of soft tissue onto the anatomically restored facial skeleton.

Functionally, there are four areas of the facial skeleton:
1. Frontal bone (supraorbital and frontal sinus areas)
2. Upper midface (zygomas and nasoethmoid)
3. Lower midface and occlusion (LeFort I maxilla and alveolar processes of the mandible and maxilla)
4. Mandible (basal horizontal and vertical sections)

Within each of the four areas, each anatomic area of the fracture may be classified as (a) minimally, (b) moderately, or (c) severely displaced and therefore treated with (a-1) no or (a-2) minimal open reduction, (b) a standard open reduction, or (c) an extended open reduction. The latter (c) is reserved for the most displaced fractures that require exposure for alignment and fixation at all buttress articulations of a particular anatomic area of the facial skeleton.

For the zygomatic portion of a pan-facial fracture, it could be so minimally displaced that reduction would not be necessary. More frequently the standard minimal displaced zygoma (a-2) (incomplete or "greensticked" at the Z-F suture) could be approached by the inferior approaches alone at the Z-M buttress. For the standard displacement (b), a more complete set of incisions, the full "anterior" approaches of the lower and upper eyelid, and gingival buccal sulcus incisions allow complete exposure and fixation of all anterior zygoma buttress articulations. The severely comminuted zygoma (c) requires a complete anterior exposure plus the zygomatic arch (anterior and posterior exposures), adding a coronal incision for the reduction and fixation at each zygomatic buttress and within the orbit laterally and inferiorly.[14]

Similarly, for the nasoethmoid area,[15] the simplest fractures would be nondisplaced or "greensticked" at the articulation with the internal angular process of the frontal bone, and like the "greensticked" zygoma, would be amenable to inferior approaches alone where the infraorbital rim and piriform aperture fractures are aligned and stabilized through a gingival buccal sulcus incision. With increasing displacement and comminution of the nasoethmoidal orbital area, the lower eyelid and coronal approaches must be added to permit more complete exposure and perhaps also to provide for detachment and reattachment of the medial canthal ligament in extremely comminuted cases.

The approaches specified for each individual anatomic area involved in the fracture would then be summed over all the areas of fracture, permitting a comprehensive treatment plan for all areas to be developed, and an order of treatment could be specified for the entire case. In this way the treatment is the least (but still effective) for each anatomic area. Such approaches were first described in the article, "Toward CT-Based Facial Fracture Treatment."[13]

Generally my preference, if no neurosurgical urgency is present, is to begin with stabilization of the occlusion by reduction of a split palate[16,17] and any maxillary or mandibular alveolar fractures and then to address the vertical and horizontal mandible or perhaps the frontal bone.[18,19] I first use wires for temporary fracture segment positioning and then proceed to rigid fixation after the multiple areas of provisional reduction are confirmed as accurate. Finally, I stabilize the upper midface and then complete the reduction of the lower midface at the LeFort I level.

Several comments about soft tissue bear repeating:
1. Every facial fracture has an injury to the soft tissue,[20,21] which may be minimal, moderate, or severe. How the soft tissue responds (and therefore the ultimate quality and position of the soft tissue) depends on when and what you do to the bone and whether the soft tissue can respond by healing and remodeling over a precisely reconstructed facial skeleton. Early bone reduction, the layered repair of the soft tissue incisions, and the replacement of the repaired soft tissues on to a reduced skeleton become the method of "soft tissue reduction."
2. Regarding timing and facial fracture management, because the soft tissue has an initial injury, it makes good sense to confine the incisions, dissection, and repair of the fractures to this initial injury period rather than to create a second set of fracture reduction injuries to the soft tissue in the vulnerable period of soft tissue healing 1 to 2 weeks after the initial soft tissue injury.

   Although many isolated, simple fractures may be operated on at any time after the injury with little compromise in the ultimate quality of the soft tissue, true high-energy facial injuries begin to develop soft tissue scarring and contracture from the point of the initial injury.[22,23] The soft tissue becomes stiffened, thicker, discolored, and less pliable with each day of initial healing. The placement of reduction incisions and dissection in this vulnerable period 1 to 2 weeks after the initial injury create a second set of soft tissue injuries from the bone reduction surgery, further damaging the soft tissue, whereas confining the incisions to the initial injury period combines the two soft tissue injuries into a single tissue reaction. The soft tissue reacts to a single insult, yielding the best result one could achieve in soft tissue quality and position.
3. Regarding dehiscence and displacement of the soft tissue, the layered closure of the incisions prevents soft tissue dehiscence. Reattaching the repaired soft tissue to the facial skeleton places the soft tissue correctly over the reconstructed and realigned facial skeleton and allows the soft tissue to heal in the correct position and with the correct contour. The shape and position of the bone are the pattern for the remodeling and repair by an internal scarring of the soft tissue injury. In some cases, such as the nasoethmoidal orbital area, placing external

soft tissue bolsters to mold the soft tissue to the facial skeleton creates the proper contours and angles in the soft tissue conforming to the shape of the bone, prevents hematoma (excess fibrosis and thickness of soft tissue), and keeps the soft tissue stretched to length over the entire curving surface of the bone.

These considerations allow a comprehensive plan for the treatment of any facial injury—both for the bone and the soft tissue. Of course, immediate bone grafting and microvascular flap transfer[24,25] may be added where necessary to replace critical missing areas of the facial skeleton and soft tissue. Mismatched cutaneous soft tissue islands from microvascular transfer may be removed secondarily by serial excision or standard facial cutaneous flap reconstruction.[26]

EDITORIAL PERSPECTIVE

C. Scott Hultman, MD, MBA, FACS

A book such as this—an attempt to identify and highlight the top 50 studies every plastic surgeon should know—is destined to fall short. Because the scope and depth of plastic surgery is so wide and rich, selecting only 50 articles is really an impossible task. Hundreds of papers and authors will inevitably be left out despite strong arguments for inclusion in this book.

However, if forced to choose a single surgeon who has made seminal, lasting contributions to the treatment of facial trauma over the course of a career, I would not hesitate to pick Paul Manson, former Chief of Plastic Surgery at Johns Hopkins Medical School. Thus our only paper on craniofacial trauma is a review article authored by Dr. Manson, a summary of his approach to the treatment of pan-facial fractures.

Similar to what William Halsted did for the treatment of breast cancer, so too has Dr. Manson done for the management of major facial injuries. Both Manson and Halsted orchestrated a change in the way we approached these problems and taught generations of surgeons, who became leaders in their own fields. Manson and Halsted incorporated new techniques and technologies into their practices, yielding both incremental and sometimes disruptive improvements in their outcomes. Whereas Halsted warned to "beware the surgeon with the plastic operation," Manson appreciated the need to restore form and function—not afraid of the plastic surgery operation. Quality of life is not just measured by mean survival, time to recurrence, and tumor burden. Real quality of life involves a successful return to school and work, reintegration back into society, and the ability to have a fulfilling existence. Paul Manson appreciated these long-term, sometimes distant goals, and I believe that this is why he was driven to restore what nature had taken away. His clinical, educational, and scientific accomplishments in the area of facial trauma, and specifically pan-facial injuries, are unlikely to be matched by anyone else.

Comparison of Radical Mastectomy With Alternative Treatments for Primary Breast Cancer. A First Report of Results From a Prospective Randomized Clinical Trial

Fisher B, Montague E, Redmond C, Barton B, Borland D, Fisher ER, Deutsch M, Schwarz G, Margolese R, Donegan W, Volk H, Konvolinka C, Gardner B, Cohn I Jr, Lesnick G, Cruz AB, Lawrence W, Nealon T, Butcher H, Lawton R.
Cancer 39(6 Suppl):2827-2839, 1977

Reviewed by Michelle C. Roughton, MD

> [The findings] presently indicate that the concept of en bloc dissection with removal of the breast, pectoral muscles and axillary nodes in continuity is without special merit.[1]

Research Question   For women with clinically node-negative axillae, is total mastectomy alone (followed by axillary lymph node dissection if the axilla becomes clinically positive in the future) versus total mastectomy with regional radiation equivalent to radical mastectomy? In addition, for women with clinically node-positive axillae, is total mastectomy and regional radiation equivalent to radical mastectomy?

Funding   Breast Cancer Task Force Contract (NIH), U.S. Public Health Service, and American Cancer Society

Study Dates   July 1971 to September 1974

Publishing Date   June 1977

Location   34 institutions in the United States and Canada

Subjects   Women with potentially operable, potentially curable breast cancer; more specifically, this study included patients with tumors confined to the breast or breast and axilla, tumors mobile relative to the underlying chest wall, and those with mobile axillary lymph nodes who lacked arm edema and were willing to participate.

Exclusion Criteria   Women who were either pregnant or lactating, those previously treated for their current cancer, those who had a prior or concomitant cancer except for well-managed basal cell or squamous cell skin cancer, those with bilateral breast cancers, tumors other than carcinomas, inflammatory tumors, those with skin ulceration >2 cm, those with peau d'orange involving more than one third of the breast, those with satellite or parasternal nodules, fixation of axillary lymph nodes (>2 cm), those with lymph nodes elsewhere suspected to contain tumor and not disproven, those with poor surgical risks precluding randomization to any treatment option, or if the presence of other preexisting disease made prolonged follow-up unlikely

Sample Size   1765 total patients, 1159 to the three node-negative groups and 606 to the two node-positive groups

Overview of Design   The study design overview can be seen in Fig. 21-1.[2]

Intervention   Three groups of women with clinically negative axillary lymph nodes were randomly assigned to either radical mastectomy, total mastectomy and regional radiation therapy, or total mastectomy alone. Those with total mastectomy alone would undergo axillary node dissection only if those nodes became clinically positive. Patients with clinically positive axillary lymph node were randomly assigned to radical mastectomy or total mastectomy with radiation therapy.

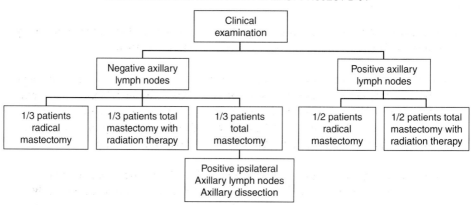

Fig. 21-1   The incidence of lung carcinoma after surgery for breast carcinoma with and without postoperative radiotherapy. (Data from Deutsch M, Land SR, Begovic M, et al. The incidence of lung carcinoma after surgery for breast carcinoma with and without postoperative radiotherapy. Cancer 98:1362-1368, 2003.)

Follow-up   Patients were examined at least every 3 months during the first 3 years and every 6 months thereafter. Blood work was drawn every 3 months for the first year, and chest radiographs were obtained every 6 months.

Endpoints
1. Treatment failure, which was defined by the presence of a tumor in local, regional, or distant sites (Note: patients who developed clinically positive axillary lymph nodes after total mastectomy alone, who then received axillary lymph node dissection in a second stage, were not considered treatment failures.)
2. Survival
3. Morbidity

Results   No statistically significant differences were found in regard to treatment failure (disease-free survival) between the three groups with negative lymph nodes, that is, radical mastectomy, total mastectomy with regional radiation, and total mastectomy with axillary lymph node dissection once the axilla became clinically positive. Furthermore, no significant differences were found in the two groups with clinically positive axillae, that is, radical mastectomy and total mastectomy with regional radiation.

Of the 344 patients with clinically negative lymph nodes who received total mastectomy alone, 49 (14.2%) developed positive nodes and underwent axillary lymph node dissection. Of those 49 patients, 26 (53%) developed a recurrence.

The rates of regional recurrence versus distant metastases were the same for all three node-negative and both node-positive treatment groups. However, local recurrence rates were lower for both groups receiving radiation therapy and those with and without clinically positive lymph nodes (Fig. 21-2). Survival within the node-negative treatment groups was equivalent as it was between the two node-positive treatment groups (Fig. 21-3).

Criticisms/Limitations   This prospective, randomized, controlled trial is limited only in its average follow-up at the time of publication, that is, 36 months.

Relevant Studies   This study was ongoing, and the 25-year follow-up was published in 2002.[3] The long-term data support those of the original National Surgical Adjuvant Breast Project (NSABP) B-04 publication in that disease-free and overall survival rates were no different among either the randomized node-negative groups or the two node-positive groups. Again, radical mastectomy offered no advantage.

A subsequent study by the same authors, NSABP B-06,[4] compared another three groups of patients, those with early stage (I or II) breast cancer who were randomly assigned to either total mastectomy, lumpectomy alone, or lumpectomy followed by radiation therapy. Overall survival at 20 years was the same among the three groups. Local recurrence was equivalent between the total mastectomy group and those who had a lumpectomy combined with radiation therapy. However, local recurrence rates were higher in the group who underwent lumpectomy alone.

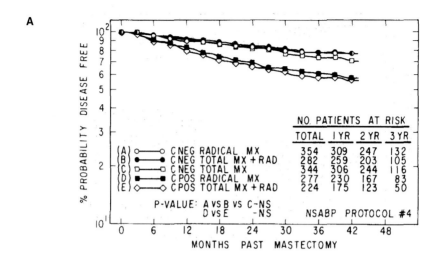

A

B

	Clinically Negative Nodes								Clinically Positive Nodes				
	Radical Mastectomy (RM)		Total Mastectomy + Radiation (TMR)			Total Mastectomy (TM)			Radical Mastectomy (RM)		Total Mastectomy + Radiation (TMR)		
	A	C	A	B	C	A	C		A	C	A	B	C
Number of patients	361	354	351	314	282	363	344		292	277	294	256	224
Failures	21.3	20.9	19.4	19.4	19.1	23.7	23.8		36.3	37.9	38.1	38.7	38.4
Local recurrences	3.0	3.1	0.3	0.3	0.0	5.0	4.9		5.1	5.1	1.0	1.2	1.3
Regional recurrences	2.5	2.5	2.3	1.9	2.1	2.8	2.9		4.5	4.7	6.8	7.0	6.7
Distant metastases	13.3	12.7	14.0	14.3	14.2	12.7	12.8		19.2	20.2	24.1	24.6	24.6
Combinations	2.6	2.6	2.9	2.8	2.9	3.5	3.3		7.5	7.9	6.2	6.0	5.7

Fig. 21-2 A, Probability (%) of survival without disease. *MX,* Mastectomy; *NSABP,* National Surgical Adjuvant Breast Project; *RAD,* radiation. **B,** NSABP Protocol No. 4: site of first reported treatment failure (% of patients). *A,* Eligible for protocol; *B,* patients per protocol, including radiation variations; *C,* patients per protocol with follow-up. (From Fisher B, Montague E, Redmond C, et al. Comparison of radical mastectomy with alternative treatments for primary breast cancer. A first report of results from a prospective randomized clinical trial. Cancer 39[6 Suppl]:2827-2839, 1977.)

The lead author of the aforementioned trials, Dr. Bernard Fisher, is quoted, "There are two aims in the management of patients with primary breast cancer. In order of importance, the first is related to achieving a disease-free life, and the second is directed toward attaining the best cosmesis possible without compromising the patient's chance of cure."[5] The wisdom in this remark seems to be the impetus for first abandoning the deeply disfiguring technique of radical mastectomy and the subsequent acceptance of breast conservation for early stage breast cancers. For patients for whom breast conservation is not an option, the concept of skin-sparing mastectomy, that is, to remove the nipple-areola complex but otherwise preserve the breast skin, has become increasingly popular.[6] Furthermore, the concept of oncologic safety in nipple-sparing mastectomy has gained traction.[7] Thus the surgical technique for mastectomy alone has fundamentally changed over the past 30 years.

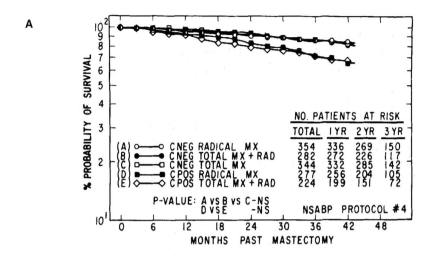

Fig. 21-3 A, Probability (%) of survival. *MX,* Mastectomy; *NSABP,* National Surgical Adjuvant Breast Project; *RAD,* radiation. **B,** NSABP Protocol No. 4: percent of deaths and average monthly death rate. *A,* Eligible for protocol; *B,* patients per protocol, including radiation variations; *C,* patients per protocol with follow-up. (From Fisher B, Montague E, Redmond C, et al. Comparison of radical mastectomy with alternative treatments for primary breast cancer. A first report of results from a prospective randomized clinical trial. Cancer 39[6 Suppl]:2827-2839, 1977.)

However, for women who are able to conserve their breasts, the disfigurement has not been entirely eliminated. Approximately one third of patients after breast-conserving surgery will develop significant breast asymmetry.[8,9] The disfigurement is worse with larger tumor volumes relative to breast size and tumors in the lower quadrants of the breast.[10] From these findings, a new field was introduced, termed *"oncoplastic surgery."* Oncoplastic techniques are used to create a solid breast mound (rather than a breast with a hollow portion) after tumor resection and before the initiation of radiation therapy. This may be accomplished with breast reduction techniques or volume replacement techniques. Volume replacement is most commonly derived from the latissimus muscle with overlying soft tissue. The field of oncoplastic surgery has not only improved cosmesis,[11] but may expand the indication for breast conservation because it allows the oncologic surgeon to resect an even larger margin than he or she perhaps otherwise would.[12] With the ongoing attempt to preserve cosmesis and symmetry while maintaining oncologic safety, Dr. Fisher's message remains relevant today.

Summary   Radical mastectomy conferred no advantage in either local control or survival. Furthermore, local control was equivalent for women who underwent total mastectomy and radiation therapy and those who had total mastectomy and axillary lymph node dissection only when their axillae became clinically positive.

Implications   This study essentially abolished any indication for radical mastectomy other than tumor invasion into the pectoral muscles. It paved the way for skin-sparing mastectomy first, then breast conservation, and finally oncoplastic surgery as an expanding spectrum in cancer control and cosmesis.

REFERENCES

1. Fisher B, Montague E, Redmond C, et al. Comparison of radical mastectomy with alternative treatments for primary breast cancer. A first report of results from a prospective randomized clinical trial. Cancer 39(6 Suppl):2827-2839, 1977.
2. Deutsch M, Land SR, Begovic M, et al. The incidence of lung carcinoma after surgery for breast carcinoma with and without postoperative radiotherapy. Cancer 98:1362-1368, 2003.
3. Fisher B, Jeong JH, Anderson S, et al. Twenty-five year follow-up of a randomized trial comparing radical mastectomy, total mastectomy, and total mastectomy followed by irradiation. N Engl J Med 347:567-575, 2002.
4. Fisher B, Anderson S, Bryant J, et al. Twenty-year follow-up of a randomized trial comparing total mastectomy, lumpectomy, and lumpectomy plus irradiation for the treatment of invasive breast cancer. N Engl J Med 347:1233-1241, 2002.
5. Fisher B, Wolmark N. New concepts in the management of primary breast cancer. Cancer 36:627-632, 1975.
6. Toth BA, Lappert P. Modified skin incisions for mastectomy: the need for plastic surgical input in preoperative planning. Plast Reconstr Surg 87:1048-1053, 1991.
7. de Alcantara FP, Capko D, Barry JM, et al. Nipple-sparing mastectomy for breast cancer and risk-reducing surgery: the Memorial Sloan-Kettering Cancer Center experience. Ann Surg Oncol 18:3117-3122, 2011.
8. Bajaj A, Kon PS, Oberg KC, et al. Aesthetic outcomes in patients undergoing breast conservation therapy for the treatment of localized breast cancer. Plast Reconstr Surg 114:1442-1449, 2014.
9. Wang HT, Barone CM, Steigelman MB, et al. Aesthetic outcomes in breast conservation therapy. Aesthet Surg J 28:165-170, 2008.
10. Clough KB, Nos C, Salmon RJ, et al. Conservative treatment of breast cancers by mammaplasty and irradiation: a new approach to lower quadrant tumors. Plast Reconstr Surg 96:363-370, 1995.
11. Clough KB, Lewis JS, Couturaud B, et al. Oncoplastic techniques allow extensive resections for breast-conserving therapy of breast carcinomas. Ann Surg 237:26-34, 2003.
12. Kaur N, Petit JY, Rietjens M, et al. Comparative study of surgical margins in oncoplastic surgery and quadrantectomy in breast cancer. Ann Surg Oncol 12:1-7, 2005.

13. Rizzo M, Wood WC. The changing field of locoregional treatment of breast cancer. Oncology (Williston Park) 25:813-816, 2011.

14. Lukuabi AE, Hunt KK, Ballman KV, et al. Axillary dissection vs no axillary dissection in women with invasive breast cancer and sentinel node metastasis: a randomized clinical trial. JAMA 305:569-575, 2011.

15. Fisher B, Jepang JH, Anderson S, et al. Twenty-five year follow up of a randomized trial comparing radical mastectomy, total mastectomy, and total mastectomy followed by irradiation. N Engl J Med 347:567-575, 2002.

EXPERT COMMENTARY

Albert Losken, MD, FACS

We have made significant strides in breast reconstruction over the past few decades. Patient satisfaction, quality of life, and aesthetic outcomes have improved because of refinements in our surgical techniques and better technology. However, one of the more dramatic changes that directly impact our reconstructive results is the extent of tumor resection. The days of radical Halstedian mastectomies are long gone, and we have shifted more toward an era of surgical conservatism in breast cancer management. This paper by Fisher et al in 1977 is one of the landmark studies that paved the way for future refinements in cancer management. It was not only a well-designed, multi-institutional, prospective evaluation of lesser resection, but it also reinforced what we hoped to hear—that more radical resections confer no local control or survival advantage. Suddenly the surgical dogma of radical resection was no longer gospel, and the next generation of breast surgeons started to look for ways to improve cosmesis and maintain survival in the management of breast cancer.[13] What followed was a barrage of randomized clinical trials, with more recently, the Z11 study, which showed once again that patients do better when we do less.[14] This has all been thanks to this initial Fisher paper, which was updated at 25 years without survival benefit to radical resections.[15]

For plastic surgeons, this has dramatically impacted out practice. Less radical mastectomies also spurred lumpectomy-type resections. With the popularity of breast conservation therapy, we started to see fewer mastectomies and more breast conservation therapy–type deformities, which then paved the way for partial breast reconstruction techniques after radiation therapy and at the time of mastectomy. When mastectomies are done, we have seen more skin-sparing–type mastectomies and now nipple-areola–sparing mastectomies. This has improved not only cosmetic results but has also allowed many direct-to-implant or one-stage breast reconstructions. Patients with breast cancer now have many choices and are definitely in a better place today than they were 50 years ago. I predict refinement in respective and reconstructive techniques will likely continue, and as a result, outcomes will continue to improve.

CHAPTER 22

Breast Reconstruction After Mastectomy Using the Temporary Expander

Radovan C. Plast Reconstr Surg 69:195-208, 1982

Reviewed by Michelle C. Roughton, MD

> *The principal [sic] problem in breast reconstruction after mastectomy is the absence of adequate skin coverage. The needed amount of skin for breast reconstruction is regained by expanding the remaining chest wall skin.[1]*

Research Question A new technique for breast reconstruction, which is performed in two stages, is described, that is, the novel use of tissue expansion

Funding Not described

Study Dates 1976 to 1982

Publishing Date February 1982

Location Encino, CA

Subjects Female patients undergoing delayed breast reconstruction

Exclusion Criteria Not described

Sample Size 68 patients

Overview of Design A prospective trial of tissue expansion for delayed breast reconstruction

Intervention Women with a previous mastectomy had a subcutaneous tissue expander placed through a 5 cm lateral/axillary incision. Expansion was then performed both during surgery and at outpatient visits to 150 to 200 cc larger than the planned permanent implant. In a second stage the expander is removed, the capsule is adjusted as necessary, and a permanent implant is placed. Commonly, a symmetry procedure on the contralateral breast (for example, mastopexy, reduction, or subcutaneous mastectomy with direct-to-implant reconstruction) was performed at the time of the second stage.

Follow-up   The average follow-up was 1 to 2 years: 18 patients, less than 6 months; 21 patients, 1 year; 14 patients, 2 years; 15 patients, 3 years.

Endpoints   Complications were recorded: hematoma (n = 3), infection (n = 5; two expanders were removed), skin necrosis (n= 3; one expander was removed), deflation (n = 1; the expander was removed and exchanged), and Baker III capsular contracture (n = 8). In all cases of expander removal, the expander was eventually exchanged for a new device.

Results   All 68 patients had successful tissue expansion and exchange for a permanent prosthesis.

Criticism   This prospective, nonrandomized trial was the first to describe the use of tissue expansion for breast reconstruction. A comparison with other techniques, specifically the use of one-stage implant reconstruction, serial placement of implants increasing in size, and latissimus flaps, would be helpful to ascertain the benefits of this new technique, including patient satisfaction, the volume of the permanent prosthesis, and even the cost. However, over 30 years later, this technique with only a slight modification of pocket placement (most surgeons will expand the subpectoral versus subcutaneous pocket) is the most commonly used method of breast reconstruction today.

Relevant Studies   Before Dr. Radovan's paper,[1] breast reconstruction was commonly performed with the addition of autologous tissue, such as Millard's tubed pedicled flaps,[2] latissimus muscle or myocutaneous flaps first described by Tansini,[3] Hartrampf's transverse rectus abdominis myocutaneous flap (TRAM),[4] or single-stage implant-based techniques.[5,6]

Dr. Radovan was the first to report the use of a temporary tissue expander to recruit native breast skin, which allowed the placement of larger volume implants in a second stage. Although he described a subcutaneous pocket, this was later modified to submuscular placement (pectoralis major, serratus, and rectus abdominis)[7] because of complications such as the exposure of the expander, rippling, and capsular contracture. In time, the popularity of immediate breast reconstruction has overtaken that of delayed.[8] Today immediate breast reconstruction with tissue expanders often involves the use of acellular dermal matrix,[9] which is secured both to the inferior edge of the pectoralis major muscle and the inframammary fold. This may afford more rapid expansion and a lower immediate position of the implant on the chest wall. The superior pole of the implant remains covered by the pectoralis major, whereas the lower pole is covered by the acellular dermal matrix. This is described for both single-stage (direct-to-implant placement) and two-stage (tissue expander placement and later exchange for permanent implant) approaches and is arguably the most commonly performed technique of implant-based breast reconstruction.

Single-stage implant reconstruction and the avoidance of the expander altogether are becoming increasingly popular, especially in patients for whom nipple-sparing mastectomy is an option.[10]

Elsewhere in the body, tissue expansion was developed and championed by Manders et al,[11] who described the successful use of tissue expanders in the reconstruction of scalp, extremity, and trunk defects. Not only did Dr. Manders pioneer the clinical work that led to this alternative method of reconstruction, but he performed detailed histochemical analyses of cellular activity within these tissues. Stretching muscle, nerves, and fascia lengthens these structures more than would be predicted with conventional models of elasticity, and the skin reacts to tissue expansion through increased numbers of keratinocytes despite the thinning of the dermis. Much like distraction, osteogenesis generates new bone, tissue expanders generate new skin.

Summary   Dr. Radovan's groundbreaking work, which represents the marriage of tissue expansion and breast reconstruction, was a landmark in breast reconstruction. With his novel technique, women could choose to avoid longer operations and increased surgical/donor sites while achieving larger volume implants for their breast reconstruction.

Implications   His technique, although now modified to a submuscular pocket and frequently involving the use of acellular dermal matrix, is the most popular method of breast reconstruction in the United States today.

REFERENCES

1. Radovan C. Breast reconstruction after mastectomy using the temporary expander. Plast Reconstr Surg 69:195-208, 1982.
2. Millard DR Jr. Breast reconstruction after a radical mastectomy. Plast Reconstr Surg 58:283-291, 1976.
3. Tansini I. Sopra il mio nuovo processo di amputazione della mamella. Riforma Medica (Palermo, Napoli) 12:757, 1906.
4. Hartrampf CR, Scheflan M, Black PW. Breast reconstruction with a transverse abdominal island flap. Plast Reconstr Surg 69:216-225, 1982.
5. Guthrie RH Jr. Breast reconstruction after radical mastectomy. Plast Reconstr Surg 57:14-22, 1976.
6. Hartwell SW Jr, Anderson R, Hall MD, et al. Reconstruction of the breast after mastectomy for cancer. Plast Reconstr Surg 57:152-157, 1976.

7. Apfelberg D, Laub DR, Maser MR, et al. Submuscular breast reconstruction—indication and techniques. Ann Plast Surg 7:213-221, 1981.

8. Losken A, Carlson GW, Bostwick J III, et al. Trends in unilateral breast reconstruction and management of the contralateral breast: the Emory experience. Plast Reconstr Surg 110:89-97, 2002.

9. Salzberg C. Nonexpansive immediate breast reconstruction using human acellular tissue matrix graft (AlloDerm). Ann Plast Surg 57:1-5, 2006.

10. Salzberg CA, Ashikari AY, Koch RM, et al. An 8-year experience of direct-to-implant immediate breast reconstruction using human acellular dermal matrix (AlloDerm). Plast Reconstr Surg 127:514-524, 2011.

11. Manders EK, Schenden MJ, Furrey JA, et al. Soft tissue expansion: concepts and complications. Plast Reconstr Surg 74:493-507, 1984.

EXPERT COMMENTARY

Ernest K. Manders, MD, FACS

Think it, do it, teach it!

What a pleasure it is to resurrect the memory of a long-departed dear friend who was a significant contributor to the art and craft of plastic surgery. Today Ched Radovan's technique of breast reconstruction after mastectomy with the use of tissue expansion is well established as the dominant reconstructive method used around the world. To be sure, the operation as he described it has changed in important ways: the expander is routinely placed under the pectoralis major; acellular dermal matrix has become a valuable adjunct in obtaining a better ultimate shape; and skin-sparing mastectomies are becoming more common. However, the fundamental idea of expansion lives on robustly and has proved its worth.

Perhaps just as important as commenting on Ched Radovan's idea of controlled tissue expansion is a brief reflection on Dr. Radovan, the man, and other lessons we can learn from his life. First, Ched was an American success story. Emigrating from Serbia as Chedomir Radovanovich, he made his way through medical school and residency supporting himself with his musicianship. He was a virtuoso on the accordion and played in a Serbian band. He developed his idea of controlled tissue expander reconstruction with the help of another immigrant from then West Germany, Mr. Rude Schulte, a founder of Mentor Corporation. Times were different then. Ched enjoyed regaling us with stories of how he took Linda, the chief laboratory technician, out to lunch to get her to tell Dr. Hufnagel, Chief of Surgery, that "it worked in dogs." Mr. Schulte obliged with the delivery of the first device within 10 days of the disclosure of the idea in a parking lot. One of Ched's first cases was expansion of the dorsum of a foot in a diabetic patient with an open wound adjacent to the expander. This is an absolute no-no today! But, thank God, it worked and the idea gained momentum. It has proved its worth many times over.

Readers and especially younger readers should note that good ideas often come from people who are "wild and crazy guys." We must identify and support these innovative leaders among us. For 3 years in a row Ched was denied a place on the podium at the annual meeting of the American Society of Plastic and Reconstructive Surgeons by people I knew, who informed me they would never allow such "a crazy idea" on the program. They also told me that "It will never happen in my hospital." But, of course, it did! Ched and the eventual recognition of his good idea were certainly facilitated by Dr. William C. Grabb, Chief of Plastic Surgery at the University of Michigan, who was an established figure in plastic surgery. Dr. Eric Austad, who worked with him at Michigan, had demonstrated expansion with an osmotic expander and had prepared Dr. Grabb for his being an early champion of the new idea. Everyone needs a friend with connections.

Ched died in a drowning accident near Miami in 1986. I have often wondered what else this innovative, exuberant colleague would have contributed had he been with us to march through the last 30 years of plastic surgery together.

CHAPTER 23

Meta-analyses of the Relation Between Silicone Breast Implants and the Risk of Connective-Tissue Diseases

Janowsky EC, Kupper LL, Hulka BS. N Engl J Med 342:781-790, 2000

Reviewed by Michelle C. Roughton, MD

> *On the basis of the research to date, no association is evident between breast implants and any of the individual connective-tissue diseases, all connective-tissue diseases combined, or the other autoimmune or rheumatologic conditions . . .*[1]

Research Question A series of meta-analyses was performed to assess any possible relationship between silicone breast implants and connective tissue or autoimmune disease.

Funding Contract with the Administration Office of the U.S. Courts

Study Dates Studies from 1966 to 1998 were collected.

Publishing Date March 2000

Location Meta-analyses performed at the University of North Carolina at Chapel Hill; studies from the United States, Canada, Europe, and the United Kingdom were included.

Subjects Female patients who had silicone gel–filled breast implants described in previous reports were included in this meta-analysis.

Exclusion Criteria Patients who had direct injection of silicone (or any material) into the breasts were excluded. Studies describing only the symptoms and frequency of symptoms were excluded. Publications in languages other than English were also excluded.

Sample Size   9 cohort studies, 9 case-controlled studies, and 2 cross-sectional studies

Overview of Design   Studies were selected through literature searches for key words regarding breast implants and connective tissue diseases. A total of 757 citations were found. For inclusion, studies must have included an internal comparison group and have provided adequate data for two-by-two table construction in regard to the presence of disease and implants. If multiple studies on the same group of patients were published, only the most recent study was included.

Intervention   Because the studies included were retrospective by design, the intervention or variable was the presence or absence of silicone breast implants.

Follow-up   Not applicable in meta-analysis

Endpoints   The authors measured disease presence or absence (of five individual connective tissue diseases, connective tissue diseases combined, or any rheumatologic or autoimmune diagnosis) when exposed to the presence or absence of any breast implant. A separate analysis was performed for studies describing "silicone-gel–filled breast implants."

Results   Twenty studies were included, 4 of which relied on patient-reported diagnoses, whereas 16 studies extracted data directly from the medical records. All diseases in all studies except for two had 95% confidence intervals that crossed 1. In one of these two papers, Goldman et al,[2] the adjusted relative risk was less than 1, 0.52. The other, Hennekens et al,[3] was a larger study, including 395,000 patients, that used patient-reported data (not substantiated by the medical records) in which the adjusted relative risk for any connective tissue disease was 1.24. The authors then performed two estimates of summary adjusted relative risk for each condition, one with and one without the large study containing only self-reported data.

When the Hennekens et al study was included, the estimates of summary adjusted risks were elevated for all connective tissue diseases combined (1.14), rheumatoid arthritis (1.15), scleroderma or systemic sclerosis (1.30), Sjögren's syndrome (1.47), and other autoimmune or rheumatic conditions (1.15). However, the 95% confidence intervals included 1 except for all connective tissue diseases combined (1.01 to 1.28) and Sjögren's syndrome (1.01 to 2.14). When the Hennekens et al study[3] was excluded, all estimates of summary adjusted relative risks were lower and associated with 95% confidence intervals that included 1.

Criticisms/Limitations   The authors made a point to perform two separate meta-analyses with and without the large study by Hennekens et al because this data, which was unsubstantiated by the medical records, were considered unreliable. In fact, in the authors' discussion, they included a reference that described the self-reported diagnoses of rheumatoid arthritis to have only a 20% positive predictive value.[4] Furthermore, the risk of Sjögren's syndrome remained higher than that of other connective tissue

Table 23-1 Estimates of the Summary Adjusted Relative Risks of an Association Between Breast Implants and Connective-Tissue Diseases

Disease and Studies Included Analysis	Number of Studies	Summary Adjusted Relative Risk (95% CI)*	p Value for Homogeneity	Weight of Hennekens et al[3] in Summary Adjusted Relative Risk	p Value†
All Connective-Tissue Diseases Combined					
All studies	14	1.14 (1.01-1.28)	0.34	0.80	0.003
All studies, excluding Hennekens et al[3]	13	0.80 (0.62-1.04)	0.92	—	
Rheumatoid Arthritis					
All studies	8	1.15 (0.97-1.36)	0.90	0.79	0.56
All studies, excluding Hennekens et al[3]	7	1.04 (0.72-1.51)	0.87	—	
Systemic Lupus Erythematosus					
All studies	5	1.01 (0.74-1.37)	0.33	0.77	0.12
All studies, excluding Hennekens et al[3]	4	0.65 (0.35-1.23)	0.53	—	
Scleroderma or Systemic Sclerosis					
All studies	5	1.30 (0.86-1.96)	0.55	0.42	0.16
All studies, excluding Hennekens et al[3]	4	1.01 (0.59-1.73)	0.80	—	
Sjögren's Syndrome					
All studies	4	1.47 (1.01-2.14)	0.98	0.77	0.92
All studies, excluding Hennekens et al[3]	3	1.42 (0.65-3.11)	0.90	—	
Dermatomyositis or Polymyositis					
All studies	1	1.52 (0.97-2.37)	—	1.00	—
All studies, excluding Hennekens et al[3]	—	—	—	—	
Other Autoimmune or Rheumatic Conditions					
All studies	7	1.15 (0.97-1.36)	0.11	0.59	0.08
All studies, excluding Hennekens et al[3]	6	0.96 (0.74-1.25)	0.19	—	

From Janowsky EC, Kupper LL, Hulka BS. Meta-analyses of the relation between silicone breast implants and the risk of connective-tissue diseases. N Engl J Med 342:781-790, 2000.
*CI denotes confidence interval.
†p values for grouped data were obtained with a chi-square test; this test assessed whether the estimate of the adjusted relative risk for the study by Hennekens et al[3] was significantly different from the estimate of the summary adjusted relative risk for the other studies.

diseases in both analyses. The authors postulated that because the gold standard for the diagnosis of Sjögren's syndrome is a salivary gland biopsy, it is possible that many of these patients were improperly diagnosed.

Relevant Studies The silicone breast implant "crisis" occurred predominantly within the popular press rather than in scientific journals. Perhaps most well remembered is an episode of "Face to Face with Connie Chung," which aired on Dec. 10, 1990.[5] In this episode doctors and patients were interviewed on national television and claimed several ill effects related to silicone breast implants. Most of these complaints were autoimmune or rheumatologic. The link between silicone gel and disease causation was not substantiated in the medical literature, and silicone itself is ubiquitous in both the environment and in medical devices.[6] However, in April 1992, silicone gel–filled breast implants were placed under a strict moratorium by the U.S. Food and Drug Administration.[7]

Exceptions were made for their use in reconstruction and for women undergoing revision of existing gel-filled implants who were participating in clinical trials.

The American Society of Plastic Surgeons released a consensus statement on the relationship between breast implants and connective tissue disease in December 1992. Their recommendations were as follows:

1. "There is insufficient information to determine whether silicone in the form of a breast implant can be implicated as a cause of scleroderma-like disorders or any other autoimmune disease. Judging from the paucity of reported cases in the very large population of implanted women, if a casual association were to be established, the statistical risk would likely be very low. The presence of risk and magnitude thereof can be determined only by appropriate epidemiologic research."

2. "At present, there is no reason to discourage women from considering breast augmentation on the basis of the risk of acquiring or exacerbating a connective-tissue disorder. Until the question is answered by further research, patients should be informed that a theoretical risk might exist, especially if they already have a connective-tissue disorder, idiopathic Raynaud's phenomenon, or an affected first-degree relative."

3. "There is currently insufficient evidence to state that the removal of the implants and their surrounding scar capsule will alter the course of existing disease or prevent the occurrence of new disease . . ."[8]

Subsequently, many clinical trials and meta-analyses have revealed no link between implants and systemic disease.[9,10]

Importantly, the silicone gel implant crisis of the early 1990s was avoided in the more recent reports of non-Hodgkin's lymphoma associated with breast implants. In 1997 Keech and Creech[11] described the first known case of anaplastic large cell lymphoma (ALCL) associated with a breast implant. Subsequently, 42 cases of non-Hodgkin's lymphoma of the breast have been described, including 35 cases of ALCL.[12] All reported cases of implant-associated ALCL, save one,[13] are relatively indolent and present most commonly with a late-onset seroma around the implant and are without constitutional "B" symptoms. The treatment of affected patients has ranged from explantation of the implant and capsule only to combinations of surgery, chemotherapy, and radiation therapy.[14] A population-based study in the Netherlands calculated that the odds ratio of developing ALCL in the presence of breast implants was 18.2. The authors caution that this number, although significantly elevated, must be balanced by the absolute incidence of the disease, which is extremely rare (all sites 0.1/100,000 per year; 0.1 to 0.3/100,000 primary breast incidence in implanted women per year).[15] The response of the plastic surgery community to the creation of a breast implant registry[16] and the expedited online publication of all ALCL-relevant articles in *Plastic and Reconstructive Surgery*[17] indicate a collaborative effort between the Food and Drug Administration and the plastic surgery society that perhaps was not seen during the initial implant "crisis." Implants have remained available, and appropriate patient counseling is encouraged as we continue to learn more about this new disease phenomenon.

In addition, a new generation of implants is now available on the U.S. market: shaped, cohesive, form-stable silicone gel implants. Long-term data have not been collected on their incidence of rupture and capsular contracture; however, the initial reports suggest findings similar to other round implants.[18]

Summary There is no association between breast implants and connective tissue disease.

Implications All medical interventions must be assessed for the relevant risks and benefits. This includes the use of breast implants for both augmentation and reconstruction. As plastic surgeons and innovators, the onus is on us to diligently collect data and review the available scientific literature for ourselves and with our patients, including the risks of connective tissue disease, ALCL, and more benign complications, such as capsular contracture, infection, extrusion, and rupture.

REFERENCES

1. Janowsky EC, Kupper LL, Hulka BS. Meta-analyses of the relation between silicone breast implants and the risk of connective-tissue diseases. N Engl J Med 342:781-790, 2000.
2. Goldman JA, Greenblatt J, Joines R, et al. Breast implants, rheumatoid arthritis, and connective tissue diseases in a clinical practice. J Clin Epidemiol 48:571-582, 1995.
3. Hennekens CH, Lee IM, Cook NR, et al. Self-reported breast implants and connective-tissue diseases in female health professionals. A retrospective cohort study. JAMA 275:616-621, 1996.
4. Star VL, Scott J, Sherwin R, et al. Validity of self-reported physician-diagnosed rheumatoid arthritis for use in epidemiologic studies [abstract]. Arthritis Rheum 36(9 Suppl):S100, 1993.
5. CBS, "Face to Face with Connie Chung, Dec. 10, 1990.
6. Fisher JC. The silicone controversy—when will science prevail? N Engl J Med 326:1696-1698, 1992.
7. Food and Drug Administration. Available at *http://www.fda.gov/MedicalDevices/Products andMedicalProcedures/ImplantsandProsthetics/BreastImplants/ucm064461.htm.* Accessed March 22, 2013.
8. Brody GS, Conway DP, Deapen DM, et al. Consensus statement on the relationship of breast implants to connective tissue disorders. Plast Reconstr Surg 90:1102-1105, 1992.
9. Muzaffar AR, Rohrich RJ. The silicone gel-filled breast implant controversy: an update. Plast Reconstr Surg 109:742-747, 2001.
10. Hölmich LR, Lipworth L, McLaughlin JK, et al. Breast implant rupture and connective tissue disease: a review of the literature. Plast Reconstr Surg 120(7 Suppl 1):62S-67S, 2007.
11. Keech JA, Creech BJ. Anaplastic T-cell lymphoma in proximity to a saline-filled breast implant. Plast Reconstr Surg 100:554-555, 1997.
12. Taylor KO, Webster HR, Prince HM. Anaplastic large cell lymphoma and breast implants: five Australian cases. Plast Reconstr Surg 129:610e-617e, 2012.
13. Carty MJ, Pribaz JJ, Antin JH, et al. A patient death attributable to implant-related primary anaplastic large cell lymphoma of the breast. Plast Reconstr Surg 128:112e-118e, 2011.

14. Jewell M, Spear SL, Largent J, et al. Anaplastic large T-cell lymphoma and breast implants: a review of the literature. Plast Reconstr Surg 128:651-661, 2011.

15. de Jong D, Vasmel WL, de Boer JP, et al. Anaplastic large-cell lymphoma in women with breast implants. JAMA 300:2030-2035, 2008.

16. American Society of Plastic Surgeons. ASPS collaborates with the FDA to establish breast implant registry. Available at *http://www.plasticsurgery.org/news-and-resources/press-release-archives/2011-press-release-archives/asps-collaborates-with-fda-to-establish-breast-implant-registry.html.* Accessed April 26, 2013.

17. Eaves FE, Haeck PC, Rohrich RJ. Breast implants and anaplastic large cell lymphoma: using science to guide our patients and plastic surgeons worldwide. Plast Reconstr Surg 127:2501-2503, 2011.

18. Lista F, Tutino R, Khan A, et al. Subglandular breast augmentation with textured, anatomic, cohesive silicone implants: a review of 440 consecutive patients. Plast Reconstr Surg 132:295-303, 2013.

19. U.S. Food and Drug Administration. FDA Update on the Safety of Silicone Gel-Filled Breast Implants. Center for Devices and Radiological Health, June 2011.

EXPERT COMMENTARY

Albert Losken, MD, FACS

We learned some important lessons from the silicone breast implant moratorium in 1990. That crisis changed how we approach medical devices and patient safety and how we interact with industry, the media, and the public. Although we recognize as physicians that patient safety is of paramount importance, we also understand that some unanticipated "associations/outcomes" are inevitable that might not be known when we initiated a particular treatment plan. All medications have side effects, and many of these are known and discussed. It is up to physicians to disclose this information either before prescribing or immediately once it becomes apparent. The "Face to Face with Connie Chung"[5] episode is a classic example of why appropriate channels must be established for this type of concern. Media hype, patient concern, and the legal world took on a life of its own before the true facts were available. This paper was one of the major scientific articles that demonstrated no association between breast implants and connective tissue diseases. However, it is obvious that no amount of scientific evidence can correct the now "unproven association" that became public fear in the 1990s. I had a patient in clinic this morning, and probably one in every clinic, question me about the safety of silicone breast implants based on their concerns from the 1990s. Despite recent Food and Drug Administration approval of probably the most scrutinized device in medical history,[19] the perception that silicone implants are unsafe remains. Hopefully, studies like this one, continued patient education, and documented safety records moving forward will help lift the fear and stigmata associated with silicone breast implants.

CHAPTER 24

Breast Reconstruction With a Transverse Abdominal Island Flap

Hartrampf CR, Scheflan M, Black PW. Plast Reconstr Surg 69:216-225, 1982

Reviewed by Michelle C. Roughton, MD

> *Reconstructing the breast, which is largely a fat gland, with vascularized fat seems desirable. It is an attractive concept to take fat from where it is present in excess and transpose it to a chest wall defect where it is absent and needed.*[1]

Research Question A new concept for breast reconstruction without the use of implants or the latissimus muscle is introduced.

Funding Not mentioned

Study Dates September 1980

Publishing Date February 1982

Locations Emory University, Atlanta, GA, and Medical College of Virginia, Richmond, VA

Subject A single case report of a 52-year-old moderately obese woman who had undergone a right radical mastectomy and on examination had a denervated right latissimus dorsi muscle

Exclusion Criteria Not applicable

Overview of Design Cadaver dissection (n = 2), case report (n = 1), and case series (n = 8)

Intervention Excess upper abdominal tissue, left attached to the ipsilateral right rectus muscle, was transposed into the mastectomy defect after detaching the muscle from its insertion on the costal margin. Two costosternal cartilages were resected to lengthen the internal thoracic pedicle, avoiding damage to the pleura. A portion of the abdominal skin was deepithelialized and buried underneath the mastectomy flaps. Finally, the lower abdominal skin was mobilized up to the donor site in "reverse abdominoplasty fashion" and the umbilicus was transposed.

Follow-up   The authors note that the postoperative recovery was uneventful.

Endpoints   Flap survival

Results   Single case flap survival; in the discussion the authors describe a flap success rate of 100% in a total of 16 patients.

Criticisms/Limitations   A single case report alone does not carry much weight or authority. However, this was a feasibility study and introduced a completely new concept into the field of autologous breast reconstruction. In their discussion the authors note that they performed 16 procedures and had success with both vertical and low transverse skin islands. Although they describe that both are feasible, they prefer the low transverse donor site for cosmesis. Furthermore, they describe the concept of a 2-week "delay" in which the inferior epigastric vessels are ligated before the formal reconstructive procedure. These techniques are still in practice today and help improve blood supply to the flap from the superior system and thus avoid fat necrosis, a not-uncommon complication of this procedure.

Relevant Studies   This paper introduced the procedure now known as the pedicled transverse rectus abdominis myocutaneous (TRAM) flap. Just before Hartrampf's landmark paper, Dr. Bostwick published and began to popularize the latissimus flap for breast reconstruction,[2] which was first described by the Italian surgeon Tansini.[3] Bostwick et al, however, combined this musculocutaneous flap with an implant. The pedicled TRAM flap was the first popular approach to total autologous breast reconstruction since tubed pedicled flaps.

As previously mentioned, the pedicled TRAM flap is still in use today. It was initially described as an ipsilateral flap harvest but then became more popular as a contralateral transfer.[4] Arguments still exist over the preferred approach, ipsilateral versus contralateral flap harvest.[5-7] Fat necrosis, a sequela of inadequate blood supply, is a relatively common complication of this flap with either donor site. Plastic surgeons have sought to improve this procedure by seeking a more robust alternative blood supply. With the advent of microsurgical techniques, the free TRAM flap (based off the inferior rather than the superior epigastric pedicle) was initially described by Holmstrom[8] and popularized by Shaw[9] and Grotting et al.[10] Although this technique significantly improved blood supply and the incidence of fat necrosis,[11] abdominal wall hernia and/or bulge[12] remained a concern. Thus the deep inferior epigastric artery perforator (DIEP) flap,[13] which spares the muscle and fascia, became increasingly popular.[14,15] In fact, the superior inferior epigastric artery (SIEA) flap,[16] based on the superficial epigastric vessels, avoids fasciotomy altogether and thus has no risk of abdominal hernia or bulge.

Moreover, for patients who have an inadequate abdominal donor site either because of habitus, previous abdominoplasty, or other abdominal surgery, several other donor sites for autologous tissue have been described. Most popular are the inner thigh and buttock donor sites, free transverse upper gracilis (TUG),[17] and gluteal artery perforator (GAP)[18] flaps, respectively.

Summary   Dr. Hartrampf's paper, as a single case report of delayed breast reconstruction, popularized the concept of using excess abdominal tissue to perform breast reconstruction. This procedure has been only subtlety refined since its inception and remains the standard of care for many plastic surgeons worldwide.

Implications   This paper led to a fundamental change in autologous breast reconstruction and made it possible to avoid implants altogether. Subsequent studies have described an evolution of technique from the use of microsurgery and free TRAMs to perforator flaps, such as the DIEP, to spare increasing amounts of the abdominal wall. Given that these procedures are associated with increased operative time and case complexity, arguments within the literature abound to date regarding whether Dr. Hartrampf's pedicled TRAM flap should remain the preferred technique.

REFERENCES

1. Hartrampf CR, Scheflan M, Black PW. Breast reconstruction with a transverse abdominal island flap. Plast Reconstr Surg 69:216-225, 1982.
2. Bostwick J III, Nahai F, Wallace JG, et al. Sixty latissimus dorsi flaps. Plast Reconstr Surg 63:31-41, 1979.
3. Tansini I. Sopra il mio nuovo processo di amputazione della mammella. Riforma Medica (Palermo, Napoli) 12:757, 1906.
4. Hartrampf CR, Bennett GK. Autogenous tissue reconstruction in the mastectomy patient. A critical review of 300 patients. Ann Surg 205:508-519, 1987.
5. Clugston PA, Lennox PA, Thompson RP. Intraoperative vascular monitoring of ipsilateral vs. contralateral TRAM flaps. Ann Plast Surg 41:623-628, 1948.
6. Clugston PA, Gingrass MK, Azurin D, et al. Ipsilateral pedicled TRAM flaps: the safer alternative? Plast Reconstr Surg 105:77-82, 2000.
7. Olding M, Emory RE, Barrett WL. Preferential use of the ipsilateral pedicle in TRAM flap breast reconstruction. Ann Plast Surg 40:349-353, 1998.
8. Holmstrom H. The free abdominoplasty flap and its use in breast reconstruction. An experimental study and clinical case report. Scand J Plast Reconstr Surg 13:423-427, 1979.
9. Shaw W. Microvascular free flap breast reconstruction. Clin Plast Surg 11:333-341, 1984.
10. Grotting JC, Urist MM, Maddox WA, et al. Conventional TRAM versus free microsurgical TRAM flap for immediate breast reconstruction. Plast Reconstr Surg 83:828-841; discussion 842-844, 1989.
11. Kroll SS, Gherardini G, Martin JE, et al. Fat necrosis in free and pedicled TRAM flaps. Plast Reconstr Surg 102:1502-1507, 1998.
12. Man LX, Selber JC, Serletti JM. Abdominal wall following free TRAM or DIEP reconstruction: a meta-analysis and critical review. Plast Reconstr Surg 124:752-764, 2009.

13. Koshima I, Soeda S. Inferior epigastric artery skin flaps without rectus abdominis muscle. Br J Plast Surg 42:645-648, 1989.

14. Allen R, Treece P. Deep inferior epigastric perforator flap for breast reconstruction. Ann Plast Surg 32:32-38, 1994.

15. Blondeel P, Boeckx W. Refinements in free flap breast reconstruction: the free bilateral deep inferior epigastric perforator flap anastomosed to the internal mammary artery. Br J Plast Surg 47:495-501, 1994.

16. Grotting JC. The free abdominoplasty flap for immediate breast reconstruction. Ann Plast Surg 27:351-354, 1991.

17. Wechselberger G, Schoeller T. The transverse gracilis myocutaneous free flap: a valuable tissue source in autologous breast reconstruction. Plast Reconstr Surg 114:69-73, 2004.

18. Allen R, Tucker C Jr. Superior gluteal artery perforator free flap for breast reconstruction. Plast Reconstr Surg 95:1207-1212, 1995.

EDITORIAL PERSPECTIVE

C. Scott Hultman, MD, MBA, FACS

In June 2006, Carl Hartrampf returned to Chapel Hill, 50 years after starting his surgical training at the University of North Carolina, to serve as the Ethel and James Valone Visiting Professor of Plastic Surgery. In his lecture entitled, "The History of Breast Reconstruction with Living Tissue," he recounted the early days of Gillies and waltzing, tubed pedicled flaps; the early attempts by P.G. Arnold and Josh Jurkiewicz to use the omentum; and finally John McCraw's and John Bostwick's success with extended latissimus adipofascial myocutaneous flaps. Despite practicing mostly hand surgery in private practice in Atlanta, his epiphany for the transverse abdominal island flap came during an abdominoplasty case, when he wondered if the periumbilical perforators that were cauterized could be used to perfuse the tissue in the mid-lower abdomen to reconstruct a breast.

Of course, he was correct, and he unveiled his first series of transverse abdominal island flaps at the American Association of Plastic Surgeons in 1981. Although the flap was modified considerably in the decades to follow, the pedicled TRAM flap remains one of the most powerful operations in plastic surgery. Thanks to the refinements of John Bostwick, we no longer resect rib; we base the flap more caudad on the rectus, we prefer an ipsilateal arc of rotation, and we harvest just a strip of muscle carrying the superior epigastric vessels (or none at all, for those surgeons who now perform perforator flap breast reconstruction). Perhaps Bostwick's most endearing contribution is the naming of this flap, with TRAM in the middle of *harTRAMpf*. The acronym was worked backward to create the "transverse rectus abdominis myocutaneous" flap in homage to a great hand surgeon who developed one of the greatest procedures in all of plastic surgery.

CHAPTER 25

Vertical Mammaplasty and Liposuction of the Breast

Lejour M. Plast Reconstr Surg 94:100-114, 1994

Reviewed by Michelle C. Roughton, MD

> . . . *Vertical mammaplasty has many advantages: 1. The markings are adjustable to all patients; 2. the upper pedicle of the areola is larger in larger breasts, making the procedure safe for all sizes of breasts; 3. the skin is not relied on to support the breast; 4. stable results are produced because the gland is strongly sutured; 5. few postoperative complications occur; 6. limited scars are created; and 7. the procedure is easy to learn and perform.*[1]

Research Question This is a feasibility study of "(1) the applicability of value of this modified vertical mammaplasty technique in all sizes of breasts and in patients of all ages and (2) the proportion of patients with large breasts who can benefit from the adjunctive use of liposuction. . ."[1]

Funding Not described

Study Dates 1990 to 1992

Publishing Date July 1994

Location Brussels, Belgium

Subjects All women undergoing mastopexy or breast reduction surgery in Dr. Lejour's private practice from 1990 to 1992

Exclusion Criteria Not described

Sample Size 100 patients and 192 breasts

Overview of Design   A prospective case series of female patients undergoing masto-pexy or breast reduction surgery with a modified vertical technique

Intervention   All patients' breasts were evaluated for the possible benefit of lipo-suction before mastopexy or reduction. If the patient was a candidate for liposuction (for example, did not have obviously nodular breasts with scant adipose tissue), this technique was used at the beginning of the surgical case and everywhere except the planned superior pedicle. After liposuction, a modified vertical breast reduction or mastopexy was performed.

Specifically, this technique involves the following components, as demonstrated in Fig. 25-1:
- Design of freehand markings before surgery with the patient standing to delineate how much excess skin and parenchyma to remove
- Creation of a superior dermoglandular pedicle for the nipple-areola complex (NAC)
- Limited undermining of the medial and lateral skin from the gland
- Discard of the central inferior breast parenchyma previously marked
- Undermining of the medial and lateral breast pillars from the underlying chest wall
- Suturing of these pillars together to support the NAC
- Suturing the superior pedicle to the pectoralis fascia as needed
- Skin redraping with attention to shortening the nipple-to-fold distance with gath-ering of the suture line

Follow-up   Not addressed

Endpoints   Rate of complication and its correlation to the use of liposuction and weight of the tissue excised

Results   Patient results can be found in Table 25-1 and Table 25-2.

Mastopexy was performed on 21 patients and 39 breasts and no complications were seen. Modified vertical breast reduction was performed in 79 patients and 153 breasts with an average weight of 480 g of tissue removed per breast. Liposuction was at-tempted in 120 breasts and accomplished in 86 (the remainder did not have adequate adipose tissue for aspiration at the time of surgery) for an average of 300 cc per breast. Complications were noted in 20 of 153 (13%) patients undergoing breast reduction. Larger reductions (>500 g) represented 19 of the 20. Excluding eight seromas and two hematomas, 10 patients had wound healing problems, two of which involved partial areolar necrosis. One of these patients required operative revision. The incidence of complications did not correlate with the use of liposuction.

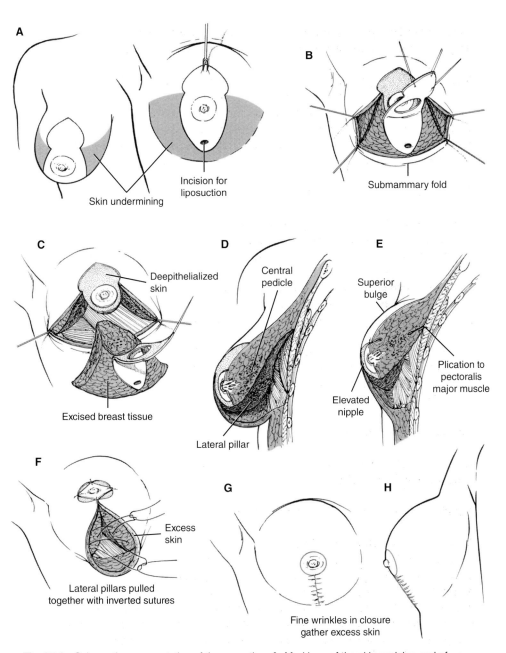

Fig. 25-1 Schematic representation of the operation. **A,** Markings of the skin excision and of the lateral skin undermining *(gray areas)* and incision for liposuction above the lower marking. **B,** Deepithelialization and incision of the gland from the upper parts of the vertical markings diverging to the lower breast. **C,** Excision of the excess tissue below and, if necessary in large breasts, behind the areola. **D,** Final resection of glandular tissue. **E,** Plication of the pedicle to the areola and fixation of the gland to the pectoralis muscle. **F,** Suture of the areola in its new site and suture of the lateral pillars of breast tissue. **G,** Gathering of the skin inferiorly, from the nipple to the inframammary fold. **H,** Final inverted appearance immediately after surgery. (From Lejour M. Vertical Mammaplasty and Liposuction. St Louis: Quality Medical Publishing, 1994.)

Table 25-1   Complications After Vertical Mammaplasty in 100 Patients (192 Breasts)

Complication	Total Breasts		
	Number	Percent	Number of Breasts With Liposuction
Seroma	8	4.2	—
Hematoma	2	1	—
Partial areolar necrosis	2	1	1
Wound dehiscence			
Superficial	4	2.1	3
With glandular necrosis	4	2.1	2

From Lejour M. Vertical mammaplasty and liposuction of the breast. Plast Reconstr Surg 94:100-114, 1994.

Table 25-2   Healing Complications (192 Breasts)

Complication	Case	Fat Suctioned (cc)	Tissue Excised (g)
Partial areolar necrosis	1	0	900
(n = 2)	2	400	1200
Superficial wound dehiscence	3	0	200
(n = 4)	4	150	600
	5	500	500
	6	1100	1500
Superficial wound dehiscence	7	0	1350
with glandular necrosis	8	0	1400
(n = 4)	9	400	900
	10	400	1600

From Lejour M. Vertical mammaplasty and liposuction of the breast. Plast Reconstr Surg 94:100-114, 1994.

Criticisms/Limitations   Dr. Lejour's modification of the vertical breast reduction stresses the importance of glandular suturing to reshape breast parenchyma and the elimination of the inframammary scar, which can be a source of much dissatisfaction for the patient. Her case series is limited in the lack of follow-up standardization and a comparison group. She stresses the improvement in breast shape long-term but offers no objective data to that effect. However, her work remains an extremely important contribution to the evolution of breast reduction and is in use today.

Relevant Studies   During the 1960s and 1970s, plastic surgeons sought to improve the techniques for breast reduction by simultaneously reducing the size and volume of the breast while preserving the blood supply and sensation to the NAC. Inferior pedicles with Wise-pattern skin reduction (producing an anchor-shaped scar) became very popular in the United States.[2,3] In 1970 a French surgeon, Dr. Claude Lassus,[4] described a vertical breast reduction with a superior pedicle. In time, however, he grew frustrated with the vertical midline scar's extension beyond the inframammary fold and returned to the use of a horizontal component. Dr. Lejour's work popularized this technique and modified his description to limit the length of the vertical scar and eliminate any transverse component, emphasizing the importance of glandular sutures for long-term shape and support. In addition to her 1994 paper, she published a follow-up study 5 years later in which she tracked her complications further and in a larger patient series of 250 patients and 476 breasts.[5] In that paper she stresses the correlation between an increase in the rate of complications and larger reduction volumes. She recommends limiting her procedure to those patients undergoing reductions smaller than 1000 g.

Interestingly, in that same journal, another surgeon, Dr. Elizabeth Hall-Findlay,[6] describes a modification of the Lejour technique to increase the applicability to larger breasted women. This study modifies the vertical reduction further to incorporate a medial dermoglandular pedicle (rather than superior), avoids skin undermining, only rarely uses liposuction, and avoids sutures to the pectoralis fascia. She argues that this allows an easier inset of the pedicle and an improvement in skin perfusion, thus decreasing the complications from wound healing. She believes that it is applicable to even the largest of reduction volumes.

Furthermore, Dr. Lejour's emphasis on using the parenchyma of the breast for reshaping rather than on skin excision alone has also had effects on mastopexy. Perhaps she inspired Dr. Rubin's approach[7] to mastopexy in massive weight loss. In this technique, the excess dermal-adipofascial components of the breast, typically excised in a Wise-pattern reduction, are rotated over the central gland to auto-augment these patients.

Summary   Dr. Lejour's description of vertical skin pattern reduction, which relied on parenchymal rather than skin sutures to reshape the breast, was a landmark paper in breast reduction surgery. Her technique, which built on the work of previous surgeons, eliminated scarring at the inframammary fold, which reduced the potential for delayed wound healing at the T-junction, often seen in traditional Wise-pattern reductions.

Implications   Although the inferior pedicle, the Wise-pattern reduction remains popular, especially in the United States. Vertical breast reductions, which were popularized by Drs. Lejour and Hall-Findlay, were revolutionary at the time and are currently still considered cutting edge in reduction surgery. In addition, techniques that are devoid of the vertical scar[8] and the use of liposuction alone[9] are other less common surgical options used for breast reduction today.

REFERENCES

1. Lejour M. Vertical mammaplasty and liposuction of the breast. Plast Reconstr Surg 94:100-114, 1994.
2. Wise R. A preliminary report on a method of planning the mammaplasty. Plast Reconstr Surg 17:367-375, 1956.

3. Robbins T. A reduction mammaplasty with the areola-nipple based on an inferior dermal pedicle. Plast Reconstr Surg 59:64-67, 1977.
4. Lassus C. A technique for breast reduction. Int Surg 53:69-72, 1970.
5. Lejour M. Vertical mammaplasty: early complications after 250 personal consecutive cases. Plast Reconstr Surg 104:764-770, 1999.
6. Hall-Findlay E. A simplified vertical reduction mammaplasty: shortening the learning curve. Plast Reconstr Surg 104:748-759, 1999.
7. Rubin JP. Mastopexy after massive weight loss: dermal suspension and total parenchymal reshaping. Aesthetic Surg J 26:214-222, 2006.
8. Schleich AR, Black DM, McCraw JB. The aesthetic correction of the ptotic breast by the procedure of nipple-areola transposition—a contemporary translation and commentary. J Plast Reconstr Surg 63:1136-1141, 2010.
9. Matarasso A, Courtiss EH. Suction mammoplasty: the use of suction lipectomy to reduce large breasts. Plast Reconstr Surg 87:709-717, 1991.

EDITORIAL PERSPECTIVE

C. Scott Hultman, MD, MBA, FACS

My 2 years of residency training were 2 of the best years of my life. Honest! Can you imagine the excitement, walking into conference on your first day as a plastic surgery resident and being greeted by Josh Jurkiewicz, John Bostwick, Grant Carlson, Jack Culbertson (we loved Jack so much that it hurt), and Glyn Jones? Foad Nahai, Rod Hester, and Monte Eaves had just left Emory, but their lingering presence was palpable—and so was Madeline Lejour's, who had just come to the university as a visiting professor. We were so impressed with vertical reduction mammaplasty that all of the attendings and all of the residents at Grady Memorial Hospital were completely entranced with learning this new technique. I would argue that Nahai climbed the learning curve the fastest, and there is no need to argue that the results of the Emory attendings far exceeded the results of the Grady residents.

After decades of inferior-pedicle, inverted-T, Wise-pattern reduction mammaplasties, plastic surgeons were again excited to perform breast reductions. Suddenly breast reduction surgery became an innovative niche for many of our finest surgeons to pursue. Of course, Lejour did not invent the vertical reduction—that was Claude Lassus—but she is the teacher who propagated the technique and showed everyone else how compelling, challenging, and rewarding this operation could be. Later in my learning curve as an attending, I also discovered that one size does not fit all. The most successful plastic surgeons have many different ways of doing the same operation; aligning patient goals with one's technical skill set may be the greatest predictor of a successful outcome. I do not perform vertical reductions on everyone with macromastia, but this is always my first option to consider.

CHAPTER 26

Thumb Replacement: Great Toe Transplantation by Microvascular Anastomosis

Buncke HJ Jr, McLean DH, George PT, Creech BJ, Chater NL, Commons GW.
Br J Plast Surg 26:194-201, 1973

Reviewed by Amita R. Shah, MD, PhD

A successful microsurgical great toe to thumb transplant has been presented.[1]

Research Question   The development of a method for one-stage toe-to-thumb transfer with the use of microvascular techniques

Funding   Grants from the Microsurgical Unit, Ralph K. Davies Medical Center, San Francisco, CA, and the Microsurgical Transplantation Research Foundation and Clinical Investigation Center, Naval Hospital, Oakland, CA

Study Dates   February 1972

Publishing Date   1973

Location   San Francisco, CA

Subject   A single case study of a 30-year-old man who amputated the right thumb of his dominant hand with a power saw and failed replantation

Exclusion Criteria   Not applicable

Sample Size   A single case study

Overview of Design   Not applicable

Intervention   One-stage transplantation of the great toe to the hand with microvascular anastomosis

Follow-up   6 months after surgery

Endpoints   Survival of transplanted toe and functionality as a thumb

Results   A 30-year-old fireman who amputated his right thumb with a power tool underwent a successful great toe-to-thumb transfer. The first metatarsal artery, medial and lateral digital nerves, and two dorsal veins were identified and taken when the toe was disarticulated and amputated at the metatarsophalangeal joint. A bone peg was used to attach the osseous structures. The vessels from the toe were anastomosed to the hand dorsal veins and palmar artery. The digital nerves and tendons were then repaired, and the area was closed with skin flaps from the hand (Fig. 26-1).[1]

The patient's postoperative course was complicated by arterial thrombosis at 8 and 48 hours. Both times the patient was taken back to the operating room and a thrombus was removed. At his 6-month follow-up, he was using power and hand tools. He had intact protective sensation and 30 degrees of flexion at the interphalangeal joint. His grip strength was 80% of the uninjured hand. No morbidity from the donor site was reported.

Limitations   The manuscript is a single case study and lacks extensive details about the operative technique or postoperative rehabilitation regimen. Although the transfer was ultimately successful, it was complicated twice by arterial thrombosis. Aspirin was used; its antiplatelet effects were described only a few years earlier.

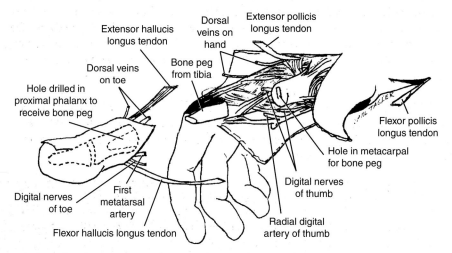

Fig. 26-1   Successful great toe-to-thumb transfer after right thumb was amputated by a power tool. (From Buncke HJ Jr, McLean DH, George PT, et al. Thumb replacement: great toe transplantation by microvascular anastomosis. Br J Plast Surg 26:194-201, 1973.)

Relevant Studies   Before the development of the great toe-to-hand technique for the reconstruction of the thumb, prostheses, osteoplastic procedures, and pollicization were used.[1] The first use of the toes for thumb reconstruction was by Nicoladoni[2] in 1902, during which a pedicled second toe was used as a thumb. This procedure was limited because the patient had his foot sutured to his hand in an awkward position until the vasculature was set up and then underwent a second-stage procedure for release.[3] With the maturation of microsurgery, ways to advance the procedure to one stage were developed to eliminate the need to keep the donor attached to the site. Buncke et al[4] first developed the methods for microvascular anastomosis of the great toe to reconstruct the thumb in rhesus monkeys.

After the publication of this work, initial attempts of great toe-to-thumb transfers in humans failed secondary to venous thrombosis and poor arterial flow. During Dr. Buncke's first attempt in 1967, they were unable to achieve sufficient arterial flow. The first reported successful transplant of the great toe to hand was by Cobbett in 1968.[3] Although the transplant survived and was eventually functional, the postoperative course was complicated, and the patient required multiple revisions for arterial thrombosis and skin necrosis. Anastomosis of the digital nerves was successful, but the patient regained only protective sensation and poor two-point discrimination. Flexion of the thumb interphalangeal joint was limited to 10 degrees, and the patient could adequately perform pinch functions.[3] The first successful great toe-to-thumb transplant in the United States was performed by Dr. Buncke in 1971 as described above.[1]

Since 1968, the procedure has been improved. Early attempts were often compromised by venous and arterial thrombosis. A better understanding of coagulation and advances in microsurgical techniques have mitigated the problem. The anatomy and use of the vasculature of the foot have been further defined. O'Brien[5] described the use of the dorsalis pedis artery as the main pedicle, and Gilbert[6] described the anatomic variants of the dorsal metacarpal artery. Partial toe procedures have been developed so that the transplant more closely matches the size and shape of a native thumb,[7] but Buncke et al[8] reported that over time, the transplanted toe will start to resemble a thumb more than a toe.

In 2007 Buncke et al[8] reported that from 1972 to 2004, they performed 161 great toe transplants. They had only four failures over 34 years and no failures from 1997 to 2007. Two-point discrimination has improved to 5 to 8 mm and the average interphalangeal joint motion is 40 degrees.

Summary   The work of Dr. Buncke's group in 1965 on monkeys defined the technique for great toe-to-hand transplant for the reconstruction of the thumb, leading to the first successful great toe-to-thumb transfer in humans in 1968 and the first great toe-to-thumb transfer in the United States in 1971.

Implications   The work of Dr. Buncke advanced microsurgical techniques for the hand and set the stage for replantation of the hand.

REFERENCES

1. Buncke HJ Jr, McLean DH, George PT, et al. Thumb replacement: great toe transplantation by microvascular anastomosis. Br J Plast Surg 26:194-201, 1973.
2. Gurunluoglu R, Shafighi M, Huemer GM, et al. Carl Nicoladoni (1847-1902): professor of surgery. Ann Surg 239:281-292, 2004.
3. Cobbett JR. Free digital transfer. Report of a case of transfer of a great toe to replace an amputated thumb. J Bone Joint Surg Br 51:677-679, 1969.
4. Buncke HJ Jr, Buncke CM, Schulz WP. Immediate Nicoladoni procedure in the Rhesus monkey, or hallux-to-hand transplantation, utilising microminiature vascular anastomoses. Br J Plast Surg 19:332-337, 1966.
5. O'Brien B. Microvascular Reconstructive Surgery. London: Churchill Livingstone, 1977.
6. Gilbert A. Composite tissue transfer from the foot: anatomic basis and surgical technique. In Daniller AJ, Strauch B, eds. Symposium on Microsurgery. St Louis: CV Mosby, 1976.
7. Loda G. Atlas of Thumb and Finger Reconstruction. New York: Thieme Medical Publishers, 1999.
8. Buncke GM, Buncke HJ, Lee CK. Great toe-to-thumb microvascular transplantation after traumatic amputation. Hand Clin 23:105-115, 2007.

EXPERT COMMENTARY

Gregory M. Buncke, MD, FACS

I was a high school student at the time of the great toe transplantation, and I remember this period well. While growing up, I assumed everyone had a makeshift microsurgical operating room in their garage. We also had pet rabbits with missing ears, and I often walked into the garage to see my father, a surgeon, and my mother, a dermatologist, transplanting a toe to thumb on a sleeping rhesus monkey.

The toe transplant described in this article was performed on a Friday. We were anxious to hear the outcome that night, but my father came home the next morning after the first take back. He was very happy to have noticed the arterial thrombosis in time to redo the artery and salvage the toe. Unfortunately, shortly after dinner on Sunday night, he had to rush back to the hospital because the signal was gone and the toe was white. He arrived home the next morning dejected. He had done everything he could, but the toe would not pink up. He was sure the next step would be removal of the toe. We were crushed, but miraculously the toe pinked up within a few hours.

Microsurgery continues to be a demanding but very rewarding field. We are grateful for the vision and determination of microsurgical pioneers like Harry J. Buncke.

CHAPTER 27

Early Microsurgical Reconstruction of Complex Trauma of the Extremities

Godina M. Plast Reconstr Surg 78:285-292, 1986

Reviewed by Amita R. Shah, MD, PhD

> *The planning of the microvascular free-tissue transfer and the transfer itself are much easier immediately after the injury*[1]

Research Question   When is the optimal time to perform microvascular free tissue transfer for posttraumatic wounds?

Funding   Not applicable

Study Dates   1976 to 1983

Publishing Date   September 1986

Location   Ljubljana, Slovenia

Subjects   Patients with posttraumatic extremity defects treated by the author's microsurgical team

Exclusion Criteria   Not discussed

Sample Size   532 total patients: 134 in the early group, 167 in the delayed group, and 231 in the late group

Overview of Design   A retrospective

Intervention   Patients who underwent microsurgical reconstruction of extremity injuries were divided into three groups: those who underwent free flap transfer within 72 hours of injury (early), those treated between 72 hours and 3 months (delayed), and patients treated between 3 months and 12.6 years (late). The outcomes analyzed were

167

Table 27-1   Results

Group of Patients	Early	Delayed	Late	Together
Number of patients (%)	134 (25.5)	167 (31.4)	231 (43.4)	532 (100)
Number of microsurgical procedure failures (%)	1 (0.75)	20 (12)	22 (9.5)	43 (8)
Number of postoperative infections (%)	2 (1.5)	29 (17.5)	14 (6)	45 (8.45)
Bone healing time (average)	6.8 mo (n = 33)	12.3 mo (n = 95)	29 mo (n = 78)	17.7 mo (n = 206)
Hospitalization time (average)	27 days	130 days	256 days	159 days
Number of anesthesias (average)	1.3	4.1	7.8	5

From Godina M. Early microsurgical reconstruction of complex trauma of the extremities. Plast Reconstr Surg 78:285-292, 1986.

flap failure, infection, bone healing time, the length of the hospital stay, and the number of operative procedures.

Follow-up   Patients were followed to the endpoints of bone healing, which was determined to be when full weight-bearing was started and to the time of discharge from the hospital.

Endpoints   Bone healing and length of hospitalization

Results   The early group showed a decrease in flap failure rates, infections, bone healing time, the length of the hospital stay, and the number of operative procedures (Table 27-1).[1] Statistics were performed on the data for free tissue transfer failure and bone healing time. Statistically significant improvement in both groups was seen in the early group compared with both the delayed and late groups.

The only early free flap failure was an arterial thrombosis, which was the result of a "mistake in planning," in which a small groin flap artery was anastomosed to a larger anterior tibial artery. There were 20 flap failures in the delayed group and 22 failures in the late group. Most of the flap failures in these groups were caused by venous thrombosis (85% and 91%, respectively). Free flap failure rates and operating times for the first 100 flaps and the last 100 flaps were also compared. There were 26 flap failures in the first 100 cases compared with 4 failures in the last 100 cases. None of the first 100 flaps were completed in 2 to 4 hours, and 73 required 6 to 8 hours for completion. Ten were completed in 8 to 10 hours. In contrast, 24 flaps of the last 100 flaps were completed in 2 to 4 hours, 68 were completed in 4 to 6 hours, and only 2 flaps required 8 to 10 hours.

Criticisms/Limitations   This manuscript is one of the largest series of free flaps by a single center for its time, and the descriptions of the evolution of the treatment protocols and the observations by the author are invaluable. The study is limited by its retrospective nature and the limited data analysis. In addition, it was published posthumously, and therefore limited in its discussion and follow-up by the original author. Dr. Graham Lister, a friend and colleague of Dr. Godina, submitted the paper posthumously and served as its corresponding author.

Relevant Studies   One of the early studies describing improved outcomes with early flap coverage of posttraumatic wounds was done by Cierny et al[2] 3 years before the publication of this article. In this study 36 traumatic tibial wounds were serially debrided and underwent fasciocutaneous flap coverage. Wounds that underwent flap coverage in 0 to 7 days (early) were compared with those that were covered in 8 to 30 days (late). The late group had a higher percentage of wound complications and nonunions compared with the early group.[2]

After the publications of Dr. Godina's case series, his findings were further validated by multiple studies, which also showed decreased complications and infections with early soft tissue coverage.[3] Wounds that are left open for an extended period are at increased risk of nosocomial infection as seen by the evaluation of bacterial organisms in delayed wounds. This revealed that 34% of the infected wounds were infected with organisms not seen on initial cultures, which suggested infection obtained in the hospital while the wound was open.[4] With aggressive debridement, stabilization of bone, and early coverage of the soft tissue defect with flaps, the rate of limb salvage has been reported as high as 93%.[5,6]

Collaboration between the microsurgical team and orthopedics and plastic surgery was further developed at other institutions after the publication of Dr. Godina's manuscript.[5,7] Early flap coverage was possible when orthopedic and plastic surgery services were coordinated, and delays in wound coverage beyond 72 hours were determined by the patient's condition rather than by surgeon availability. The creation of a combined orthopedic and plastic microvascular surgery group is not possible at all hospitals, and it has been recommended that patients with complex extremity trauma injuries be expeditiously transferred to a hospital with a microvascular surgery group.[5]

Current trends in lower extremity reconstruction for severe open fractures show a decrease in the number of free flaps performed. The increased use of negative-pressure therapy and the development of new local flaps have decreased the necessity for free flaps.[8]

Summary   Marko Godina's article was one of the first papers to introduce the idea of the "emergency free flap," in which traumatic wounds are aggressively debrided, bone was stabilized, and the wound was closed early with free flaps. It also further emphasized the concept of this treatment "triad" at the initial surgery for traumatic wounds, which made it possible for the first surgery to be the only surgery.[9] It is his observation that the presence of fibrosis is what complicates the planning of microvascular free tissue transfer and is responsible for the higher rate of venous thrombosis seen in delayed cases.

Implications   This study showed that early microvascular free flap coverage of posttraumatic wounds by a microsurgical team, coupled with aggressive debridement, result in improved outcomes. This changed the paradigm of traumatic wound treatment from serial debridements with delayed reconstruction to primary reconstruction.

REFERENCES

1. Godina M. Early microsurgical reconstruction of complex trauma of the extremities. Plast Reconstr Surg 78:285-292, 1986.
2. Cierny G, Byrd HS, Jones RE. Primary versus delayed soft tissue coverage for severe open tibial fractures. A comparison of results. Clin Orthop Relat Res 178:54-63, 1983.
3. Wood T, Sameem M, Avram R, et al. A systematic review of early versus delayed wound closure in patients with open fractures requiring flap coverage. J Trauma Acute Care Surg 72:1078-1085, 2012.
4. Patzakis MJ, Wilkins J. Factors influencing infection rate in open fracture wounds. Clin Orthop Relat Res 243:36-40, 1989.
5. Naique SB, Pearse M, Nanchahal J. Management of severe open tibial fractures: the need for combined orthopaedic and plastic surgical treatment in specialist centres. J Bone Joint Surg Br 88:351-357, 2006.
6. Francel TJ, Vander Kolk CA, Hoopes JE, et al. Microvascular soft-tissue transplantation for reconstruction of acute open tibial fractures: timing of coverage and long-term functional results. Plast Reconstr Surg 89:478-487; discussion 488-489, 1992.
7. Gopal S, Giannoudis PV, Murray A, et al. The functional outcome of severe, open tibial fractures managed with early fixation and flap coverage. J Bone Joint Surg Br 86:861-867, 2004.
8. Parrett BM, Matros E, Pribaz JJ, et al. Lower extremity trauma: trends in the management of soft-tissue reconstruction of open tibia-fibula fractures. Plast Reconstr Surg 117:1315-1322; discussion 1323-1324, 2006.
9. Lister G. Many Changeful Years. Bloomington, IN: Xlibris, 2005.
10. Lister G. Commentary in Godina M. A thesis on the management of injuries to the lower extremity. Ljubljana, Slovenia: Presernova druzba, 1991.
11. Lister G. Marko Godina, M.D. (1943-1986). Plast Reconstr Surg 78:443-444, 1986.
12. Morrison commentary in Godina M. A thesis on the management of injuries to the lower extremity. Ljubljana, Slovenia: Presernova druzba, 1991.
13. Arnez commentary in Godina M. A thesis on the management of injuries to the lower extremity. Ljubljana, Slovenia: Presernova druzba, 1991.
14. Godina M. A thesis on the management of injuries to the lower extremity. Ljubljana, Slovenia: Presernova druzba, 1991.

STUDY AUTHOR REFLECTIONS

Graham D. Lister, MD

The editors have chosen well; this paper is unique, a word often loosely used, but here appropriate. It is unique for several ways: the 532 patients, a number unsurpassed "for such a juxtaposition of technical advances, clinical opportunity and a man of boundless energy, innovative genius and charismatic leadership is unlikely to recur."[10] These were only a portion of the 826 free tissue transfers performed between 1976 and 1983 by one man before the age of 40 years; most poignantly, the paper was published post-humously.

Born in 1943, Godina was separated from his partisan parents the day after his birth. He took an assumed name, Stanko Rozman; he was a baby pursued by the SS from foster family to foster family. When he was finally located after World War II, he was in the day care—unbeknown to her—of his own grandmother.

He became a surgeon "distinguished by his tireless energy, his impeccable logic, his boundless optimism and his constant good humor and courtesy."[11] He traveled widely, at first to visit and learn from, among others, Cobbett in England, Acland in Scotland, Skoog in Sweden, Buck-Gramcko in Germany, and Kleinert in Kentucky, but later to lecture on his innovative techniques in 11 countries. His lectures were inspiring, al-ways extemporaneous, with "boldness and conviction . . . that separated Marko as the true missionary."[12] "Everything good which he saw throughout the world he trans-ferred to the motherland; everything which we did better he was able to convey to oth-ers."[13] His innovations were many: routine end-to-side anastomosis, arterial autografts, immediate mobilization after replantation, emergency free flap coverage, the tailored latissimus flap, preferential use of the posterior approach to vessels of the lower leg, and ectopic implantation of parts for temporary storage.

It was a delight to operate with Marko. He taught as he worked, happy that observ-ers crowded around him. A student once jostled his elbow, causing him to divide the pedicle he was dissecting. He did not break his sentence, placing a clamp above the spurting artery. He marked with a fine suture the partial division that he later repaired during flap transfer. Always direct and precise, he worked quickly—it was said in Ljubljana that this was because he craved a cigarette every hour.

"He always found great joy among the simple people he loved best."[13] At an official dinner for the International Hand Course in Ljubljana, he was seated with the lecturers. He excused himself, saying he would be "right back." He did not return, but could be seen from afar throughout the evening smoking, drinking, and chatting with different groups of hospital workers.

How did this paper come to be published posthumously? In late 1985 Godina spent 4 weeks in Louisville with the primary purpose of writing the thesis necessary for his full professorship because he found no time in Slovenia. After dinner each day, he settled to collate the data from Ljubljana and to write. In the morning he was gone; he was back at the hospital to participate in the morning conferences and surgery sched-ules. However, the overflowing ashtrays where he had worked bore witness not merely to his continued addiction, but also to the many overnight hours he had spent at his desk. It was never clear when he slept. It was as though he had intimations of mortality. In that he was sadly correct. He was killed instantaneously with his wife Vesna less than 2 months later on the notorious two-lane highway from Zagreb to Ljubljana.

The fruits of those nights of labor were presented in three papers, of which this is one—in the September 1986 issue of *Plastic and Reconstructive Surgery*[1] and in his thesis published in 1991 in both English and Slovenian.[14]

That Marko Godina "became an irreplaceable stone in the history of surgery"[13] has been confirmed by the immediate contribution to a scholarship fund from donors worldwide including icons such as Harry Buncke and Susumu Tamai. Their contributions still fund the Marko Godina Lecture at each annual meeting of the American Society for Reconstructive Microsurgery.

CHAPTER 28

The Radial Forearm Flap: A Versatile Method for Intra-oral Reconstruction

Soutar DS, Scheker LR, Tanner NS, McGregor IA. Br J Plast Surg 36:1-8, 1983

Reviewed by Amita R. Shah, MD, PhD

> *. . . the radial forearm flap appears to offer a safe, reliable, versatile, and convenient method of intra-oral reconstruction.*[1]

Research Question Description of the radial forearm flap for reconstruction

Funding Not applicable

Study Dates Unspecified

Publishing Date January 1983

Location Glasgow, Scotland

Subjects Patients who underwent intraoral reconstruction with the forearm flap by the authors

Exclusion Criteria Not discussed

Sample Size 10 patients

Overview of Design A clinical case series

Intervention The radial forearm flap was successfully used for intraoral reconstruction in 10 patients. The proximal, mid, or distal forearm was used, and the intraoral defects included the retromolar trigone, buccal mucosa, palate, lateral tongue, floor of the mouth, alveolus, and symphysis. One flap included a portion of the radius for the reconstruction of the mandible.

The forearm fasciocutaneous flap is based on the radial artery. The recipient arteries are most commonly the facial artery or superior thyroid artery, and the recipient veins are branches of the internal jugular, external jugular, or anterior jugular veins. The flap is dissected deep to the deep fascia of the volar aspect of the arm, and the subcutaneous veins and radial artery are elevated with the flap. After the flap is removed from the donor site, the radial artery is repaired with an interpositional vein graft and the donor defect is closed with a skin graft.

Follow-up   All 10 flaps were successful. Complications were not discussed, but it was reported that there was no postoperative disability of the hand on the side of the donor. In the footnote, it was mentioned that after submission of the manuscript, 13 additional radial forearm flaps were performed with 2 flap failures.

Endpoints   Flap survival

Limitations   This paper describes the design, dissection, and use of the radial forearm flap based on their experience with 10 patients with intraoral defects. There were no flap failures reported with the 10 patients, but there were 2 flap failures that occurred in additional flaps performed between the time of submission and publication of the manuscript, which were mentioned but not expounded on. The complications and follow-up of the patients are not discussed, and therefore this manuscript serves as a technical paper. The group's follow-up paper in 1986 provides the analysis of the flap results that are absent in this paper.[2]

Relevant Studies   In 1973 Daniel and Taylor[3] described the first successful free flap in a human, which was an iliofemoral island flap based off the superficial inferior epigastric artery to the right posterior tibial region. Since then, many types of free flaps have been developed that balance the size and composition of the flap, functionality, length of the pedicle, and donor-site morbidity.

The forearm flap was first known as the "Chinese" flap because it was first described by Yang et al.[4,5] In their paper 60 radial forearm flaps were performed with only 1 flap loss. Forty seven of the flaps were performed in the head and neck region. This study was published in the *National Medical Journal of China* in Chinese and was formally translated into English and published in the *British Journal of Plastic Surgery* in 1997. Other studies on the forearm flap published before 1983 by Shaw[6] and Song et al[7] used the forearm free flap for nasal reconstruction and neck burn contractures, respectively. The featured manuscript is the first study that specifically looked at the use of the radial forearm flap for intraoral reconstruction.[1] In 1986 the group[2] published a follow-up study, which examined the results of 60 consecutive radial forearm flaps, including the 10 flaps from the first paper. In this study the flap success rate was 90%. The six flap failures were from arterial thrombosis (two patients) or venous thrombosis (four patients) and occurred in areas difficult to monitor (the posterior third of the tongue/tonsil region and the posterior aspect of the lateral tongue and lower alveolus). In the first paper all 10 patients had reconstruction of the radial artery with a reverse vein graft, but the subsequent 50 patients did not routinely undergo radial artery reconstruction. These patients did not suffer complications related to hand ischemia. Thirty-nine of the 60 patients underwent postoperative radiation, and there were no problems with wound breakdown or flap ischemia. Seven patients had their donor sites closed primarily and no wound healing complications were encountered. The remaining patients required skin grafts. They found that complete graft take was difficult and the flexor carpi radialis tendon was often exposed. One patient required an additional skin graft. Seven patients received an osteocutaneous forearm flap for the reconstruction of the mandible. These patients were placed in a full-length plaster splint for 3 to 4 weeks and there were no incidences of radial fractures after surgery. It is recommended that no more than 40% of the cross section of the radius should be removed.[2] The outcomes of the osteocutaneous free flap with the radius were also reported by Soutar and Widdowson[8] in 1986. Twelve of 14 immediate mandible reconstructions were successful, even with postoperative radiation therapy.

Summary   The radial forearm flap is a reliable free flap for the reconstruction of intraoral defects, even in the setting of postoperative radiation. It has consistent, predictable anatomy and can be easily tailored for a variety of defects, including those that require bone. The flap can also be raised at the same time as the intraoral resection without changing the position of the patient.

Implications   The radial forearm flap is presented as a solution for intraoral reconstruction. Before this, the pectoralis major and trapezius myocutaneous flaps and jejunal flaps were used, but were too bulky for smaller reconstructions and had high donor-site morbidity.[9,10] Although other flaps, including the anterolateral thigh flap, have been introduced for intraoral reconstructions since then, the radial forearm flap has remained one of the workhorse flaps for these defects.

REFERENCES

1. Soutar DS, Scheker LR, Tanner NS, et al. The radial forearm flap: a versatile method for intra-oral reconstruction. Br J Plast Surg 36:1-8, 1983.
2. Soutar DS, McGregor IA. The radial forearm flap in intraoral reconstruction: the experience of 60 consecutive cases. Plast Reconstr Surg 78:1-8, 1986.
3. Daniel RK, Taylor GI. Distant transfer of an island flap by microvascular anastomoses. A clinical technique. Plast Reconstr Surg 52:111-117, 1973.
4. Yang GF, Chen P, Gao X, et al. Forearm free skin flap transplantation. Natl Med J China 61:139-141, 1981.
5. Yang GF, Chen PJ, Gao YZ, et al. Forearm free skin flap transplantation: a report of 56 cases. 1981. Br J Plast Surg 50:162-165, 1997.
6. Shaw WW. Microvascular reconstruction of the nose. Clin Plast Surg 8:471-480, 1981.
7. Song R, Gao Y, Song Y, et al. The forearm flap. Clin Plast Surg 9:21-26, 1982.

8. Soutar DS, Widdowson WP. Immediate reconstruction of the mandible using a vascularized segment of radius. Head Neck Surg 8:232-246, 1986.

9. Ariyan S. The pectoralis major myocutaneous flap. A versatile flap for reconstruction in the head and neck. Plast Reconstr Surg 63:73-81, 1979.

10. Robinson DW, MacLeod A. Microvascular free jejunum transfer. Br J Plast Surg 35:258-267, 1982.

EDITORIAL PERSPECTIVE

C. Scott Hultman, MD, MBA, FACS

My first major case as a plastic surgery resident was a reverse radial forearm flap to cover a distal defect of the palm, in which we had repaired several flexor tendon and digital nerve injuries after electrical damage to the hand. As the junior resident assisting, I remember with complete clarity how the anatomy made sense, even though it did not: creating the skin island over the brachioradialis and flexor carpi radialis muscles, harvesting the septum and perforators that traveled down obliquely between the brachioradialis and flexor carpi radialis, and elevating the flap from proximal to distal down to the wrist where the density of perforators increased exponentially.

The patient did well, with excellent perfusion of the flap and restoration of finger flexion and sensation. This case gave me the confidence to do the "anterograde" forearm flap, even with the added complexity of microsurgery. The radial forearm flap with all of its variants (free versus pedicle, reverse flow, adipofascial turnover, and composite with bone) remains one of the most versatile flaps in all of plastic surgery. In fact the extended, innervated radial forearm flap is the ideal flap for total penile reconstruction, given the thinness and pliability of the skin paddle.

CHAPTER 29

Conventional TRAM Flap Versus Free Microsurgical TRAM Flap for Immediate Breast Reconstruction

Grotting JC, Urist MM, Maddox WA, Vasconez LO. Plast Reconstr Surg 83:828-841; discussion 842-844, 1989

Reviewed by Cindy Wu, MD

Transfer of the tissue as a free flap offers additional advantages that may eventually make this technique the preferred method of transfer of the lower abdominal tissue for breast reconstruction.[1]

Research Question The authors studied the transverse rectus abdominis myocutaneous (TRAM) flap in the setting of immediate breast reconstruction, which was a novel idea at the time. After the first successful transfer of the TRAM as a free flap for immediate reconstruction,[2] the authors proposed certain advantages for the microsurgical flap.[3] This paper compares the conventional versus the free TRAM flap for the very first time in the literature.

Funding None

Study Dates July 1985 to April 1988

Publishing Date 1989

Location University of Alabama at Birmingham, Birmingham, AL

Subjects Fifty-four patients underwent immediate breast reconstruction—44 had pedicled TRAM flap reconstruction and 11 had microsurgical free TRAM flap reconstruction.

Exclusion Criteria Patients who underwent implant-based breast reconstruction

Sample Size   54

Overview of Design   A retrospective review of a single institution's experience

Intervention   The authors performed conventional TRAM in 44 patients and free TRAM in 10 patients.

Follow-up   3 years

Endpoints   Any complications

Results   In the pedicled TRAM group, there were no complete flap failures. Two patients had partial flap loss, six had delayed healing of the mastectomy flaps, and one patient had abdominal relaxation with no true hernia treated with bilateral external oblique advancement flaps.

The average age was 44 years in the pedicled TRAM group and 47 years in the free TRAM group. Most patients had stage I or II breast cancer. Two patients in the pedicled TRAM group had stage III cancer. The total time for the mastectomy and pedicled unilateral TRAM reconstruction averaged 6 hours 50 minutes. The unilateral free TRAM group averaged 1 hour longer. There was a difference in transfusion requirements; 2.62 units were replaced in the pedicled TRAM group versus 2 units in the free TRAM group. The authors state that this difference reflects the more limited dissection needed for the free flap donor site. The average length of stay was 8.56 days for the pedicled TRAM group compared with 8 days in the free TRAM group. This is the result of less abdominal wall dissection in the free TRAM group, which allowed more rapid return to functional baseline. There were no local recurrences. In one patient pathologic evaluation revealed a tumor at the deep margin. She was treated by radiation through the reconstructed breast without complications. Three patients developed metastases, and two patients died of metastatic disease at 16 months. In the pedicled TRAM group, one patient had partial flap loss and ultimately required latissimus dorsi reconstruction. There were no complete flap losses in this group. One patient had abdominal relaxation that required bilateral external oblique advancement flaps. Six patients had delayed healing of the mastectomy flaps, one of which required operative debridement and closure. In the free TRAM group, there were no flap losses and no donor site complications. One patient had delayed mastectomy flap healing that resolved without surgery. Most patients did not require revision of the reconstructed breast as a secondary procedure, and for those requiring revision, it was accomplished under local anesthesia at the time of nipple-areola reconstruction.

Conclusions   The TRAM flap, whether pedicle or free, is a reasonable option for immediate reconstruction that compares favorably with other techniques. The microsurgical free TRAM offers the advantage of more limited donor site dissection, which subsequently decreases blood loss, length of stay, and abdominal wall morbidity.

Criticisms/Limitations   This study had a small sample size, with unequal sizes between the conventional and free TRAM groups.

Summary and Implications   Grotting et al[1] were the first to compare pedicled versus free TRAM flaps for immediate breast reconstruction. In this eloquently described paper, the authors first described the rationale behind why they were "taking a technically difficult operation and making it more complex by adding the risk of microsurgery."[1] The rationale behind undertaking the more involved procedure was to preserve abdominal wall function. They described that "carrying the lower abdominal tissue on the inferior epigastric pedicle could be done without sacrificing the full length or width of the rectus abdominis muscle."[1] By publishing this, the authors were the first ones to describe the muscle-sparing free TRAM flap.

The additional advantages of the free flap include less undermining required to create the tunnel into the breast wound, a more direct inflow and venous drainage through large donor and recipient vessels, no pedicle rotation, and readily available recipient vessels (thoracodorsal vessels). When the serratus branch is left intact, the latissimus flap is still a viable backup option via retrograde flow.

In conclusion, the authors make an accurately prescient forecast of the future of microsurgical breast reconstruction, perhaps stimulating further exploration of muscle-sparing free flaps: "Transfer of the tissue as a free flap offers additional advantages that may eventually make this technique the preferred method of transfer of the lower abdominal tissue for breast reconstruction."[1]

REFERENCES

1. Grotting JC, Urist MM, Maddox WA, et al. Conventional TRAM flap versus free microsurgical TRAM flap for immediate breast reconstruction. Plast Reconstr Surg 83:828-841; discussion 842-844, 1989.
2. Hartrampf CR Jr, Scheflan M, Black PW. Breast reconstruction with a transverse abdominal island flap. Plast Reconstr Surg 69:216-225, 1982.
   This landmark article introduced the pedicle TRAM flap for breast reconstruction.
3. Grotting JC. The free abdominoplasty flap for immediate breast reconstruction. Ann Plast Surg 27:351-354, 1991.
   This was the first description of the superficial inferior epigastric artery (SIEA) free flap used for immediate breast reconstruction. The author described a single case of a woman in whom they performed unilateral immediate reconstruction with the SIEA flap. He stated that the advantage is complete rectus abdominis sparing; the disadvantage was difficult pedicle dissection. He concluded that the SIEA flap may be suitable for the reconstruction of a smaller breast in a woman with large superficial epigastric vessels.
4. Holmstrom H. The free abdominoplasty flap and its use in breast reconstruction: an experimental study and clinical case report. Scand J Plast Reconstr Surg 13:423-427, 1979.
   The author described the use of a free TRAM flap in a woman who had a radical mastectomy, skin grafting, and postoperative radiation. After a delay procedure, the author trans-

ferred a free TRAM flap to the chest wall. Two months later, this flap was revised by spreading out the flap, placing a silicone implant underneath it, and performing a contralateral reduction.

5. Friedman RJ, Argenta LC, Anderson R. Deep inferior epigastric free flap for breast reconstruction after radical mastectomy. Plast Reconstr Surg 76:455-460, 1985.

6. Georgaide GS, Riefkohl R, Cox E, et al. Long-term clinical outcome of immediate reconstruction after mastectomy. Plast Reconstr Surg 76:415-420, 1985.

   This study was a comparison of relapse-free survival between 101 patients who had immediate tissue expander reconstruction and 377 who had mastectomy without reconstruction. After multivariate analysis, there was no significant difference between the two groups. The authors concluded that immediate reconstruction had no adverse effect on disease-free survival in patients who have undergone mastectomy for breast cancer.

7. Ishii CH Jr, Bostwick J III, Raine TJ, et al. Double-pedicle transverse rectus abdominis myocutaneous flap for unilateral breast and chest wall reconstruction. Plast Reconstr Surg 76:901-907, 1985.

8. Hartrampf CR Jr, Bennett GK. Autogenous tissue reconstruction in the mastectomy patient. A critical review of 300 patients. Ann Surg 205:508-519, 1987.

   This was a retrospective, 6-year review of 300 patients who received pedicle TRAM flap reconstruction. In 58% the breast was reconstructed in a single operation. Eighteen of 383 breast reconstructions required modification after 1 year. Symmetry was achieved without contralateral balancing procedures in 52% of the 217 unilateral reconstructions. Complications included 1 total (0.3%) and 18 partial flap losses (6%). There was one hernia (0.3%), two small defects in the upper anterior rectus sheath (0.8%), and lower abdominal laxity in two patients (0.8%), one of whom required repair.

STUDY AUTHOR REFLECTIONS

James C. Grotting, MD, FACS

This paper was significant because it was the first to describe the free transverse rectus abdominis myocutaneous (TRAM) flap for breast reconstruction as immediate treatment and was the largest series of conventional TRAM flaps for immediate reconstruction up until that time. In the past TRAM flaps were generally reserved for the salvage of cases in which the implants had failed and in delayed reconstruction. We were unaware that Hans Holmstrom had described the microsurgical transfer of the lower abdominal flap.[4] Single delayed cases had been published by Friedman et al[5] and mentioned by Bill Shaw. In subsequent conversations with Dr. Holmstrom, I learned that his concept was to resurface the chest wall with the lower abdominal free flap in heavy scar conditions such as radiation to allow the placement of an implant and not to actually make a breast out of the tissue alone. Subsequently, we also learned that others, such as Zoran Arnez and Bob Allen, were working in this area, but we were unaware of their work at the time.

We also described how the free TRAM flap is amenable to immediate breast reconstruction because back when axillary dissections were common, the thoracodorsal vessels were always dissected out and available for use as recipient vessels.[5-7] This made anastomosis to these vessels more convenient than the internal mammary vessels. The free TRAM also lent itself to immediate reconstruction because the breast and plastic surgeons could work simultaneously in a two-team approach.

We were the first to describe the preservation of a medial and lateral strip of muscle (muscle-sparing free TRAM). In this paper there is a reference to preserving additional mastectomy skin and the use of the flap when possible as a "buried autogenous implant"—the so-called "skin-sparing mastectomy." We also emphasized for the first time closure of the abdominal donor site as an aesthetic abdominoplasty in contradistinction to the teachings of Carl Hartrampf.[1,8] We were also the first to compare the outcomes between pedicled and free TRAM flaps.

CHAPTER 30

Have We Found an Ideal Soft-Tissue Flap? An Experience With 672 Anterolateral Thigh Flaps

Wei FC, Jain V, Celik N, Chen HC, Chuang DC, Lin CH. Plast Reconstr Surg 109:2219-2226; discussion 2227-2230, 2002

Reviewed by Amita R. Shah, MD, PhD

[The anterolateral thigh flap] is a versatile soft-tissue flap in which thickness and volume can be adjusted for the extent of the defect and it can replace most soft-tissue free flaps in most clinical situations.[1]

Research Question   The use of the anterolateral thigh flap in various clinical situations is demonstrated and its anatomy and variants are described.

Funding   Not mentioned

Study Dates   June 1996 to August 2000

Publishing Date   June 2002

Location   Chang Gung Memorial Hospital, Medical College, and University, Taipei, Taiwan

---

Subjects   660 patients who underwent a total of 672 anterolateral flaps

Exclusion Criteria   None described

Overview of Design   A retrospective review

Intervention   The anterolateral thigh flap as a cutaneous, fasciocutaneous, musculo-cutaneous, chimeric, or flow-through flap was used for oncologic and traumatic reconstruction of the head and neck, lower extremity, upper extremity, and trunk.

Follow-up   Patients were followed to donor-site and recipient-site healing.

Endpoints   Flap survival

Results   The anterolateral thigh flap was successfully used for the reconstruction of traumatic and oncologic wounds in various locations on the body. The success rate was 95.68% for all flaps, with 29 of the 672 (4.3%) flaps experiencing either complete or partial failure. Twelve of the 29 flaps failed completely, and 11 of the 12 were reconstructed with another flap. A patient with a failed flow-through flap required a below-knee amputation after flap failure. The eight patients with partial failure were treated with skin grafting, primary closure, and conservative measures.

Primary closure of the donor site was possible in 403 cases and 269 required split-thickness skin grafts. Most of the anterolateral flaps were used in the head and neck region (484 flaps), followed by 121 flaps for the lower extremity. Nine flaps were used for the trunk and 58 anterolateral flaps were used for upper extremity reconstruction. The anterolateral flap was used most often as fasciocutaneous and cutaneous flaps (350 and 154 flaps, respectively). Eighty-seven percent of these flaps were musculocutaneous perforator flaps and 12.9% were septocutaneous perforator vessel flaps. The remaining flaps were musculocutaneous flaps, which included part of the vastus lateralis muscle.

The anterolateral's primary pedicle is the lateral circumflex femoral artery, which comes off the profunda femoris artery. It has a reliable anatomic position in the groove between the rectus femoris and vastus lateralis. Septocutaneous perforators were found between the rectus femoris and vastus lateralis, and musculocutaneous perforators traversed the vastus lateralis and deep fascia to the skin. The perforators were within a 3 cm radius circle that was centered between the anterior superior iliac spine and the superolateral corner of the patella. Adequate skin vessels were found and traced back to the main pedicle in all but six flaps.

The harvest and use of the anterolateral flaps as cutaneous, fasciocutaneous, musculo-cutaneous, chimeric, or flow-through flaps were described. The suprafascial dissection technique for the elevation of cutaneous and fasciocutaneous flaps was used for 22.9% of all anterolateral flaps in this study. The cutaneous flap can be thinned to as much as 5 mm, and this flap, along with fasciocutaneous flaps, are often used for head and neck reconstruction. For defects requiring more soft tissue bulk, a musculocutaneous flap that contains the vastus lateralis muscle was described. The chimeric flaps used for three-dimensional defects were combinations of the rectus femoris, tensor fasciae latae, anteromedial thigh skin, and vastus lateralis. The flow-through flap was elevated by dissecting the pedicle from the vastus lateralis and then interposing it in a vascular defect, thus achieving a one-stage reconstruction for ischemic extremities.

Criticisms/Limitations   This study is limited by its retrospective nature and serves more as a descriptive study of the anatomy and applications of the anterolateral flap than as a comparison study. The operative technique of a variety of anterolateral flaps, anatomy, and management of complications are discussed, but a description of the types of wounds treated is lacking. The factors leading to the 29 flap failures were not evaluated.

Relevant Studies   The anterolateral flap has been used for various applications but most often for head and neck reconstruction. The advantage of this flap is that it can be harvested with the patient in the supine position so its dissection can be done simultaneously and therefore shorten the operative time. It has a long pedicle with large-diameter pedicle vessels, and the flaps can be made thick or thin. It can be used as a cutaneous, fasciocutaneous, myocutaneous, chimeric, or flow-through flap.[2]

The first lateral thigh flap was reported by Baek,[3] who described a posterolateral thigh skin flap based on the third cutaneous perforator off the profunda femoris. The first reported anterolateral flap as it is known today was by Song et al[4] in 1984. This flap was based on the descending branch of the lateral circumflex femoral artery and was described as having mainly musculocutaneous perforators. Further studies to define the anatomy of the anterolateral flap perforators have classified them into proximal, middle, and distal perforators, which were named A, B, and C, respectively, by Yu.[5] The study shows that the middle perforators were present most often and were usually musculocutaneous. Proximal perforators were found in only 49% of cases and were often septocutaneous.

Wei continued to define anterolateral anatomy and applicability, and in 2004 Wei and Mardini[6] described the freestyle anterolateral flap. The freestyle flap is designed and harvested based on preoperative Doppler signals.[6] The freestyle anterolateral flaps from this study were cutaneous flaps, which used the suprafascial dissection technique for elevation. By using the freestyle flap approach, many of the difficulties of dealing with anatomic variability in this area of the body are circumvented.

Summary   The anterolateral thigh flap is a versatile flap with a long and relatively reliable pedicle. It can supply sensate coverage, does not sacrifice major vessels of the lower extremity, and has low donor-site morbidity.

Implications   In their paper Wei et al showed that the anterolateral flap is a versatile flap with reliable anatomy for the head and neck, lower extremity, upper extremity, and trunk reconstruction. This is the largest study that has examined the use of the anterolateral flap all over the body and its variations in anatomy, thus expanding the known use of the flap. The paper is often cited in manuscripts about anterolateral flaps, and at the time of this publication, had more than 650 citations.

Before the publication of the paper, the use of the anterolateral flap was not widespread because of concerns about variable anatomy. Because of their experience with 672 anterolateral flaps, they further defined the anatomy, which has resulted in this flap becoming a workhorse flap for soft tissue reconstruction.

REFERENCES

1. Wei FC, Jain V, Celik N, et al. Have we found an ideal soft-tissue flap? An experience with 672 anterolateral thigh flaps. Plast Reconstr Surg 109:2219-2226; discussion 2227-2230, 2002.
2. Lee YC, Chiu HY, Shieh SJ. The clinical application of anterolateral thigh flap. Plast Surg Int 2011:127353, 2011.
3. Baek SM. Two new cutaneous free flaps: the medial and lateral thigh flaps. Plast Reconstr Surg 71:354-365, 1983.
4. Song YG, Chen GZ, Song YL. The free thigh flap: a new free flap concept based on the septo-cutaneous artery. Br J Plast Surg 37:149-159, 1984.
5. Yu P. Characteristics of the anterolateral thigh flap in a Western population and its application in head and neck reconstruction. Head Neck 26:759-769, 2004.
6. Wei FC, Mardini S. Free-style free flaps. Plast Reconstr Surg 114:910-916, 2004.

EDITORIAL PERSPECTIVE

C. Scott Hultman, MD, MBA, FACS

The anterolateral free flap has become the workhorse flap for the coverage of large defects of the head and neck. Admittedly, I do not have much experience with this flap except as a pedicle flap for groin coverage, but the anterolateral flap has replaced the free radial forearm flap at our institution when a large surface area is required for reconstruction. Although not quite as thin as the radial forearm flap, the donor site of the thigh has substantially less morbidity, and the distant site of the flap facilitates the two-team approach when head and neck extirpation and reconstruction must be performed. In addition to serving as a primary flap for head and neck reconstruction, the anterolateral flap has other interesting indications: a former resident of ours used this as a backup for breast reconstruction after a pedicled latissimus flap failed because of venous congestion. Sometimes starting out at the top of the reconstructive ladder provides our best solutions.

"Components Separation" Method for Closure of Abdominal-Wall Defects: An Anatomic and Clinical Study

Ramirez OM, Ruas E, Dellon AL. Plast Reconstr Surg 86:519-526, 1990

Reviewed by Patrick Mannal, MD

This study suggests that large abdominal-wall defects can be reconstructed with functional transfer of abdominal-wall components without the need for resorting to distant transposition of free-muscle flaps.[1]

Research Question   When the closure of a large abdominal wall defect or hernia is attempted, could separation of the individual muscular components allow mobilization over a greater distance compared with mobilization of the abdominal wall as a single unit?

Funding   Unknown

Study Dates   Late 1980s

Publishing Date   1990

Location   Johns Hopkins University School of Medicine, Baltimore, MD

Subjects   Ten fresh cadavers were used to define the anatomic dissection; the findings were then used to repair abdominal wall defects in 11 patients.

Exclusion Criteria   None

Sample Size   11 patients

Intervention   Abdominal wall component separation for the repair of large ventral defects is accomplished through the dissection of the external oblique muscle from the underlying internal oblique in an avascular plane. The internal oblique and transversus abdominis muscles are left adherent to each other, thus reducing blood loss and preserving the neurovascular bundle that enters the rectus muscle just lateral to the axis of the inferior and superior epigastric vessels. The rectus muscle is dissected free from the posterior rectus sheath but left adherent to the anterior rectus sheath through the tendinous inscriptions. With the rectus muscle released from its posterior sheath and still attached to the internal oblique, bilateral advancement of 10 cm (epigastrium), 20 cm (waistline), and 6 cm (suprapubic) can be achieved.

Follow-up   4 months to $3\frac{1}{2}$ years

Endpoints   Adequate reconstruction of the abdominal wall with dynamic muscular support

Results   None of the 11 patients developed abdominal wall hernias or weakness at the time of follow-up.

Criticisms/Limitations   Before the anatomically based technique outlined by Ramirez et al,[1] the surgeon was faced with trying to reapproximate the rectus muscle primarily for the repair of abdominal wall defects. The failure of the primary closure of the rectus muscle indicated the need to place synthetic mesh in the wound. This was usually followed either by granulation or skin grafting. However, if the mesh became infected or had to be removed, the result was catastrophic. Although both local and distant fasciocutaneous flaps have been used, their ability to tolerate the dynamic movement of the abdominal wall is less than desirable. The use of innervated muscle to repair abdominal wall hernias helps create a more robust support structure than the use of fascial flaps or mesh. The process of separating the various muscles of the abdominal wall, with careful attention to preserving neurovascular structures, allows a more sustainable construct.

Discussion   With the modern era of general anesthesia, the ability to perform complex procedures within the abdomen (and the rest of the body) has provided surgeons a way to push the boundaries of physiology and anatomic knowledge. From this marriage of exploration and science, a petulant and vexing dilemma has emerged: the ventral hernia. The repair of ventral hernias whether from trauma or iatrogenic has been the topic of great debate and consternation for generations of surgeons. Early techniques were less than optimal in restoring abdominal domain and protecting internal organs from injury. Early in the twentieth century, Gibson[2] described a technique in which large abdominal wall hernias could be closed by means of relaxing incisions at the lateral anterior rectus sheath. His idea was the precursor to the subsequent work of Young,[3] who in 1961 recognized that the lateral retraction of the rectus muscles was the primary issue to overcome in the closure of large midline ventral hernias of the abdominal wall.[4] He also stated what is now taken as common knowledge in our era of abdominal wall reconstruction: the freeing of fascial attachments between abdominal muscles laterally allows the medial movement of such muscles to cover midline defects.

There was little implementation or improvement on Young's ideas until the sentinel work by Ramirez et al in 1990.[1] Through Ramirez's work with cadavers and the subsequent knowledge which he applied to a series of patients, the field of plastic surgery has helped delineate what is possible when confronted with difficult defects of the abdominal wall. His description of the anatomic relationships of the rectus abdominis and internal and external oblique muscles in the lateral abdominal wall has helped define the basis for the medial advancement (up to 10 cm) of healthy tissue to help re-create the anterior abdominal wall. By recognizing the fascial planes and innervation inherent in the lateral abdomen, Ramirez et al started a revolution of surgeons conquering a once daunting problem. Whereas previously inadequate coverage options such as skin grafts were used with little success, innervated and robust tissue can now resolve ventral hernias with near uniform success.

However, there is always room for improvement, and not all hernias can be repaired with one technique alone. Since Ramirez's work, the boom in surgical technology has helped provide alternatives for recalcitrant cases and more elegant dissection to minimize the morbidity of the surgery. One such advancement has been the use of laparoscopic techniques to perform the lateral component separation.[5] The ability to avoid further injury to the abdominal wall by avoiding a repeat laparotomy and extensive dissection is certainly appealing. The surgeons in training today are familiar with minimally invasive surgical techniques, helping make laparoscopy the standard of care in many procedures.

Another modern surgical tool that has found a place in the execution of Ramirez's concept is the endoscope. Once again the idea of a minimally invasive method of performing the fascial separation of the external oblique from the internal oblique is appealing. By confining the incisions and dissection to just the lateral abdominal wall, the ability to reduce episodes of repeated trauma in the midline is a great advantage.[6] This is especially true in cases in which the ability to access the lateral abdominal wall is compromised because of scar tissue and the obliteration of tissue planes.

One of the main concerns of Ramirez's component separation technique has been maintaining adequate vascularity of the tissue as they are advanced toward the midline. The mobilization of large muscle flaps can compromise the arterial supply and result in wound breakdown and infection. Borrowing from another technique in modern plastic surgery, the concept of perforator-sparing component separation evolved to help reduce such issues.[7] Through careful dissection and preservation of periumbilical arterial perforators, the overlying tissue can retain a robust vascular supply, thus reducing the risk of ischemic injury to the repair.

Regardless of the blood supply to the abdominal wall, there will always be defects that are too large to fix with native tissue alone. The repair of hernias with mesh has proved superior to primary closure because of the ability to obtain tension-free closure.[8] Whether the mesh is used in an underlay versus overlay manner is still subject to debate, but no repair will last if challenged by excessive tension. The addition of mesh to a component separation can help achieve a tension-free final result by adding additional length to the repair. The use of biologic mesh or acellular dermal matrix has added another dimension to the repair of ventral hernias, especially those with active or resolving infection in which synthetic material will only continue to harbor bacteria.[9]

Progress, however, comes at a price and the field of surgery is no exception. Often the cost of innovation and progress are the moments of failure and reevaluation. It has been only 25 years since Ramirez et al published their work on component separation, and surgeons are only beginning to understand the long-term results of their actions. As new techniques are adopted and incorporated into clinical practice, there will be periods of increased complications as the methodology is refined.[10,11] Overall, however, the results are promising. In fact the results of abdominal hernia repairs at some academic institutions have indicated that not only was Ramirez (and Gibson and Young) correct in his theory, but that component separation will continue to define ventral hernia repair for future generations of surgeons.

REFERENCES

1. Ramirez OM, Ruas E, Dellon AL. "Components separation" method for closure of abdominal-wall defects: an anatomic and clinical study. Plast Reconstr Surg 86:519-526, 1990.
2. Gibson CL. Post-operative intestinal obstruction. Ann Surg 63:442-451, 1916.
3. Young D. Repair of epigastric incisional hernia. Br J Surg 48:514-516, 1961.
4. Halvorson EG. On the origins of components separation. Plast Reconstr Surg 124:1545-1549, 2009.
5. Milburn ML, Shah PK, Friedman EB, et al. Laparoscopically assisted components separation technique for ventral incisional hernia repair. Hernia 11:157-161, 2007.
6. Lowe JB, Garza JR, Bowman JL, et al. Endoscopically assisted "components separation" for closure of abdominal wall defects. Plast Reconstr Surg 105:720-729, 2000.
7. Saulis AS, Dumanian GA. Periumbilical rectus abdominis perforator preservation significantly reduces superficial wound complications in "separation of parts" hernia repairs. Plast Reconstr Surg 109:2275-2280, 2002.
8. Luijendijk RW, Hop WC, van den Tol MP, et al. A comparison of suture repair with mesh repair for incisional hernia. N Engl J Med 343:392-398, 2000.
9. Rosen MJ. Biologic mesh for abdominal wall reconstruction: a critical appraisal. Am Surg 76:1-6, 2010.
10. Hultman CS, Tong WM, Kittinger BJ, et al. Management of recurrent hernia after components separation: 10-year experience with abdominal wall reconstruction at an academic medical center. Ann Plast Surg 66:504-507, 2011.
11. Hultman CS, Clayton JL, Kittinger BJ, et al. Learning curves in abdominal wall reconstruction with components separation: one step closer toward improving outcomes and reducing complications. Ann Plast Surg 72(Suppl 2):S126-S131, 2014.

STUDY AUTHOR REFLECTIONS

Oscar M. Ramirez, MD

The most important features of any new technique or technology that is introduced into the body of knowledge are the principles. After the student or researcher understands those principles, it is easier to modify, improve, or expand on that knowledge. Here I emphasize the principles of the *components separation technique* so new surgeons embarking on this type of reconstruction can understand the advances that have been made in this technique and have a better grasp of further improvements or the applications to other body areas. The most important principles are:

- The translation of the muscular layer of the abdominal wall to enlarge its tissue surface.
- The separation of muscle layers that allows maximal individual expansion of each muscle unit.
- This expansion is facilitated by its disengagement of some muscle unit from its fascial sheath envelope that restricts its horizontal mobilization.
- The abdominal wall musculature in around 70% of its surface is covering hollow viscous. This can be more easily compressed than solid structures, particularly after a good bowel preparation. Likewise, false and floating ribs can be pushed to some extent by the action of the muscle pull.
- Provided that all the muscle elements (although retracted or scarred down) are in place, bilateral mobilization works more effectively than unilateral advancements. This will also equilibrate the forces of the entire abdominal wall and centralize the midline.

Any technique has its logistic limitations. The components separation is not without its shortcomings. The main limitations are:

- Size of the defect.
- Blood supply to the abdominal skin.
- Its applicability in all acute cases; with these in mind, the surgeon should use a graduated approach to abdominal wall mobilization.
- Minor defects can be closed by muscle approximation after mobilization of the medial borders of the recti muscle and its elevation from the posterior rectus sheath only. This requires skin separation from the abdomen similar to an abdominoplasty procedure. To minimize skin separation from the muscles, the abdominoplasty component should be done vertically only.
- Medium-sized defects may require significant lateral-to-medial traction of the external oblique/internal oblique/transversus muscle complex, which will require anterior recti/muscle separation from its posterior sheath up to near the junction to the linea semicircularis and in some cases minor interrupted releasing incisions of the fascia of the external oblique muscle.

- Large defects will require varying degrees of longer fascia release of the external oblique muscle. In either case of fascial release, particularly in the lower quadrants, Vicryl or Prolene mesh can be applied to restore the continuity of the muscle layer and to avoid areas of muscle wall weakness or potential "hernias." Because this mesh will be covered internally by a muscle and externally by a thick panniculum, there is no risk of exposure to bowels or extrusion to the skin surface. In repairing small areas of relaxing incisions, Vicryl mesh may be enough because the collagen deposition will provide a structural support similar to a fascial layer after its absorption; however, larger relaxing incisions will require a more permanent material.

The "loss of domain" of the abdominal cavity creates conditions that can produce respiratory and vascular compromise after the repair. To prevent these conditions in cases of elective reconstruction, the following ancillary steps should be followed:
- An abdominal binder should be used to gradually compress the abdominal cavity. The patient should perform chest-breathing exercises for at least 4 to 6 weeks while wearing the binder.
- In patients with large defects with significant "loss of domain," a pulmonary consult and spirometric evaluation should be done with the abdomen at maximal compression.
- The patient should be placed on a liquid diet for 2 or 3 days before surgery and have a good bowel preparation that includes antibiotics to diminish the formation of gas and stool. These allow easier closure, less tension on the diaphragm, and less tension on the vena cava. These last two effects will decrease the risk of pulmonary complications and venous thrombosis, respectively. They will also diminish postoperative pain, discomfort, and the risk of ileus paralyticus.

The advent of biologic materials has expanded the use of the components separation, which decreases tension during closure and avoids respiratory compromise by a tight closure. It has also helped close larger and irregular defects. In cases of acute conditions, the biologic mesh has been a great addition to convert a potential exposed abdomen to a closed one. In some cases this type of approach can be considered a two-stage procedure in which final closure with complete muscle continuity can be done after the inflamed tissues are allowed to settle and relax.

CHAPTER 32

Multivariate Predictors of Failure After Flap Coverage of Pressure Ulcers

Keys KA, Daniali LN, Warner KJ, Mathes DW. Plast Reconstr Surg 125:1725-1734, 2010

Reviewed by Patrick Mannal, MD

> *Confirmation of adequate nutritional status and strict preoperative management of blood glucose may improve operative success rates [after flap coverage of pressure ulcers]. Operative management should be approached with trepidation, if at all, in young patients with recurrent ischial pressure ulcers.[1]*

Research Question Are there specific, identifiable factors associated with postoperative failure of flap coverage of pressure sores?

Funding Unknown

Study Dates 1993 to 2008

Publishing Date 2010

Location Seattle, WA

Subjects Patients from the Puget Sound Veterans Affairs (VA) Hospital from August 1993 to April 2008

Exclusion Criteria Patients treated with conservative management, primary closure, or skin grafting

Sample Size A multiyear, retrospective review of 135 sequential patients (227 flap operations); four patients were excluded because of death within 6 months of the surgery.

Intervention   Variables evaluated included age, gender, body mass index, smoking (within 30 days before surgery), mobility, mental capacity, level of malnutrition (assessed by VA dieticians), use of a Foley catheter, presence of fecal diversion, cardiac risk factors (based on Adult Treatment Panel III modification of the Framingham Risk Score), presence of peripheral vascular disease, presence of diabetes mellitus, presence of depression, albumin, prealbumin, C-reactive protein, hemoglobin A1c (if diabetic), number of previous same-site flaps, total number of previous flaps, number of previous failed flaps, ulcer location, ulcer size at the level of the skin, size of the ulcer cavity, presence of sensation at the level of the ulcer, a recent decrease in wound size with conservative management, presence of osteomyelitis (imaging or bone biopsy), procedure length, flap tissue composition, donor location, flap motion (advancement/rotation/pedicled), time to range of motion at the flap site, time to initiate seating, wound complications (infection/hematoma), need for reoperative intervention, and recurrence of ulcers at the same or other sites (including length of time to recurrence).

Follow-up   Average: 4.4 years; 7.7 months to 12.3 years, confidence interval = 95%

Endpoints   Primary outcome was the recurrence of the pressure ulcer at the site of the flap. This was defined as a skin break at the surgical site after the completion of the postflap mobilization protocol with intact skin. Secondary outcomes were suture line dehiscence (any recorded break in the skin, excluding the donor site, at any point before or during the mobilization protocol), infection, or hematoma. Dehiscence requiring a return to the operating room for flap repair was considered separate from suture line dehiscence left to heal without intervention.

Results   Sixty-one flaps (27%) healed without complication; these flaps were used as the control group by the authors. In the postoperative period, 110 flaps (49%) had a suture line dehiscence. Of the 110 flaps, 36 (16% of the total, 33% of the dehiscence group) required a return to the operating room for repair. Of the dehiscence group, 74 flaps (77%) healed without reoperation. Eighty-eight flaps (39% of the total) within the dehiscence group developed same-site recurrence. This group of 88 flaps with same-site recurrence was further divided into "early" versus "late" if the recurrence occurred within 1 year of the flap surgery.

The composition of the flap (myocutaneous versus fasciocutaneous) was not associated with a difference in outcomes; gluteal muscle or fascial flaps were the most commonly used (56%).

A history of previous same-site recurrence or dehiscence requiring intervention increased the rate of flap failure from 40% to 52%. The need for operative revision increased from 13% to 21% for flaps performed on sites that had previous dehiscences/flap suture line failure.

Regarding individual factors associated with flap failure, variables with likelihood ratios of less than 0.1 were used in the multivariate logistic regression analysis. With the use of generalized estimating equations to control each patient's unique effect on flap recurrence while adjusting for confounding variables, the following were potential confounders in the analysis: age <45 years old, wound location, fecal diversion, hemoglobin A1c >6 (poor glycemic control), albumin <3.5 g/dL, and prealbumin <20 mg/dL. The results of the multivariate analysis indicated that ischial ulcers, any previous same-site failure, and poorly controlled diabetes correlated with increased recurrence of the ulcer.

Criticisms/Limitations   The population of the VA system is not representative of the patient population with pressure sores. The elderly patient, debilitated from chronic disease, is an area unrepresented in the current study. In addition, any retrospective study has limitations with regard to follow-up and the accuracy of data when collected.

Summary   Pressure sores and ulcers represent a significant burden to the delivery of health care in the United States and around the world. Tremendous amounts of time and energy are spent on the care of these wounds with little measurable success. In many ways, the adage "an ounce of prevention equals a pound of cure" applies to the management of pressure sores. Through prevention, many patient populations prone to the development of these lesions can be protected from the long-term morbidity associated with their care. Despite the best care, however, some sores progress to ulcers and require surgical intervention for the eradication of infection and protective coverage. Because the pathology leading to ulcer development is not dealt with by surgery, plastic surgeons often find that these patients are challenging, lifelong patients. Because of this, many investigators have attempted to answer the simple question of why some patients' ulcers heal and others continue to fail surgical therapy.

Data on the incidence of pressure sores in the United States are approximately 2.5 million, with the cost of treating these sores increasing to more than $11 billion per year.[2] The study by Mathes et al examines the population of patients who were enrolled in the VA's health care system between 1993 and 2008. Although this may not represent the full breadth and width of the patients who present with pressure sores, it certainly allows the examination of certain factors that may contribute to the success or failure of flap surgery for the coverage of pressure ulcers. However, most plastic surgeons caring for pressure sores and ulcers will have a significant percentage of their patients who are older, more frail, and less than optimal surgical candidates for large flap procedures. Flap selection for the coverage of a pressure sore can contribute greatly to the success or failure of the procedure.[3] In fact, some have evaluated whether surgery is needed at all or warranted in patients with pressure ulcers given the propensity for flap failure or recurrence.[4]

Continued

In this study, Mathes et al[1] were able to cull out the characteristics of patients who were eventual successful candidates for pressure sore surgery. Despite the abundance of evidence indicating that many factors contribute to the development of pressure ulcers,[5] Mathes was able to show how the patients fell into three distinct categories with regard to wound issues or dehiscence: no dehiscence, early dehiscence, or late dehiscence/recurrence. In short, almost half of the patients had some degree of suture line disruption and 39% had a same-site recurrence. Among the many previously held parameters that contributed to the failure of surgical therapy for pressure sores, multivariate analysis revealed three predictive factors: previous same-site flap failure, poorly controlled diabetes, and ulcer location over the ischial tuberosity. These three identifiers were the result of the evaluation of 31 variables from 227 operations in patients at the VA Hospital in Puget Sound, WA.

The surgeon's choice of flap in covering a pressure ulcer is of significant importance. Although many choices exist in theory, not all are equally suited (or available) for all patients. Certain factors must be taken into account, such as the location of the sore or ulcer, the quality of available tissues, the functional deficits certain flaps create, and patient disease limitations. In addition, the use of newer surgical techniques such as perforator flaps has led to an increased selection of flap choices for surgeons.[6] The omission of muscle from the flap design can help tailor the flap to the individual patient and reduce donor-site morbidity. Some authors have observed that fasciocutaneous flaps may have better outcomes than musculocutaneous flaps because of their greater tissue durability.[7]

Regardless of the availability or durability, certain flaps continue to dominate the discussion of the surgical treatment of pressure ulcers. Most are located in the lower truck or proximal lower extremity. Perhaps the most commonly used, the gluteal transposition (rotation) flap is able to cover most of the sacral pressure ulcers with adequate adipose, muscle, and/or facial tissue. Its use is best suited to patients who are still ambulatory. The gluteal V to Y advancement flap is another commonly used flap and is often used for patients without the use of their lower extremities because of its proximity, ease of advancement, and reliable vascularity. It can also be modified into a bilateral design to help fill larger midline defects.

Surgeons have also used the biceps femoris flap for help with sores of the perineal region. The proximally based blood supply of the flap makes the arc of rotation quite large, and its relatively diminutive thickness allows for pliability and insetting in difficult locations. Caution must be exercised when the most distal portion of the flap is incorporated into the reconstructive design because it may be prone to vascular compromise.

Another option for the repair of decubitus ulcers is the tensor fascia lata flap, which can be quite useful in the coverage of the trochanteric region. It is readily available, contains fascia and skin, and can be mobilized to cover a great territory of the thigh and groin. The use of the tensor fascia lata flap should be personalized because it is not indicated in all patients, and alternative flaps may be better suited to specific locations.

When considering the success of any pressure ulcer surgery, the postoperative period is arguably more important than the surgery itself. If the flap is not given adequate time to heal through offloading, a reduction in suture line tension, optimizing nutrition, proper patient equipment, control of muscle spasm,[8] and careful skin integrity monitoring, then no surgery will provide satisfactory outcomes. In the study by Mathes et al, they adhered to a postoperative mobilization protocol that included the following: the use of an air fluid bed for 5 weeks; starting passive range-of-motion exercises at 4 weeks; and increased time lying on the flap starting at 5 weeks, with progression to sitting on the flap at 6 weeks. If there was an observed break in the skin in the area of the flap, the protocol was halted and only restarted once complete healing had been observed.

As the population of the United States ages and medical treatments of many diseases allow longer lifespans with coexistent medical illnesses, the treatment of pressure ulcers will become more challenging. Not all patients with ulcers will be the victims of spinal trauma but rather may be increasingly elderly, frail, and debilitated. The ability to tolerate surgery will be diminished, and the quality of tissue available for reconstruction will be less than optimal. It is of the greatest importance that the plastic surgeon understands the medical, surgical, and psychological issues[9] that contribute to the formation of pressure ulcers before any treatment is enacted. Even more than previously, prevention and avoidance will be the best surgical strategies.

REFERENCES

1. Keys KA, Daniali LN, Warner KJ, et al. Multivariate predictors of failure after flap coverage of pressure ulcers. Plast Reconstr Surg 125:1725-1734, 2010.
2. Reddy M, Gill SS, Rochon PA. Preventing pressure ulcers: a systematic review. JAMA 296:974-984, 2006.
3. Foster R, Anthony J, Mathes S, et al. Flap selection as a determinant of success in pressure sore coverage. Arch Surg 132:868-873, 1997.
4. Disa J, Carlton J, Goldberg N. Efficacy of operative cure in pressure sore patients. Plast Reconstr Surg 89:272-278, 1992.
5. Byrne D, Salzberg C. Major risk factors for pressure ulcers in the spinal cord disabled: a literature review. Spinal Cord 34:255-263, 1996.
6. Coskunfirat OK, Ozgentas HE. Gluteal perforator flaps for coverage of pressure sores at various locations. Plast Reconstr Surg 113:2012-2017; discussion 2018-2019, 2004.
7. Yamamoto Y, Tsutsumida A, Murazumi M, et al. Long-term outcome of pressure sores treated with flap coverage. Plast Reconstr Surg 100:1212-1217, 1997.
8. Cushing CA, Phillips LG. Evidence-based medicine: pressure sores. Plast Reconstr Surg 132:1720-1732, 2013.
9. Anderson T, Andberg M. Psychosocial factors associated with pressure sores. Arch Phys Med Rehabil 60:341-346, 1979.

STUDY AUTHOR REFLECTIONS

David W. Mathes, MD, FACS

In this study we examined the question of what factors lead to the failure of flap coverage of pressure-induced ulcers. Our goal was to provide patients with an assessment of the likelihood of success after surgical treatment of these wounds. The patient population at the Veterans Affairs hospital often presents with multiple medical comorbidities, and we hoped that this study would clarify those factors that could be modified to improve outcomes.

Our study demonstrated a significant failure rate of 39%. Factors that increased the risk of failure were young age, diabetes, poor nutrition (albumin <3.5), and the treatment of a recurrent pressure sore. The results presented in this paper should not be used to deny a patient the option of surgical coverage of a pressure sore. Rather, the outcome data can provide the patient with information that can guide the patient and surgeon to make an informed decision regarding the next step in the treatment of these wounds.

EDITORIAL PERSPECTIVE

C. Scott Hultman, MD, MBA, FACS

David Mathes, the new Chief of Plastic Surgery at the University of Colorado (he is literally flying there as I write this), is a rising star in plastic surgery, primarily known for his basic science work in composite tissue allotransplantation. Along the way, however, he wrote a great clinical article about pressure sores, in which he identified the predictors of flap failure through a robust, multivariate statistical model. As we enter the era of evidence-based medicine, this paper provides real-time guidance for plastic surgeons like me who are considering pressure ulcer surgery in patients with sacral, trochanteric, and ischial wounds. This important document clarifies who is (and is not) a good candidate for flap reconstruction.

CHAPTER 33

High-Lateral-Tension Abdominoplasty With Superficial Fascial System Suspension

Lockwood T. Plast Reconstr Surg 96:603-615, 1995

Reviewed by Patrick Mannal, MD

> *Although the surgical principles of classic abdominoplasty certainly have stood the test of time, they are based on two theoretical assumptions that may be proved to be inaccurate: 1. Wide direct undermining is essential for flap advancement, and 2. Abdominal skin relaxation occurs in the vertical direction from xiphoid to pubis . . . Discontinuous undermining allows effective loosening of the abdominal flap while preserving vascular perforators, . . . [and] significant lateral truncal skin resection results in epigastric tightening.[1]*

Research Question   Can a more natural aesthetic contour be achieved through the modification of traditional abdominoplasty techniques and the addition of truncal liposuction?

Funding   Unknown

Study Dates   Early 1990s

Publishing Date   1995

Location   University of Kansas, Kansas City, KS

Subjects   Patients undergoing aesthetic surgery with moderate-to-severe soft tissue laxity of the anterior trunk with rectus muscle diastasis with or without abdominal and truncal fat deposits

Exclusion Criteria   Patients requiring liposuction alone or those requiring minimal skin resection techniques

Sample Size   50 patients, 36 (72%) of whom received truncal liposuction

Intervention   Modification of the traditional abdominoplasty technique to include the highest tension wound closure and significant lateral tissue resection, limiting the amount of direct undermining of the superior abdominal tissue flaps to preserve vascular perforators, liposuction as needed in the areas of truncal adiposity, and superficial fascial system suspension with permanent sutures during closure

Follow-up   4 to 16 months; average 10 months

Endpoints   Patient and surgeon satisfaction with the aesthetic outcome

Results   Good to excellent (per the author)

Criticisms/Limitations   The study is a single surgeon's experience with a modified surgical technique. There was no control group; the author only states that the complications seen in the series of 50 patients compared favorably with historic control subjects who had been previously reported. Complications in this series included dog-ear deformities (n = 3), seroma (n = 2), suture granuloma (n = 2), minor umbilical or incisional necrosis (n = 2), major flap necrosis (n = 1), and postoperative anemia (n = 1). The technique described was modified for certain patients based on physical examination findings, such as the location of skin laxity and the presence or absence of truncal adipose deposits. Neither the application of the modified technique nor the use of liposuction was uniformly applied to all patients.

Summary   Most abdominoplasties performed are based in some form on the early work of Pitanguy[2] and his description of raising abdominal flaps followed by resection of excessive skin and soft tissue. His work helped create the modern concepts of body contouring, including the patient population with massive weight loss. As these techniques were adopted and tested over time, Dr. Lockwood realized that some of the assumptions inherent in traditional abdominoplasty techniques were flawed. He identified two such issues and addressed them in his paper, "High-Lateral-Tension Abdominoplasty with Superficial Fascial System Suspension."[1]

The first issue Lockwood challenged was that wide undermining of the abdominal flaps to the costal margin was critical for the surgeon to advance the abdominal tissue inferiorly, allowing adequate resection. His second point of contention was that skin laxity in the aging abdominal wall manifests in primarily vertical skin relaxation, and as such the vertical vector (xiphoid to pubis) should be the major component of tissue resection. In the scope of a series of 50 patients, Lockwood helped redefine the technique of the abdominoplasty and better understand the anatomy so superior results can be obtained.

When Lockwood's critique of the abdominoplasty technique is examined, his assessment of the classic dogma is the natural evolution of technology and experience. Although the idea and practice of wide, direct undermining of the abdominal wall to the costal margins to allow adequate descent of the abdominal tissue flaps are sound, the introduction and widespread use of liposuction helped him develop an alternate opinion. Liposuction of the abdominal wall can help reduce the localized adipose deposits for cosmetic improvement in abdominal contour, but it also demonstrates how undermining of the abdominal wall can result in tissue mobility with preservation of vascular perforators. As one of the main complications of the classic abdominoplasty technique, tissue necrosis and wound breakdown were often the result of compromised perfusion to the tissues. Lockwood hypothesized that preservation of adequate blood flow and appropriate tissue mobility could coexist with the addition of modern liposuction techniques.

With regard to the second issue Lockwood identified in his paper, in his experience with patients presenting with abdominal tissue laxity and excess, lateral abdominal wall/trunk tissue was unrecognized as an important contributor to less than optimal aesthetic outcomes. This was mainly from the adherence of the midline tissues to deeper, stronger fascial supporting elements such as the linea alba of the rectus muscles. Indeed, the lateral tissues have no such supporting structure and tend to have greater vertical descent, requiring a greater degree of resection than previously thought to achieve the best abdominal contour. Lockwood postulated that lateral tissue resection with the tension of the incisional closure transferred laterally and to the superficial fascial system helped result in improved outcomes and patient satisfaction.

In fact, Lockwood's belief in the concept of the circumferential trunk as an aesthetic unit is a major reason for the results he achieved with posterolateral liposuction in 72% of patients in his series. This is further supported by the work of subsequent authors such as Aly et al,[3] who illustrated the benefit of belt lipectomy to help with overall abdominal contour in certain patients. Other specialists in the area of postbariatric weight loss surgery have advocated similar approaches to the excessive tissue of the lateral abdominal wall and truck such as Friedman et al,[4] who evaluated the safety of adding a vertical component to the traditional approach, or the "fleur-de-lis" abdominoplasty to help with the resection of excess upper abdominal skin.

As many investigators began to adopt the use of modified techniques to the resection of abdominal tissue, the involvement of newer technologies was only logical. The use of endoscopic techniques is an example of the application of such technology to help reduce the potential risk and morbidity associated with abdominoplasty procedures. The ability to minimize the incision while allowing dissection and repair of supporting abdominal wall structures, in addition to liposuction for additional contouring, was explored by Eaves et al[5] not long after Lockwood's work.

With the adoption of the entire trunk as an aesthetic unit, other cosmetic issues for the overweight patient have emerged as challenges to attaining the best result. For exam-

Continued

ple, after the whole abdomen is addressed and the skin laxity is removed, the flattened contour of the gluteal region becomes more apparent. Because the average patient undergoing abdominoplasty is not a candidate for implant-based gluteal augmentation to address the issue, autologous augmentation has emerged as a potential solution.[6]

Since Lockwood's paper was published, the field of plastic surgery has continued to refine the abdominoplasty. However, the procedure's continued popularity among surgeons has prompted the examination of its patient safety profile. Many surgeons have decades of experience performing the surgery, both with and without liposuction, with published reports of the outcomes, complications, and risks involved. One of the biggest arguments for avoiding the use of liposuction in combination with abdominoplasty procedures is the threat of an adverse patient safety event such as a pulmonary embolism and deep vein thrombosis. Several authors have studied the effects of abdominoplasty in high-risk groups (smokers and previous abdominal surgery) or when performed with other invasive procedures and found no increased risk of adverse outcomes.[7,8] For some authors and surgeons, conscious sedation has emerged as an option for anesthesia during abdominoplasty to help reduce the operative risk, even when it is combined with additional surgical procedures.[9] Many have refined their techniques to obtain the best outcomes through modifications of both the surgical and liposuction techniques while simultaneously reducing the risk profile for the surgery.[10] Increasingly, many of these procedures are performed in an outpatient setting, and there have been publications of evidence-based safety guidelines to help mitigate the chances of negative outcomes in such circumstances.[11] It has been a common belief that the addition of liposuction increased the risk of pulmonary embolism and deep vein thrombosis to an unacceptably high degree, but recent evidence may suggest otherwise. This is particularly true if the liposuction is limited and used as an adjunct to the abdominoplasty to obtain the best abdominal contour possible.

REFERENCES

1. Lockwood T. High-lateral-tension abdominoplasty with superficial fascial system suspension. Plast Reconstr Surg 96:603-615, 1995.
2. Pitanguy I. Abdominal lipectomy: an approach to it through an analysis of 300 consecutive cases. Plast Reconstr Surg 40:384-391, 1967.
3. Aly AS, Cram AE, Chao M, et al. Belt lipectomy for circumferential truncal excess: the University of Iowa experience. Plast Reconstr Surg 111:398-413, 2003.
4. Friedman T, O'Brien Coon D, Michaels J, et al. Fleur-de-Lis abdominoplasty: a safe alternative to traditional abdominoplasty for the massive weight loss patient. Plast Reconstr Surg 125:1525-1535, 2010.
5. Eaves FF III, Nahai F, Bostwick J III. Endoscopic abdominoplasty and endoscopically assisted miniabdominoplasty. Clin Plast Surg 23:599-616; discussion 617, 1996.
6. Centeno RF. Autologous gluteal augmentation with circumferential body lift in the massive weight loss and aesthetic patient. Clin Plast Surg 33:479-496, 2006.

7. Hester TR Jr, Baird W, Bostwick J III, et al. Abdominoplasty combined with other major surgical procedures: safe or sorry? Plast Reconstr Surg 83:997-1004, 1989.
8. Samra S, Sawh-Martinez R, Barry O, et al. Complication rates of lipoabdominoplasty versus traditional abdominoplasty in high-risk patients. Plast Reconstr Surg 125:683-690, 2010.
9. Kryger ZB, Fine NA, Mustoe TA. The outcome of abdominoplasty performed under conscious sedation: six-year experience in 153 consecutive cases. Plast Reconstr Surg 113:1807-1817; discussion 1818-1819, 2004.
10. Trussler AP, Kurkjian TJ, Hatef DA, et al. Refinements in abdominoplasty: a critical outcomes analysis over a 20-year period. Plast Reconstr Surg 126:1063-1074, 2010.
11. Haeck PC, Swanson JA, Iverson RE, et al.; ASPS Patient Safety Committee. Evidence-based patient safety advisory: patient selection and procedures in ambulatory surgery. Plast Reconstr Surg 124(4 Suppl):6S-27S, 2009.

EDITORIAL PERSPECTIVE

C. Scott Hultman, MD, MBA, FACS

Although Lockwood correctly acknowledges that "modern abdominoplasty techniques were developed in the 1960s,"[1] modern body contouring, especially for patients with massive weight loss, directly descended from the groundbreaking work that he pioneered in the 1990s. It is really hard to overstate Lockwood's influence on today's body contouring procedures, from extended abdominoplasty to lower and upper body lifts, mastopexy, and brachioplasty. Lockwood was a courageous innovator who introduced concepts that ran counter to the prevailing thinking of the surgical community in his day when laparoscopic gastric bypass was first gaining popularity. The concepts he introduced, such as high-lateral tension and repair of the superficial fascial system, allowed surgeons of the future to reconstruct the deformities that surfaced for the first time in patients with massive weight loss. Lockwood passed away from brain cancer in 2005, far too soon at the age of 59, but he gave the rest of us a legacy of surgical principles and techniques that would be used for surgical problems not yet observed. This is why Ted Lockwood is one of the greatest plastic surgeons our discipline has ever known: he anticipated surgical problems of the future and solved them for the rest of us.

CHAPTER 34

Utility of the Omentum in the Reconstruction of Complex Extraperitoneal Wounds and Defects: Donor-Site Complications in 135 Patients From 1975 to 2000

Hultman CS, Carlson GW, Losken A, Jones G, Culbertson J, Mackay G, Bostwick J III, Jurkiewicz MJ. Ann Surg 235:782-795, 2002

Reviewed by S. Tyler Elkins-Williams, MD, and Amita R. Shah, MD, PhD

The omentum can be safely harvested and reliably used to reconstruct a diverse range of extraperitoneal wounds and defects. Donor-site complications can be significant but are usually limited to abdominal wall infection and hernia.[1]

Funding None

Study Type A retrospective case series

Study Dates January 1975 to May 2000

Publishing Date June 2002

Location Emory University Hospital, Crawford Long Hospital, VA Hospital of Atlanta, Egleston Children's Hospital, and Grady Memorial Hospital, Atlanta, GA

Research Question What are the potential uses of the omentum for the reconstruction of extraperitoneal defects? What are the donor-site complications and rate of complications after harvest of the omentum for use in reconstruction?

Subjects   Patients who underwent extraperitoneal transposition or transfer of the greater omentum for reconstruction; 59% of patients were male. The mean age was 51 years old, with ages ranging from 4 to 86 years old.

Exclusion Criteria   Not discussed

Sample Size   135 patients

Intervention   The omentum was used as a primary flap in 106 patients and as a secondary "salvage" flap in 29 patients. Free tissue transfer was performed in 71 patients. The omentum was harvested by laparotomy in all but one patient in whom it was harvested laparoscopically. The mean operative time was 6.2 hours. The right gastroepiploic artery was used as the pedicle in 95 patients, the left gastroepiploic artery was used in 28 patients, and both gastroepiploic arteries were used in 5 patients (in the remaining 7 patients, there was incomplete data to determine pedicle choice).

Results   Successful free tissue transfer was achieved in 68 of 71 patients (95.8%). Three free flaps were loss because of vascular thrombosis. Eleven patients had partial flap loss, and 40 patients underwent revision of the flap, mostly for contouring. Most of the omental flaps were used for the orbit/face (24.4%) and sternum (25.2%). Some of the more unusual indications included coverage of the irradiated brachial plexus, revascularization of the brain in Moyamoya disease, soft tissue augmentation for Romberg hemifacial atrophy, and massive degloving of the upper extremity.

Donor-site complications occurred in 25 patients (18.5%); the most common complication was abdominal wall infection, followed by dehiscence and symptomatic ventral hernia. Six unplanned repeat laparotomies were performed for postoperative hemorrhage, dehiscence, or infection. Three patients had prolonged ileus, and one patient developed a partial small bowel obstruction 5 years after surgery.

Twenty-eight patients developed pneumonia, atelectasis, or prolonged ventilator dependence (20.7%). Twelve patients (8.9%) had significant cardiac complications, and 11 patients (8.1%) had neurologic dysfunction.

Patients who experienced abdominal complications were older (60.9 years old versus 48.2 years old) and were more likely to have a diagnosis of mediastinitis, have a history of prior abdominal surgeries, and require more transfusions, which indicated poorer overall condition. Intraoperative variables associated with a higher risk of complications were the use of a pedicled flap, extensive adhesiolysis, and enterotomies. Thirty-three percent of patients who received pedicle flaps experienced donor-site complications compared with 5.6% of the free flap group. Postoperative variables included the development of pulmonary complications, deep venous thrombosis, and neurologic complications.

Criticisms/Limitations   This was a retrospective case series; the study design limited the quality and reliability of the data. Although 13 different attending surgeons performed the reconstructions, all of the cases were performed within a single health care system. Only one omental flap was harvested laparoscopically, and therefore the complications related to that procedure cannot be compared with that of flaps harvested by laparotomy.

Relevant Studies   The use of pedicled omental flaps for chest wall reconstruction has been well described since the 1970s.[2] However, in many large series, an omental flap is still considered either a secondary choice or a "salvage" flap. In these series muscle and musculocutaneous flaps with latissimus dorsi, pectoralis major, rectus abdominis, serratus anterior, and others were used preferentially for chest wall reconstructions.[3-5] Several factors influence the choice of a muscle or musculocutaneous flap, including the location, previous operations, and size of the defect. For example, pectoralis major flaps are an excellent choice for anterior central chest defects, whereas a latissimus dorsi flap may be better suited for lateral or posterior defects. However, one must consider a previous thoracotomy scar in the use of the latissimus dorsi flap because the dominant thoracodorsal pedicle may have been disrupted. Likewise, a previous abdominal incision transecting the rectus muscle may rule out the use of a rectus abdominis flap. Overall, knowledge of and ability to perform a wide variety of flaps for chest wall coverage are crucial to having a proper arsenal for any clinical scenario.

The surgical technique for the omental flap is described by Hultman et al.[6] After the peritoneum is opened, adhesiolysis is performed if needed and the omentum is inspected for adequacy. Special attention is paid to the volume, surface area, and pedicle length. Typical omental dimensions are 14 to 36 cm in length and 23 to 46 cm in width.[7] The omentum is then dissected off of the transverse colon; the gastroepiploic arcade is preserved for blood supply. The short gastrics are divided, and the final blood supply to the flap can be based on the right, left, or both the right and left gastroepiploic arteries. If necessary, the omentum can be lengthened by using the arch of Barkow to "unwrap the flap." If a free tissue transfer is performed, the pedicle is then divided and the abdomen is closed. There are two options for pedicles flaps: the omentum may be transposed through a small defect in the rectus fascia or through a hole created in the diaphragm (Fig. 34-1). The omental flap can then either be buried under the flaps or covered with a split-thickness skin graft as necessary.

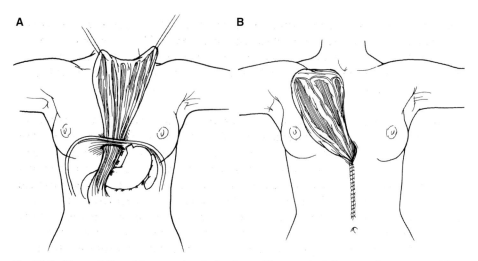

Fig. 34-1 Transposition of the omentum to the thorax. The arc of rotation permits coverage of the mediastinum, subclavian region, neck, and chest wall, via defects in the diaphragm **(A)** and the abdominal wall **(B)**. (From Hultman CS, Carlson GW, Losken A, et al. Utility of the omentum in the reconstruction of complex extraperitoneal wounds and defects: donor-site complications in 135 patients from 1975 to 2000. Ann Surg 235:782-795, 2002.)

The omental flap is especially well suited for use in an infected field, such as a deep sternal wound infection (DSWI). The omentum's robust lymphatic network and hearty vascular supply promote the transport of inflammatory cells to the area and help in fighting infection.[7,8] The mortality rate from a DSWI has been reported to range from 10% to 47% in the literature. The use of flap reconstruction for a DSWI should now be considered the standard of care; patients undergoing this treatment have significantly lower morbidity and mortality rates than patients treated with "traditional" debridement and closed drainage.[9] Stump et al[8] published data in 2010 suggesting that in diabetic patients, those patients who underwent pectoralis major flaps for DSWIs had 5.4 times increased risk of requiring reoperation for flap revision compared with those undergoing initial omentoplasty.

Laparoscopic harvest is not contraindicated in patients with prior abdominal surgery because laparoscopic adhesiolysis can be undertaken in most patients. In the technique described by Acarturk et al,[7] the omentum is separated from the greater curvature of the stomach with a harmonic scalpel before mobilization off of the transverse colon. A slit in the diaphragm is made beside the falciform ligament through the sternal defect, and the omentum is passed into the sternal cavity under laparoscopic visualization. It is then secured into place with sutures and covered either with pectoralis major flaps or a split-thickness skin graft.

The fear of potential intraabdominal complications such as infection, prolonged ileus or bowel obstruction, and ventral hernia may have limited the popularity of omental transposition in chest wall reconstructions. In this featured study, the donor-site complication rate is 18.5%.[1] However, other series have reported lower morbidity rates.[8] Although laparotomy was the historical approach for omental harvest, both laparoscopic and transdiaphragmatic omental harvests have been reported more recently, both with excellent results.[7,10]

The transdiaphragmatic approach to omental harvest promises the possibility of complete elimination of an abdominal incision. This technique has been described by Vyas et al[10] and was published in 2013. The authors describe a longitudinal incision in the anterior diaphragm large enough to admit the surgeon's hand into the peritoneal cavity (6 to 8 cm). The omentum and its attached transverse colon are then delivered into the chest, where the omentum is dissected off of the colon under direct vision. In this technique the omentum remains attached to the greater curvature of the stomach. If greater length is needed, the omentum on the left is brought into the chest, and the lateral splenic attachments and left gastroepiploic pedicle are divided. In their study the authors demonstrated a 28.3% shorter mean operating time and 44.3% lower mean blood loss compared with a standard laparotomy approach for omental harvest. In a small number of patients (nine), the omentum was tethered to a focal adhesion at the site of prior abdominal surgery. In these cases a small incision was required through the old scar for safe adhesiolysis. If there were overly extensive adhesions or any concern regarding bowel injury, a laparotomy was used instead for omental harvest.

In the reconstruction of chest wall defects, the plastic surgeon must consider both skeletal support and soft tissue coverage. Although bone and autogenous rib grafts were used historically, most authors today advocate the use of synthetic meshes (for example, Prolene, Marlex, Vicryl, polytetrafluoroethylene [PTFE], or methyl methacrylate) if needed to achieve rib cage or sternal stability.[3-5]

Summary   A wide variety of defects may be reconstructed with the omentum performed either as a pedicled flap or a free tissue transfer. The most common donor-site complications were ventral hernia, dehiscence, and abdominal wall infection. Advanced age, an impaired physiologic state, the use of a pedicled flap, previous abdominal surgery, mediastinitis, and postoperative pulmonary or neurologic complications increase the risk for donor-site complications. The recent introduction of laparoscopic and transdiaphragmatic techniques for omental harvest may ameliorate the risk of these complications.

Implications   The use of the omentum is an excellent option for a plastic surgeon confronted with a complex defect, especially of the orbit, face, or sternum. It may be used either as a primary flap in reconstruction or as a reliable option in the salvage of previously failed reconstructions with muscle or musculocutaneous flaps.

REFERENCES

1. Hultman CS, Carlson GW, Losken A, et al. Utility of the omentum in the reconstruction of complex extraperitoneal wounds and defects: donor-site complications in 135 patients from 1975 to 2000. Ann Surg 235:782-795, 2002.
2. Jurkiewicz MJ, Arnold PG. The omentum: an account of its use in the reconstruction of the chest wall. Ann Surg 185:548-554, 1977.
3. Arnold PG, Pairolero PC. Chest-wall reconstruction: an account of 500 consecutive patients. Plast Reconstr Surg 98:804-810, 1996.
4. Mansour KA, Thourani VH, Losken A, et al. Chest wall resections and reconstruction: a 25-year experience. Ann Thorac Surg 73:1720-1726; discussion 1725-1726, 2002.
5. Losken A, Thourani VH, Carlson GW, et al. A reconstructive algorithm for plastic surgery following extensive chest wall resection. Br J Plast Surg 57:295-302, 2004.
6. Hultman CS, Culbertson JH, Jones GE, et al. Thoracic reconstruction with the omentum: indications, complications, and results. Ann Plast Surg 46:242-249, 2001.
7. Acarturk TO, Schwartz WM, Luketich J, et al. Laparoscopically harvested omental flap for chest wall and intrathoracic reconstruction. Ann Plast Surg 53:210-216, 2004.
8. Stump A, Bedri M, Goldberg N, et al. Omental transposition flap for sternal wound reconstruction in diabetic patients. Ann Plast Surg 65:206-210, 2010.
9. Singh K, Anderson E, Harper JG. Overview and management of sternal wound infection. Semin Plast Surg 25:25-33, 2011.
10. Vyas RM, Prsic A, Orgill DP. Transdiaphragmatic omental harvest: a simple, efficient method for sternal wound coverage. Plast Reconstr Surg 131:544-552, 2013.
11. Kiricuta I. Use of the Omentum in Plastic Surgery. New York: Pergamon Press, 1980.

STUDY AUTHOR REFLECTIONS

C. Scott Hultman, MD, MBA, FACS

Maurice "Josh" John Jurkiewicz, Chief Emeritus when I trained at Emory, had a love affair with the omentum.

Even when other flaps were indicated based on the size or location of the wound, I knew what he was secretly thinking: "I wonder if the omentum would be a good flap for this defect?" I too shared his enthusiasm, even rapture, for this flap and for good reason. Just like we know that the omentum is "the policeman of the abdomen," the omentum can be used to reconstruct an extremely wide range of extraperitoneal defects. With its rich supply of mesenchymal stem cells, angiogenic growth factors, lymphocytes and macrophages, and lymphatic channels, the omentum is the flap I choose for the most complex of infected, irradiated, and ischemic wounds because of its large surface area, pliability, malleable volume, generous pedicle length, and redundant and reliable blood supply. Our paper, which is a summary of Dr. J's experience, demonstrated that the donor-site complication rate was real but acceptable.

Dr. J always gave credit to the Romanian surgeon Ion Kiricuta[11] for discovering so many indications for the omental flap, but Dr. J popularized this flap in the United States and demonstrated how powerful this flap could be in solving diverse surgical problems that previously had no solution. Much of the clinical work was done by Dr. J's faculty members: John Coleman, John Bostwick, P.G. Arnold, Foad Nahai, Luis Vasconez, and Rod Hester. Dr. J's success as a plastic surgeon was enormous, allowing him to rise to President of the American College of Surgeons, but he would always tell us that he was really in the business of developing and educating the next generation of surgical thinkers. He followed a basic but too often forgotten model of leadership: pick really good people, make sure they have some basic resources, and get out of their way.

John Bostwick told me perhaps the best story about Dr. J. While traveling with the boss to present a paper at a national meeting, the two boarded an airplane, sat together, and the flight attendant asked them what they did. Excited about the trip and his recent promotion to assistant professor, Bostwick proudly answered, "I am a plastic surgeon at Emory." Dr. J responded, "I am the teacher."

CHAPTER 35

Body Contouring by Lipolysis: A 5-Year Experience With Over 3000 Cases

Illouz YG. Plast Reconstr Surg 72:591-597, 1983

Reviewed by Cindy Wu, MD

> *The concept of modifying the body contour with liposuction by developing numerous subcutaneous "tunnels" with subsequent homogenous contractions of the overlying skin will add a new dimension to the plastic surgeons' armamentarium. Successful correction of these deformities can be obtained without a large amount of surgical undermining and skin resection and with minimal scar formation.[1]*

Research Question   Is there a less invasive method of body contouring other than the older methods of direct excision or curettage?

Funding   Not applicable

Study Dates   June 1977 to June 1982

Publishing Date   November 1983

Location   Paris, France

Subjects   3447 total procedures on 1326 patients, 1073 (or 81%) of whom had multiple procedures; 1140 (86%) had "saddle bags," 519 (39%) knees, 477 (36%) gluteal folds, 424 (32%) buttocks, 384 (29%) hips, 291 (22%) abdomen, 159 (12%) ankles, and 53 (4%) double chins, arms, gynecomastia, inner thighs, or thorax.

Exclusion Criteria   Patients without lipodystrophy

Sample Size   1326 patients

Study Design   Patients with localized lipodystrophies who underwent tumescence and liposuction of concerning areas

215

Procedure   Patients were marked with topographic marks while standing. General anesthesia was induced. The areas were tumesced with 100 mL of normal saline solution + 20 mL of distilled water + 100 units of hyaluronidase (to aid in solution diffusion). Patients were allowed to sit for a few minutes. A 1 cm incision was made for cannula insertion: for saddle bags, buttocks, and hips, the incision was made in the medial buttock fold; for the abdomen, the periumbilical or suprapubic area; for the knees, the popliteal fold; for the ankle, the lateral part of the Achilles tendon; for the chin, a 0.5 cm incision in the lateral fold under the chin; and for the arms, the axilla. A blunt, rounded tip cannula with the side port facing away from the skin was used for liposuction to the endpoint of bloody aspirate. Tunneling was performed at a depth of at least 1 cm under the skin but 2 cm in the saddle bag area to preserve "the natural curvature of the hips." Tunnel channels were placed in a "spokes of a wheel" pattern.

Postoperative Care   The wound was drained for 48 hours, during which the patient was hospitalized. Elastoplast bandages for compression remained on until postoperative day 7. Drains were removed after 48 hours. No hematomas were noted. The use of a blunt cannula in a "tunnel" fashion with no undermining minimized postoperative problems because the major vessels and lymphatics were preserved. Patients were out of bed on postoperative day 1 and could return to work 1 week after surgery after the bandages were removed. Patients were warned that the most painful area was the abdomen and the least painful area was the saddle bag area. Physical therapy was advised to avoid subcutaneous sclerosing. Massage therapy was continued for 3 weeks, and patients were warned that their swelling may persist for 3 to 4 weeks and gradually disappear. Ecchymosis usually resolved in 2 weeks.

Caution   The author limited the amount of fat removed at one time to no more than 6 pounds to avoid shock. As soon as more than 4 pounds of fat were aspirated, intravenous fluids, blood, or plasma may be necessary.

Follow-up   Unclear

Endpoints   Until a reasonable aesthetic contour was obtained

Results   Early in the author's experience, he noted postoperative skin excess in the saddle bag area, which did not occur in other treated areas. Illouz hypothesized that "perhaps the skin of the outer aspect of the thigh does not slide upon the subcutaneous area and adhesions create this unsightly phenomenon. This does not seem to happen in other areas of the body, such as the hips and knees, and perhaps this is due to the constant massaging of these areas with every movement and the buttocks with constant massaging from normal movement and sitting. Therefore, it is important to be most careful in 'riding breeches' deformities to make the skin tunnels deeper, a minimum of 2.5 cm beneath the skin."

Illouz noted that later in his experience, the excess skin seen in the beginning of the author's experience in the saddle bag area was not as frequent of a complication because of the use of deeper level tunnels. He attributed this smoother contour to "the scarring retraction of the numerous channels (which) gives the skin the appearance of multiple small waves that absorb all the excessive skin with a smooth contour."

Criticisms/Limitations   A single surgeon's experience, observer bias, no control group, no patient satisfaction survey, no results table, and no complications listed

Current Relevant Research   In the November 1983 issue of *Plastic and Reconstructive Surgery,* several European and American innovators presented their experience with liposuction, which had previously been performed in Europe and was being introduced in the United States.

Teimourian[2] (United States) described submental and facial liposuction before rhytidectomy for the correction of submental and facial lipodystrophy.

Fournier and Otteni[3] (France) proposed liposuction with the "dry technique" without tumescence as Illouz had described. They showed that the fat lobules from either technique were histologically identical and that the adipocytes were undamaged and not emulsified. They described several advantages, including less time, less tissue distortion, and no hyaluronidase sensitivity. The only disadvantage was that with a hasty liposuction, blood pressure can fall quickly, requiring volume replacement.

Kesselring[4] (Switzerland) reported on his experience with liposuction with the use of his "Aspiradeps" cannula.

Reed[5] (United States) discussed that the success of this procedure depended on proper patient selection. The ideal liposuction candidate is young, with well-localized fat, and has good skin tone. It cannot make a fat person thin, and it is strictly a contouring procedure. The selection of treatment site is also important. Only sites with localized fat deposits and good skin tone perform well (for example, the riding breeches deformity and the abdomen). The arms and inner thighs perform less well. Finally, the decision on how much fat to remove is important.

Grazer[6] (United States) described the evolution of liposuction. Unpublished French references that date back to the mid-1920s described attempts to curette fat from a patient's knees, which resulted in infection and amputation. No further references are found until the early 1960s. The first generation of liposuction began with Dr. Josef Schrudde, Professor of Plastic Surgery in Cologne, West Germany, who started curettage of the hips, thighs, knees, and ankles through a small incision. He presented this at the first International Society of Aesthetic Plastic Surgery in Rio de Janeiro in 1972.[7] He called this "lipexeresis." The second generation of liposuction was introduced by Kesselring[4] (Switzerland) and Fischer and Fischer[8] (Italy). Both attached suction to curettage instruments. Illouz marked the third generation of liposuction when he described "lipolysis," which referenced his injection of hypotonic solution for cell lysis before aspiration. Grazer stated[6] that the fourth generation was about to begin with the expansion of the indications for liposuction into the reconstructive realm, such as the curettage of flaps, aspiration of tumors (lipomas), and removal of liquid silicone. He suggested that instead of rushing out to try this innovative procedure without the proper patient selection, the novice surgeon should try these techniques by aspirating the abdominoplasty flap first and then performing the traditional abdominoplasty.

Robert Goldwyn,[9] the editor of the journal *Plastic and Reconstructive Surgery,* described the characteristic sequence of events after a new surgical method arises. He pointed out the advantages of liposuction but cautioned plastic surgeons to be aware of its complications. He then conjectured on possible research questions that may arise from liposuction and ended with this quote: "If being slim is easily attainable, and if everyone becomes thin, the trend will undoubtedly be in the other direction. I shall let some other editor deal with those social repercussions of liposuction."

Summary and Implications   Illouz's technique is the foundation of how liposuction is performed today. Although there were other previous techniques of fat removal with curettage and aspiration, Illouz's contribution of tumescence made liposuction safer to perform. It transformed liposuction into a less traumatizing technique with minimal hospitalization. It was shown to be a versatile technique that can be applied to lipodystrophy in the submental area, cheek, inner thighs, and arms and can treat gynecomastia.

An important discovery was that liposuction resulted in ablation of fatty deposits with no recurrence, as evidenced by no recurrence even after pregnancy. This confirmed the theory of a fixed amount of adipocytes after puberty, and after they are removed, there is no recurrence.

REFERENCES

1. Illouz YG. Body contouring by lipolysis: a 5-year experience with over 3000 cases. Plast Reconstr Surg 72:591-597, 1983.
2. Teimourian B. Face and neck suction-assisted lipectomy associated with rhytidectomy. Plast Reconstr Surg 72:627-633, 1983.
    The author describes the indications, technique, and postoperative outcomes of face and neck liposuction.
3. Fournier PF, Otteni FM. Lipodissection in body sculpturing: the dry procedure. Plast Reconstr Surg 72:598-609, 1983.
    In this article the authors compare their technique of dry liposuction with Illouz's wet technique. As a supporting statement for their technique, they state that histologically, fat lobules collected from cannulas not connected to suction are undamaged and unemulsified and have the same appearance whether the wet or dry technique is used. One could argue that the better experiment would have been to perform histology when the suction had been applied during both the wet and dry techniques.

4. Kesselring UK. Regional fat aspiration for body contouring. Plast Reconstr Surg 72:610-619, 1983.

   The author reports his experience with the Aspiradeps cannula, which is a series of straight and angled liposuction cannulas that he developed and published in Plastic and Reconstructive Surgery *in 1978.*

5. Reed LS. Some thoughts on suction-assisted lipectomy. Plast Reconstr Surg 72:624-626, 1983.

   The author warns beginning liposuction practitioners to exercise caution when implementing this new technique into their practice and that intelligent patient selection is critical to success.

6. Grazer FM. Suction-assisted lipectomy, suction lipectomy, lipolysis and lipexeresis. Plast Reconstr Surg 72:620-623, 1983.

   The author details the history of liposuction up until the current journal publication.

7. Schrudde J. Lipexeresis as a means of eliminating local adiposity. Aesthetic Plast Surg 4:215-226, 1980.

8. Fischer A, Fischer GM. Revised technique for cellulitis fat reduction in riding-breeches deformity. Bull Int Acad Cosmet Surg 2:40-42, 1977.

9. Goldwyn RM. The advent of liposuction [editorial]. Plast Reconstr Surg 72:705, 1983.

   The author gives his opinion of the then new procedure and hypothesizes about the future directions of liposuction.

STUDY AUTHOR REFLECTIONS

Yves-Gérard Illouz, MD, FACS

The article I wrote in 1983 was not my first one on liposuction. I wrote many articles published in French scientific journals in 1978, 1980, and 1981 since I discovered liposuction in 1977. Before me, others tried to remove fat. Here are the highlights:

- In 1921 Professor Charles Dujarrier in France attempted to remove subcutaneous fat from the leg of a dancer and removed too much skin. The sutures were too tight and induced compression of the tibial artery, which resulted in necrosis of the leg and ultimately amputation. This was the first trial involving cosmetic surgery in the world. Professor Dujarrier was convicted at the first trial but won on appeal because he was not doing the surgery for money but only for scientific purposes in a charity hospital. Because of that event, cosmetic surgery and especially body contouring had a bad reputation for a long time.

- In 1976 Fischer in Italy performed curettage of fat with a sharp instrument that induced huge serohematomas and the formation of a cavity with a pseudocapsule, inducing a "skippering" of the skin.

- At the same time, Kesselring in Switzerland also performed curettage with a very sharp uterine curette and had the same problems as Fischer. All these techniques were not liposuction (only Fischer used a vacuum to remove the "mud" produced by the curettage, but not to remove fat).

- In 1977 I started to do liposuction with a tunneling technique in an area infused by a solution used to soften and magnify the fat layer and to avoid bleeding. This tunneling technique respected the vessels and nerves and thus never induced any complications such as hematomas or seromas—only ecchymosis and edema.
- Fournier observed me for 5 years and had the idea to avoid the infiltration altogether. He proposed a "dry technique," which quickly became obsolete.
- In 1980 Dr. Norman Martin from the United States came to see me in Paris and was stunned to see the fat coming out like soft butter. Norman Martin was speaking about my technique in the United States at a meeting, and I received a phone call from four American plastic surgeons: Dr. Frederick Grazer from California, Dr. Gregory Hetter from Las Vegas, and two others who wanted to come to Paris to see me. When Drs. Grazer and Hetter came in 1982 and saw the fat coming out, Grazer invited me to the next meeting of the American Society of Plastic and Reconstructive Surgery in October 1982 in Hawaii (he was the chairman of a session on body contouring and told me he would give me his time to speak because the program was already set). I gave my speech in Hawaii on the last day of the meeting. I was told that the large room of 2000 seats was full, including a multitude of people standing. After my speech, the board of directors asked to speak with me and said they would come to Paris to learn my technique. The blue ribbon committee of 14 members arrived in December, and I showed them a great number of cases. They published a favorable report in January 1983. After that, I have come to the United States many times to teach my techniques.

Burn Surgery

The Treatment of the Surface Burns

Cope O. Ann Surg 117:885-893, 1943

Reviewed by Jonathan S. Friedstat, MD

> *On Saturday evening, November 28, 1942 . . . a disastrous fire occurred in the Cocoanut Grove, a Boston nightclub . . . Of the casualties, dead and living, 114 were brought to the Massachusetts General Hospital within a period of two hours.*[1]

As in many disasters, the type of injury encountered in the casualties of the Cocoanut Grove fire conformed to a pattern. The lungs and airways were severely damaged, perhaps both by heat and irritating gases. The external burns were for the most part limited to skin surfaces not covered by clothing.

The treatment used on the burns of the skin was unorthodox but the results were gratifying. Its simplicity has much to recommend when large numbers of burn are encountered in a disaster.[1,2]

Research Question   How effective is simple burn wound care and dressings during a burn mass casualty scenario?

Funding   Harvard Medical School

Study Dates   November 1942 to June 1943

Publishing Date   June 1943

Location   Massachusetts General Hospital, Boston, MA

Subjects   One hundred fourteen patients from the Cocoanut Grove Night Club fire were brought to both the public and private wards of Massachusetts General Hospital for treatment.

Exclusion Criteria   None

Interruption of Therapy Criteria   None

Sample Size   Thirty-nine of 114 patients survived the initial minutes to receive treatment of their burns at Massachusetts General Hospital.

Overview of Design   This was not a formal study but rather a case review. The treatment protocol is shown in Fig. 36-1.

Intervention   Patients underwent a simplified dressing and wound care regimen for the treatment of their surface burns. When patients arrived in the emergency department, they were placed onto sterile bedding. Their wounds were not debrided or scrubbed as was common at the time. Instead, they were given intravenous colloid plasma resuscitation, had their burn wounds covered with boric ointment, received intravenous sodium sulfadiazine, and were followed on the floor. Dressing changes were performed starting at hospital days 5 to 10 and continued with either wet boric acid or normal saline dressings until the full-thickness burn was debrided. With a healthy-appearing granulation tissue base, the wounds then underwent skin grafting.

Follow-up   None

Endpoints   None

Results   There are limited results from this paper. Thirty-nine patients were treated according to this protocol. Cope and colleagues provided the rationale for their treatments to explain why they were different from the "normal" standards. They used a

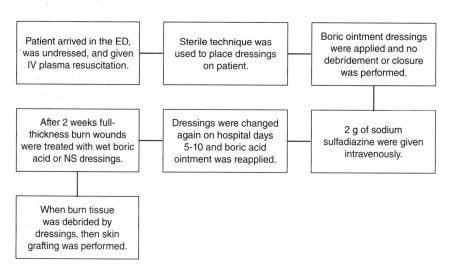

Fig. 36-1   Treatment protocol. *ED,* Emergency department; *NS,* normal saline.

simplified wound care regimen because they believed it was equivalent to traditional methods and therefore would be better in a mass casualty scenario. Wounds were not debrided, and blisters were not unroofed because they believed this would increase the risk of violating the epithelium and resulting infection.

Although extremely limited data were submitted from patients treated for the Cocoanut Grove fire, the question of whether to debride blisters in burn wounds still remains unresolved. Similarly, they described their rationale for the use of boric acid ointment because prior studies demonstrated an ability to prevent pyogenic infections. Splinting was used for some burns, and the outer layers of the splint were composed of rolled newspaper.

Patient data were limited after the fire. Sixteen patients were discharged and had their wounds healed by 15 days after the fire, which suggested they had partial-thickness wounds. One patient was transferred to a naval hospital with an ankle burn. Seven patients died of pulmonary complications, which were likely related to inhalational injury, and four patients with pulmonary complications survived and were discharged by hospital day 32. One patient suffered an anoxic brain injury and remained in the hospital until discharge on hospital day 67. Ten patients had third-degree burns that were treated, with the last patient discharged on hospital day 143.

Criticisms/Limitations   This study was performed without randomization or control subjects, much less institutional review board approval, as would be accepted practice by today's standards. This would be best described as a retrospective case series that examined whether a simplified burn dressing regimen impacted the results. Very limited data were included in this paper, but it describes important concepts in burn disaster management and wound care.

Relevant Studies   Although this study lacked much of what is considered standard for influential papers today, the publications generated from the Cocoanut Grove Night Club fire composed one of the most important collections of papers in early burn care. These papers are significant because they described study core concepts in the treatment of burn patients that at the time were either not understood well or just starting to be studied. Other important publications included key articles on inhalational injury and metabolic response to burn injuries.[3,4] The Cocoanut Grove Night Club fire created a foundation for larger changes in fire prevention with building regulations.

In my opinion, the most important paper from the Cocoanut Grove was the description of inhalational injury, which was one of the first in the literature.[4] It was the first time health care providers identified inhalational injury and its contribution to morbidity and mortality in burn patients. This manifested in part because of hypoxia and additional fluid during resuscitation.

"The pulmonary lesions in the casualties of the Cocoanut Grove disaster were unexpected and complicated the care of the shock . . . Carbon monoxide poisoning with its bright cherry-red color of the burn surfaces and mucous membranes, and the inflammation of the burned lungs and airways were quickly detected, but there was a delay in recognizing that the resulting anoxia was the cause of the mania in some of the patients."[2]

After the evaluation of the initial 15 patients, they realized that some "pulmonary pathology" occurred in burn patients from the fire. The initial thoughts were that the injuries were from a blast, but on talking to survivors from the fire with minor injuries, they learned none had occurred. They correctly concluded that "irritating fumes and heat were the cause of the pulmonary inflammation."[2]

Another key area that was already being studied at Massachusetts General Hospital was the changes in metabolism that occur during burn injury. At the time of the fire, they and other researchers were aware that after some burn injuries, there was a rise in blood glucose levels. They believed that it came from a hormone in the adrenal glands but had not yet identified it. They were also able to follow nitrogen balance in 29 patients from this fire. Cope noted that nitrogen balance correlated closely with caloric and nitrogen intake. During the initial treatment, patients experienced negative nitrogen balance, and with caloric support this pattern changed later in their hospital stay. They even considered whether testosterone supplementation would be beneficial. The description by Cope et al of the metabolic changes in burn patients and their curiosity about some steroid treatments were well ahead of its time.[3]

Today our understanding of burn resuscitation is much different than at the time of this publication. It was believed that prolonged pain contributed to burn shock, and therefore patients were given morphine early in their burn evaluation. Some of the side effects of morphine and its effect on respiratory suppression were not totally appreciated and may have contributed to some patient's respiratory complications. There were concerns that anesthesia precipitated shock in burn patients; this made the notion of avoiding anesthetics and not debriding burn wounds initially rather appealing. Also, it was not realized that the hypoxia from patients' carbon monoxide poisoning and inhalational injury could manifest as altered mental status and add additional complexity to a patient's resuscitation.[4]

Burn shock was "defined as low blood pressure shock, with hemoconcentration and diminished blood volume due to loss of plasma fluid into the burn area." They used 1:1 plasma crystalloid mixture to resuscitate patients, and the level of hemoconcentration guided the fluid rate.[4] This work established a foundation for further work on fluid resuscitation and led to one of the first published guidelines for burn fluid resuscitation in 1947 by Cope and Moore.[5]

There were other important advancements learned from this disaster that were not published by Cope. Patients at Massachusetts General Hospital were treated together on their own ward where separate areas were established for burn and wound care. Although this was a new idea at the time, in today's burn practice such treatment is considered the standard of care. Other papers published from this disaster focused on the psychiatric needs of burn survivors.[6,7] These considerations are remarkable not only because they are still in practice today, but demonstrate the tremendous breadth of knowledge gained from this disaster.[6]

Summary   The Cocoanut Grove Night Club fire was one of the most significant early burn disasters in U.S. history. From work first published at Massachusetts General Hospital and later by Boston Medical Center, this disaster introduced many concepts that are considered major pillars of burn care today. These areas include the importance of burn wound management, fluid resuscitation, metabolic response to injury, and most notably inhalational injury.

Implications   This paper demonstrated the success of a simple burn wound dressing regimen in the treatment of large numbers of burn patients after a disaster. From the larger set of publications by Cope and colleagues on the Cocoanut Grove Night Club fire, they identified inhalational injury and its challenges with fluid resuscitation. Also, they contributed to the foundation of knowledge of burn fluid administration and the understanding of metabolic changes in burn patients. The practices of isolating burn patients from other patients in the hospital, given their needs for wound care and susceptibility to infection, were noteworthy. Health care providers also identified the mental health needs of burn survivors, which still remain a challenge today. Finally, the larger epidemiologic factors of fire code regulations, disaster planning, triage, public safety, and firefighting also underwent improvements as a result of this disaster.

REFERENCES

1. Cope O. The treatment of the surface burns. Ann Surg 117:885-893, 1943.
2. Cope O. Management of the Cocoanut Grove burns at the Massachusetts General Hospital. Ann Surg 117: 801-802, 1943.
3. Cope O, Nathanson IT, Rourke GM, et al. Metabolic observations. Ann Surg 117: 937-958, 1943.
4. Cope O, Rhinelander FW. The problem of burn shock complicated by pulmonary damage. Ann Surg 117: 915-928. 1943.
5. Cope O, Moore FD. The redistribution of body water and the fluid therapy of the burned patient. Ann Surg 126:1010-1045, 1947.
6. Saffle JR. The 1942 fire at Boston's Cocoanut Grove nightclub. Am J Surg 166:581-591, 1993.
7. Stewart CL. The fire at Cocoanut Grove. J Burn Care Res. 2014 Aug 4. [Epub ahead of print]

EXPERT COMMENTARY

Robert L. Sheridan, MD, FAAP, FACS

Necessity is the mother of invention. Nowhere is that more clearly illustrated than the creative responses of surgeons to the casualties of wars and disasters. When faced with an unexpected influx of patients from the Cocoanut Grove fire, Oliver Cope and his colleagues improvised with available resources. They were able to creatively address the three major causes of acute burn mortality: burn shock, respiratory failure, and wound sepsis. They identified burn shock and began the discussion of the resuscitation interventions that evolved into the formulas of later years. They recognized inhalation injury as an important independent clinical problem and paved the way for today's respiratory interventions. They acknowledged the role of wound sepsis in late burn mortality and fashioned strategies to address this with topical and surgical interventions. Defining problems is the first step to solving them. We owe Oliver Cope and colleagues the recognition for defining the major problem set facing acutely burned patients.

CHAPTER 37

The Use of a Topical Sulfonamide in the Control of Burn Wound Sepsis

Moncrief JA, Lindberg RB, Switzer WE, Pruitt BA Jr. J Trauma 6:407-419, 1966

Reviewed by Jonathan S. Friedstat, MD

> *The determination that the waxy-white, insensitive, soft burn is indeed a very deep dermal burn may very well be the crux of the entire matter under these circumstances. Without effective topical therapy these wounds would be converted to full-thickness loss and become the site of invasive bacterial infection.[1]*

Research Question Prior animal and human studies demonstrated that 10% mafenide acetate (Sulfamylon) cream offered protection from burn sepsis. Would a prospective study of a similar treatment regimen demonstrate promising results?

Funding Department of Defense

Study Dates January 1964 to June 1965

Publishing Date May 1966

Location U.S. Army Surgical Research Unit, Brooke Army Medical Center, Fort Sam Houston, TX

Subjects During this time, 247 patients were treated at their burn center, 190 of whom received treatment with Sulfamylon. The study was a prospective, controlled before-after design comparing patients treated with Sulfamylon (1964 to 1965) with prior surgical patients as control subjects (1955 to 1963).

Exclusion Criteria None

Interruption of Therapy Criteria Treatment was held for 48 to 72 hours if patients developed metabolic acidosis from Sulfamylon's inhibition of carbonic anhydrase.

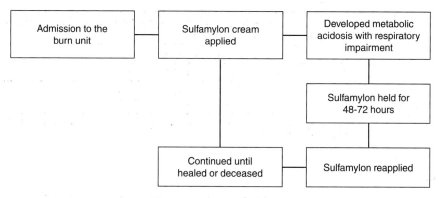

Fig. 37-1   Treatment protocol.

This time period had been studied previously in animal models by the authors, and there was no decrease in Sulfamylon's antimicrobial efficacy.

Sample Size   Two hundred forty-seven patients were treated in their burn center and 190 received Sulfamylon.

Overview of Design   The treatment protocol is shown in Fig. 37-1.

Intervention   All burn patients underwent fluid resuscitation, wound cleaning, shaving, and debridement. Wounds were covered with Sulfamylon cream and applied to completely cover the burn wound with overlap just onto normal skin. They were washed in either a Hubbard tank or whirlpool and debrided regularly, with the frequency and intensity of debridement increasing with time. Pain control was accomplished with meperidine (Demerol) or morphine.

Follow-up   Patients were followed during their hospital stay until discharge.

Endpoints   Mortality rates overall and by etiology were compared.

Results   There were 247 patients with an overall mortality rate of 20.2% in this study. This included six patients who died but never received Sulfamylon. Of the 190 patients who received Sulfamylon, the average total body surface area (TBSA) was 36.35% and the mortality rate was 17.8%. These results were compared with 474 burn patients treated from 1960 to 1963 without Sulfamylon. During this time, the average TBSA ranged from 31.69% to 40.98% and the mortality rate ranged from 35.22% to 38.5%. Mortality rates were significantly reduced in patients with 50% TBSA burns or less with the use of Sulfamylon (Table 37-1).[1]

Table 37-1   Total Body Surface Area Versus Mortality in the Pre–Sulfamylon-Treated (1960 to 1963) and Sulfamylon-Treated (1964 to 1965) Groups

	Percentage of Total Body Surface Area				
	0%-30%	30%-40%	40%-50%	60%-70%	70+%
1960-1963 (n = 474)	4.3%	42.1%	61.9%	78.3%	93.7%
1964-1965 (n = 247)	0%	3%	40.9%	86.6%	91.3%

Data from Moncrief JA, Lindberg RB, Switzer WE, et al. The use of a topical sulfonamide in the control of burn wound sepsis. J Trauma 6:407-419, 1966.

Data were also reviewed on burns with 30% to 60% TBSA from 1961 to 1965 to evaluate how overall mortality, mortality from wound sepsis, and other causes compared. In the pre-Sulfamylon time period, the mortality rate ranged from 51.7% to 56.8%, mortality from burn wound sepsis was 31.0% to 35.3%, and mortality from other causes was 20.1% to 21.5%. In the Sulfamylon treatment time period, the overall mortality rate was 22.6%, mortality from burn wound sepsis was 4.8%, and mortality from other causes was 17.9%. The authors correctly stated that "if burn wound sepsis were the primary lethal factor in the pre-Sulfamylon era, control of burn wound sepsis should result in a mortality rate the same as the due to other causes."[1]

Criticisms/Limitations   It is a dramatic example of how a successful intervention can change outcomes in a prospective before-after study design. One thing that is not mentioned in the paper is why all 247 patients did not receive Sulfamylon. One possibility is that some had superficial burns that were treated with other techniques (for example, bacitracin). Despite this, 190 patients is still a large sample size, which make the results of this intervention even more impressive.

Relevant Studies   This work represents an important time, during the early 1960s, in the development of burn surgery as a specialty. As Dr. Hartford's Presidential Address from the American Burn Association described the difficulties of treating burn patients: "Burn care was not a popular surgical sport. There were only a few organized burn care efforts and in many institutions the lot of the burned patient was rather dismal. If the patient did survive it was often in spite of the treatment rendered. Burn wards were known for the malodorous stench emanating from rotting eschar and weak, cachectic patients who displayed an air of hopelessness."[2]

In the early 1960s work by Moncrief and Teplitz[3] began to establish criteria for burn wound sepsis. Their work on postmortem tissue samples from burn patients identified quantitate features (>100,000 organisms per gram of tissue) and microscopic findings of burn wound sepsis (bacterial invasion and destruction of adjacent unburned tissue).

They also demonstrated that bacteria within burn wounds rapidly colonize the wounds and reach 10^5 colonies in 4 to 5 days.[4,5] These findings created some of the context for their search to treat burn wounds topically and control bacterial proliferation, particularly against *Pseudomonas aeruginosa*. Their search for a topical agent that could penetrate burn eschars, reach therapeutic concentrations, and remain nontoxic ultimately led to the selection of mafenide, an agent first used by Germany during World War II.[2] The initial human studies of mafenide began in 1963. From there work continued at the U.S. Army Surgical Research Unit, and the results of this paper followed shortly thereafter.

What is interesting is that while Moncrief, Pruitt, and others were doing this work, in an independent and unknown fashion Carl Moyer was also performing work that would lead to another major topical antimicrobial, 0.5% silver nitrate. It is worth noting that Moyer et al were the first to publish a paper on silver nitrate in June 1965.[6]

Moyer's work on silver nitrate was motivated by different observations. Moyer began his paper by describing the clinical observations of patients who were treated with a circulating water bath with Locke's solution, which was one of the first attempts at topical antimicrobials. He noted that patients had no pain and remained hydrated when in this isotonic salt solution. The main problem was that bacterial growth occurred rapidly in these tanks despite efforts to keep the solution clean.

From this attempted treatment, Moyer identified some important observations, which included that (1) burn wounds are painless when covered in an isotonic solution, (2) fluid and electrolyte problems seen with dry dressings and exposing burn wounds to air do not occur when patients are in the bath, (3) patients could maintain their weight with burns <60% of TBSA with oral intake alone when kept in the bath, and (4) burn eschar could be removed painlessly and without blood loss. After a safe, nontoxic, soluble salt was identified, Moyer et al[6] were able to identify 0.5% silver nitrate.

The seminal work of Moyer et al was followed by the efforts of Moncrief et al, who also developed animal sepsis models, which further supported his clinical findings. Both authors noted significant basic concepts in burn wounds as they wrote about topical antimicrobial therapy. Moncrief and his team identified quantifiable numbers of bacteria present in tissue, their rate of development, and a colony count in tissue in patients with burn wound sepsis. Moyer emphasized the need to consider the physiologic equilibrium between the patient and a topical solution. Both emphasized meticulous wound care. All of these considerations remain relevant today.

Summary This paper demonstrated the effectiveness of topical Sulfamylon cream in reducing the mortality rate from burn wound sepsis. The results were most dramatic in burns smaller than 50% TBSA, and they were able to decrease the mortality rate to that from other causes (for example, pneumonia). It also highlighted the challenges in reducing the mortality rate from other causes and in treating larger TBSA burns, which still continue to challenge burn providers today.

Implications This was one of the first large human studies to demonstrate the effectiveness of topical antimicrobial therapy in controlling burn wound sepsis. Work pioneered by Moncrief and Moyer helped establish the effectiveness of topical antimicrobial therapy in the treatment of burn wounds, which is still a fundamental component of burn care today.

REFERENCES

1. Moncrief JA, Lindberg RB, Switzer WE, et al. The use of a topical sulfonamide in the control of burn wound sepsis. J Trauma 6:407-419, 1966.
2. Hartford CE. The bequests of Moncrief and Moyer: an appraisal of topical therapy of burns—1981 American Burn Association Presidential Address. J Trauma 21:827-834, 1981.
3. Moncrief JA, Teplitz C. Changing concepts in burn sepsis. J Trauma 4:233-245, 1964.
4. Teplitz C, Davis D, Mason AD Jr, et al. *Pseudomonas* burn wound sepsis. I Pathogenesis of experimental *Pseudomonas* burn wound sepsis. J Surg Res 4:200-216, 1964.
5. Teplitz C, Davis D, Walker HL, et al. *Pseudomonas* burn wound sepsis. II Hematogenous infection at the junction of the burn wound and the unburned hypodermis. J Surg Res 4:217-222, 1964.
6. Moyer CA, Brentano L, Gravens DL, et al. Treatment of large human burns with 0.5% silver nitrate solution. Arch Surg 90:812-867, 1965.

STUDY AUTHOR REFLECTIONS

Basil A. Pruitt, Jr., MD, FACS, FCCM, MCCM

The material in this article was initially presented at the 1965 annual meeting of the American Association for the Surgery of Trauma to confirm, on the basis of 18 months of use, the effectiveness of Sulfamylon burn cream in controlling burn wound sepsis. The reviewer has perceptively used his review of this article to illustrate the differences in the contemporaneous development of Sulfamylon burn cream and 0.5% silver nitrate soaks for the topical control of invasive bacterial burn wound invasion.

The comparable effectiveness of the two agents when application can be initiated promptly after injury is cited, but no mention is made about the lesser effectiveness of silver nitrate soaks when treatment is delayed and bacteria have penetrated the eschar. Precipitation of the silver on contact with any proteinaceous material prevents eschar penetration, which makes the unaffected intraeschar bacteria potential causes of invasive infection. Conversely, the mafenide in Sulfamylon burn cream can diffuse into the eschar and exert better control of the intraeschar bacterial burden.

The reviewer has pointed out that the article includes a brief history of mafenide, cites the laboratory studies that preceded clinical use, and describes the limitations and complications related to Sulfamylon burn cream. The clinical use of Sulfamylon burn cream is detailed as are the treatment modifications used to reduce the risk of or correct complications associated with its use. In that context, the subsequent change of the sulfonamide component from mafenide hydrochloride to mafenide acetate to reduce the risk of acidosis might have been mentioned.

The reviewer questions the exclusion of 57 of the 247 burn patients admitted during the study period. To address that I recall the exclusion of patients with other than flame and scald burns, patients with toxic epidermal necrolysis syndrome, and patients admitted late with largely healed burns. There may have been other exclusions that I do not recall at this time. The reviewer also notes, as did the article, that the increased survival was most evident in patients with burns of less than 60% of the total body surface. It should be noted that the survival benefit was extended to patients with more extensive burns when early burn wound excision was combined with initial topical antimicrobial chemotherapy.

In short, the reviewer has well summarized this article, which documented the effectiveness of Sulfamylon burn cream in controlling burn wound sepsis. The review also illustrates the effectiveness of integrated clinical/laboratory research in which a problem of clinical importance is identified at the bedside, taken to the laboratory where a model was developed, and used to identify a solution to the problem, which was then returned to the bedside.

EXPERT COMMENTARY

Interview With Anthony A. Meyer, MD, PhD, FACS, FRCS, at the University of North Carolina, May 2014

Question: What are the five most important advances in burn care in the past 100 years?

Answer:
1. Fluid resuscitation to reverse burn shock
2. Ventilatory support not only for inhalation injury but also to protect the airway during resuscitation and to treat hospital-acquired pneumonia

3. Early excision of the burn wound with timely coverage
4. Application of topical antimicrobials to decrease the rate of burn wound infection
5. Regulation of metabolism through nutritional and biochemical support

Question: Why is the use of topical antimicrobials only fourth on your list?

Answer: Topical antimicrobials are absolutely critical to reduce the incidence of infection, but the acutely injured burn patient needs to be treated for shock first and have their airway protected second. The early excision of burn wounds improves outcomes by decreasing the bacterial load that burn wounds carry and by reducing translocation and subsequent infection of distant organ systems, such as the urinary tract and pulmonary tree. Before early excision was shown to be beneficial in the 1980s, we relied on topical antimicrobials to decrease colonization and subsequent infection of the burn wound.

Question: Which agent—silver nitrate, Sulfamylon, or silver sulfadiazine—had the biggest impact on reducing sepsis from burn wounds?

Answer: Sulfamylon was the most important of these topical antimicrobials because of the penetration of the burn eschar and coverage of *Pseudomonas*. Multidrug-resistant organisms, such as *Acinetobacter, Stenotrophomonas,* and methicillin-resistant *Staphylococcus aureus*, plus invasive fungal pathogens, have become our most difficult infections to treat today.

CHAPTER 38

Early Excision and Grafting vs. Nonoperative Treatment of Burns of Indeterminant Depth: A Randomized Prospective Study

Engrav LH, Heimbach DM, Reus JL, Harnar TJ, Marvin JA. J Trauma 23:1001-1004, 1983

Reviewed by Jonathan S. Friedstat, MD

Those patients who underwent early excision had a shorter hospitalization than those treated with Silvadene. Time away from work was one third that of the other group and total hospital costs were less.[1]

Research Question   Are patients with indeterminate depth burns better served with early excision and grafting or nonoperative therapy?

Funding   Unknown

Study Dates   July 1, 1979, to December 31, 1980

Publishing Date   1983

Location   Harborview Medical Center, Seattle, WA

Subjects   Burn patients with sustained flame or scald burns <20% total body surface area (TBSA) who were otherwise healthy, had no smoke inhalation, and had no other associated injuries were considered for the study. Burns were evaluated by the senior authors on the third postburn day and were felt to be indeterminate (usually mottled, red, and white in appearance with decreased sensation).

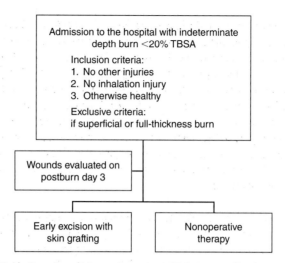

Fig. 38-1 Overview of the study method. *TBSA*, Total body surface area.

Exclusion Criteria   On the third postburn day, any patient whose wounds were judged by the senior authors to heal within 3 weeks or burns that were clearly full thickness were excluded.

Sample Size   Forty-seven patients total; 25 patients were treated nonoperatively with silver sulfadiazine (Silvadene), hydrotherapy twice daily, and debridement. Twenty-two patients were treated with early excision and grafting.

Overview of Design   The design of this study is outlined in Fig. 38-1.

Intervention   Patients who met the inclusion criteria were blindly randomized to early excision and grafting or nonoperative therapy. Nonoperative therapy occurred as described previously and surgery was performed with tangential excision. Meshed skin grafts were covered with a moist dressing soaked in mafenide (Sulfamylon, Winthrop Pharmaceuticals, Winthrop, NY) and sheet grafts were left open. The donor site received either fine mesh gauze or Opsite. Range-of-motion exercises began at 72 hours after surgery.

Follow-up   Patients underwent 3-month follow-up for approximately 1 year from surgery. Appearance and function were evaluated and photographs were taken at 3-month intervals.

Endpoints   Wounds were followed for the presence or absence of blisters and hypertrophic burn scars. Contour was evaluated for surface irregularities—how the burn wound followed their normal body contour. Extremity function was evaluated for total range of motion.

Results The two groups were similar in age, gender, TBSA, and burn distribution. Patients randomly assigned to the early excision group spent a shorter time in the hospital compared with the nonoperative Silvadene group (16.4 versus 25.0 days, $p = 0.001$), had lower hospital and physician costs ($9063 versus $12,702, $p = 0.05$), required less time off (56 versus 135 days), and had slightly higher blood requirements (1.9 versus 1.2 units of packed red blood cells). Both had comparable follow-up (12.1 versus 11.6 months). Although not statistically significant, three patients in the early excision group had hypertrophic scars only at the juncture lines compared with seven patients in the Silvadene group that involved larger areas of the burn. Surface irregularity was noted in eight patients treated with early excision and grafting compared with one treated nonoperatively.

Criticisms/Limitations The study addresses indeterminate burns limited to flame and scald burns. It does not address the role of early excision in full-thickness burns or in burns larger than 20% TBSA. Although the study suggests that earlier excision has more favorable scarring patterns as a trade-off for more surface irregularity from skin grafts, this does not achieve statistical significance.

Relevant Studies At the time of this publication,[1] burn care was in a period of rapid evolution that helped form the foundation of standard burn care today. Lessons learned from the Cocoanut Grove Night Club fire improved burn care in many areas including emergency medical responses, burn prevention, fluid resuscitation, and inhalational injury. Although it was recognized that observing a burn wound allowed one to better determine viable from nonviable tissue, the feasibility of such treatment in mass casualty settings like the Cocoanut Grove fire and World War II prompted a search for alternatives.

During the 1940s and 1950s Young,[2] Cope et al,[3] Whittaker,[4] and Jackson et al[5] explored the idea of whether early surgical excision and grafting could be applied to burn wounds. It was not until the 1970s when Janzekovic[6] demonstrated good results with surgical burn wound excision that the notion of early excision and grafting gained support. This was followed by the work of Burke et al,[7-9] who examined the role of early excision and grafting in nonrandomized, retrospective studies. There they demonstrated that early excision shortened the length of stay, decreased morbidity and mortality, and improved the functional outcomes in burned hands.

Engrav et al[1] expanded on this work by demonstrating the effectiveness of early excision and grafting in a prospective, randomized fashion. Their study proved not only what others were beginning to believe about a paradigm shift in how burns were treated, but it established this practice as a fundamental component to burn care.

Interestingly, the clinical work from Harborview preceded many of the basic and translational studies and confirmed the importance of early burn wound excision. One mechanism for improved survival was the restoration of immune function, which had the downstream effect of decreasing infection, improving metabolism, and enhancing survival after major thermal injury. The laboratory of Anthony Meyer, currently Chair of Surgery at the University of North Carolina, demonstrated that early burn wound excision, either complete or partial, restored many parameters in immune function such as B-cell production of bacterial-specific antibodies and CD-8–mediated T-cell cytotoxicity.[10-12]

The clinical studies from Harborview were followed up by Tompkins et al,[13] who examined the impact of adopting early excision and grafting into their practice. In the 10 years since its introduction and optimization at Massachusetts General Hospital and the Shriners Hospital for Children–Boston, they decreased their mortality rate from 24% to 7%.[10] Although they acknowledged the limitation that the average TBSA of burn admissions decreased and may have contributed to the decreasing trend in mortality, their retrospective statistical analysis was robust for that time. It solidified the contributions of Engrav, Heimbach, and others from Harborview and ushered in a new era in the surgical treatment of burn wounds.

Summary   Early excision and grafting are superior to nonoperative therapy for indeterminate thickness burns because it shortens hospital stays, lowers the overall cost of treatment, and shortens the time patients spend away from work.

Implications   This study provided prospective, randomized trial evidence that early excision and grafting are superior to nonsurgical therapy. It confirmed the results of other nonrandomized trials and helped establish early excision and grafting of burn wounds as the standard of care for smaller burns of indeterminate depth.

REFERENCES

1. Engrav LH, Heimbach DM, Reus JL, et al. Early excision and grafting vs. nonoperative treatment of burns of indeterminant depth: a randomized prospective study. J Trauma 23:1001-1004, 1983.
2. Young F. Immediate skin grafting in the treatment of burns: a preliminary report. Ann Surg 116:445-451, 1942.
3. Cope O, Langohr JL, Moore FD, et al. Expeditious care of full-thickness burn wounds by surgical excision and grafting. Ann Surg 125:1-22, 1947.
4. Whittaker AH. Treatment of burns by excision and immediate skin grafting. Am J Surg 85:411-417, 1953.
5. Jackson D, Topley E, Cason JS, et al. Primary excision and grafting of large burns. Ann Surg 152:167-189, 1960.
6. Janzekovic Z. A new concept in the early excision and immediate grafting of burns. J Trauma 10:1103-1108, 1970.
7. Burke JF, Bondoc CC, Quinby WC. Primary burn excision and immediate grafting: a method shortening illness. J Trauma 14:389-395, 1974.

8. Burke JF, Quinby WC Jr, Bondoc CC. Primary excision and prompt grafting as routine therapy for the treatment of thermal burns in children. Surg Clin North Am 56:477-494, 1976.
9. Burke JF, Bondoc CC, Quinby WC Jr, et al. Primary surgical management of the deeply burned hand. J Trauma 16:593-598, 1976.
10. Hultman CS, Cairns BA, deSerres S, et al. Early, complete burn wound excision partially restores cytotoxic T lymphocyte function. Surgery 118:421-429; discussion 429-430, 1995.
11. Yamamoto H, Siltharm S, deSerres S, et al. Immediate burn wound excision restores antibody synthesis to bacterial antigen. J Surg Res 63:157-162, 1996.
12. Hultman CS, Yamamoto H, deSerres S, et al. Early but not late burn wound excision partially restores viral-specific T lymphocyte cytotoxicity. J Trauma 43:441-447, 1997.
13. Tompkins RG, Burke JF, Schoenfeld DA, et al. Prompt eschar excision: a treatment system contributing to reduced burn mortality. A statistical evaluation of burn care at the Massachusetts General Hospital (1974-1984). Ann Surg 1204:272-281, 1986.
14. Janzekovic Z. Once upon a time . . . how west discovered east. J Plast Reconstr Aesthet Surg 61:240-244, 2008
15. Cole JK, Engrav LH, Heimbach DM, et al. Early excision and grafting of face and neck burns in patients over 20 years. Plast Reconstr Surg 109:1266-1273, 2002.

STUDY AUTHOR REFLECTIONS

Loren H. Engrav, MD, FACS

Now in 2014, it seems almost funny that excision of burn wounds ever needed justification. However, there were many doubters and objections. In fact, to verify and observe, burn surgeons worldwide flew to Maribor, Slovenia.[14] But that was then and now is now. Since then the procedure has been extended to almost all body parts.[15] It should be added, however, that there are still some patients with small, indeterminate burns for whom the "watch and wait" plan is indicated, such as indeterminate burns of the penis.

CHAPTER 39

Improved Net Protein Balance, Lean Mass, and Gene Expression Changes With Oxandrolone Treatment in the Severely Burned

Wolf SE, Thomas SJ, Dasu MR, Ferrando AA, Chinkes DL, Wolfe RR, Herndon DN. Ann Surg 237:801-810; discussion 810-811, 2003

Reviewed by Felicia N. Williams, MD, and Jonathan S. Friedstat, MD

> *This study demonstrates statistically significant improvement in net muscle protein synthesis, and lean body mass in severely burned patients treated with early enteral nutrition and oxandrolone. Genotypically, this was associated with increased gene expression for functional muscle proteins.*[1]

Research Question Does oxandrolone (a testosterone analog) improve net muscle protein synthesis and affect gene expression in severely burned patients?

Funding National Institutes of Health, Washington, DC, and Shriners Hospitals for Children, Galveston, TX

Study Dates January 1999 to December 2001

Publishing Date December 2002

Location Single institution, United States

Subjects This study included pediatric patients (children less than 18 years of age) who were admitted from January 1999 through December 2001 with burns over 30% total body surface area (TBSA) and had received definitive care of their burn injury within 2 weeks of injury. For inclusion patients must have required at least two operative interventions. These patients were able, willing, and consented to participate in two stable isotope studies and were nutritionally replete.

Exclusion Criteria   Pediatric patients admitted 2 weeks after injury and not during the study period who had less than a 30% TBSA burn, emaciated patients, those not requiring at least two surgical interventions, and those patients randomly assigned to other anticatabolic or anabolic agents in other metabolic studies were excluded.

Sample Size   32 total patients; 18 patients were randomly assigned to the standard of care with a placebo, and 14 patients were randomly assigned to the standard of care with oxandrolone (0.1 mg/kg) twice daily.

Overview of Design   An overview of design from the previously published study is shown in Fig. 39-1.[1]

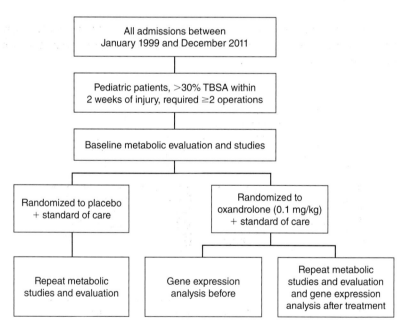

Fig. 39-1   Overview of design. *TBSA,* Total body surface area.

Intervention   All 32 patients underwent metabolic studies to evaluate their baseline weights, body composition, and muscle protein synthesis. All 32 patients were randomly assigned either to a placebo or oxandrolone. Eighteen patients were randomly assigned to the placebo group, and 14 patients were randomly assigned to receive oxandrolone (0.1 mg/kg) twice daily. Those patients who were randomly assigned to the oxandrolone group underwent gene expression analysis before and after treatment.

Follow-up   Patients were followed and studied through their acute hospitalization, at discharge, and at 6 months after injury.

Endpoints   Body composition, net muscle protein balance, and gene expression for functional muscle proteins

Results   Body composition in the group randomly assigned to a placebo and the standard of care was significantly decreased in the form of body weights and fat free mass. There was no change in body weight or fat free mass in the oxandrolone group between admission and discharge.

There was no significant difference in net muscle protein balance in the placebo group. The group randomly assigned to oxandrolone had statistically significant improvement in net muscle protein balance (Fig. 39-2).

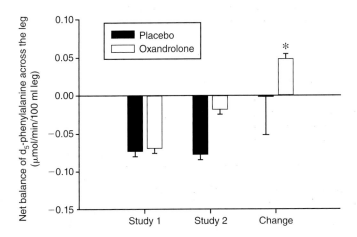

Fig. 39-2   Oxandrolone improved net muscle protein synthesis. Net balance of d_5-phenylalanine across the leg with and without therapy. There was a significant improvement in net balance in the oxandrolone-treated group ($p < 0.05$). There was no difference in the placebo group. Significance denoted by * and accepted as $p < 0.05$. (From Wolf SE, Thomas SJ, Dasu MR, et al. Improved net protein balance, lean mass, and gene expression changes with oxandrolone treatment in the severely burned. Ann Surg 237:801-810; discussion 810-811, 2003.)

Table 39-1   Changes in Gene Expression From Before and After 1 Week of Oxandrolone Treatment

Gene	Fold Change*
Down syndrome critical region	6.2
Myosin light polypeptide	3.1
Myosin light polypeptide—regulatory	2.6
Tubulin	2.3
26S proteasome	2.0
Staufen RNA-binding protein	1.6
Dynein	1.6
Guanine nucleotide-binding protein	1.6
Glutathione S-transferase	1.6
Tyrosine 3-monooxygenase	1.5
Adenylate kinase 2	1.5
Myobrevin	1.4
CALM1 gene	−2.3
Protein phosphatase 1	−3.1

Table is an adaptation of the data previously published.
From Wolf SE, Thomas SJ, Dasu MR, et al. Improved net protein balance, lean mass, and gene expression changes with oxandrolone treatment in the severely burned. Ann Surg 237:801-810; discussion 810-811, 2003. Significance denoted with * and accepted at $p < 0.05$.

There were significant changes in gene expression for 14 structural proteins involved in the regulation of protein synthesis. In Table 39-1,[1] changes in gene expression are shown from before and after 1 week of oxandrolone treatment.

Criticisms/Limitations   This prospective, randomized, controlled trial is limited by the number of patients, which may lead to a type I error and the limited follow-up of 6 months. It is also not clearly stated that oxandrolone therapy continued beyond the acute hospitalization.

Relevant Studies   This study was a follow-up to a study on the effects of oxandrolone on cachectic, malnourished, severely burned pediatric patients who had a delay to definitive therapy. These patients had not received early enteral nutrition or early excision and grafting, which is the standard of care noted at this institution.[2] The authors hypothesized that these patients may benefit from the anabolic properties of oxandrolone treatment.[2] The original study found improvement in net muscle protein synthesis in cachectic, severely burned patients. Subsequently, the authors hypothesized that oxandrolone therapy improved muscle protein synthesis even in those treated with early enteral nutrition and early excision and grafting, which led to the findings in this study. Fortunately, the study of the effects of oxandrolone in severely burned pediatric patients has continued.[2-9]

In 2003 this group studied the effects of oxandrolone on gene expression patterns specifically in the skeletal muscle of burned children. The goal was to elucidate a better fundamental understanding of muscle wasting at the molecular level and then to challenge those findings by comparing the results with burned children receiving this anabolic treatment. At this time the hypothesis was that the findings would help identify new therapeutic targets to attenuate muscle wasting in severely burned children, improving both short-term and long-term morbidity.[10]

In 2004 the authors looked at the inflammatory response with oxandrolone treatment.[5,9] Because profound derangements in the acute phase and constitutive proteins are the hallmarks of severe burn injury, this group studied the effects of oxandrolone therapy on these proteins. Patients in this particular study were randomly assigned to receive the drug for an entire year. Metabolic studies were performed at regular intervals throughout that period (on admission, at discharge, and at 6 months, 9 months, and 12 months after injury). They found that key constitutive proteins, such as albumin, prealbumin, and retinal-binding protein, significantly increased compared with patients randomly assigned to receive the standard of care alone. They found that protein levels in the acute phase significantly decreased in the treatment group.[9] The physiologic and metabolic improvements that oxandrolone treatment provided led to the investigation of body composition improvements in oxandrolone long-term. That same year they found significant improvements in lean body mass, bone mineral content, and bone mineral density that persisted even longer than just the treatment year.[5,9,11]

In 2008 the effect of oxandrolone therapy on adults during acute hospitalization was studied in a multicenter, observational trial. This trial showed promising results in the improvement in survival in the cohort of adults taking oxandrolone therapy for at least 7 days,[6] the mechanism of which is still not understood. However, this trial spearheaded continued investigations into the molecular mechanisms by which oxandrolone works.

In 2012 the authors looked at 5-year outcomes of patients randomly assigned to oxandrolone therapy for 1 year.[7] Over the past decade, Herndon's group has published multiple studies that looked at long-term follow-up from burns. They have found that the physiologic derangements after severe burn injury persist years after injury.[12-14] Thus this makes burns a chronic medical and surgical problem. To determine the long-term effects of oxandrolone therapy, this group followed patients for 5 years. The authors looked at resting energy expenditure, height, weight, lean body mass, muscle strength, bone mineral content, cardiac function, inflammatory cytokines, hormones, and hepatic function. The study period lasted up to 5 years after burn injury and 4 years after oxandrolone was stopped. Oxandrolone significantly decreased hypermetabolism.[7] It improved cardiac function in combination with exercise, and it increased lean body mass and muscle strength.[7] Compared with those receiving the standard of care alone, pediatric patients treated with oxandrolone had improved bone mineral content and height percentiles, and these changes persisted throughout the 5 years studied.

Summary   Oxandrolone therapy improves body composition and reverses the growth retardation once experienced by severely burned pediatric patients. The effects last long after therapy has stopped.

Implications   This study highlights the profound effects severe burns have on the phenotypes and genotypes of thermally injured pediatric patients. Although the mechanism remains unclear, oxandrolone therapy positively impacted gene expression and muscle protein synthesis. This study led to longer treatment regimens and improved morbidity and mortality for burn patients. The collection will be the foundation of many needed pediatric and adult multicenter trials needed to fully elucidate the effects of oxandrolone on severe burn injury.

REFERENCES

1. Wolf SE, Thomas SJ, Dasu MR, et al. Improved net protein balance, lean mass, and gene expression changes with oxandrolone treatment in the severely burned. Ann Surg 237:801-810; discussion 810-811, 2003.
2. Hart DW, Wolf SE, Ramzy PI, et al. Anabolic effects of oxandrolone after severe burn. Ann Surg 233:556-564, 2001.
   In this article, the authors intervened on the most difficult patients encountered—the severely burned cachectic patients. It became the basis of future oxandrolone studies of severely burned pediatric patients.
3. Gauglitz GG, Williams FN, Herndon DN, et al. Burns: where are we standing with propranolol, oxandrolone, recombinant human growth hormone, and the new incretin analogs? Curr Opin Clin Nutr Metab Care14:176-181, 2011.
4. Jeschke MG, Finnerty CC, Suman OE, et al. The effect of oxandrolone on the endocrinologic, inflammatory, and hypermetabolic responses during the acute phase postburn. Ann Surg 246:351-360; discussion 360-362, 2007.
5. Murphy KD, Thomas S, Mlcak RP, et al. Effects of long-term oxandrolone administration in severely burned children. Surgery 136:219-224, 2004.
6. Pham TN, Klein MB, Gibran NS, et al. Impact of oxandrolone treatment on acute outcomes after severe burn injury. J Burn Care Res 29:902-906, 2008.
   In this observational study, the authors showed a positive relationship between oxandrolone treatment and improved survival in severely burned adults.
7. Porro LJ, Herndon DN, Rodriguez NA, et al. Five-year outcomes after oxandrolone administration in severely burned children: a randomized clinical trial of safety and efficacy. J Am Coll Surg 214:489-502; discussion 502-504, 2012.
   The authors followed patients for 5 years after injury to determine the long-term effects of oxandrolone treatment and to see if the acute benefits of oxandrolone could be sustained. The positive results spawned other efficacy studies of growth hormone and propranolol treatments long-term after severe burn injury.
8. Przkora R, Herndon DN, Suman OE. The effects of oxandrolone and exercise on muscle mass and function in children with severe burns. Pediatrics 119:e109-e116, 2007.

9. Thomas S, Wolf SE, Murphy KD, et al. The long-term effect of oxandrolone on hepatic acute phase proteins in severely burned children. J Trauma 56:37-44, 2004.

10. Barrow RE, Dasu MR, Ferrando AA, et al. Gene expression patterns in skeletal muscle of thermally injured children treated with oxandrolone. Ann Surg 237:422-428, 2003.

11. Przkora R, Jeschke MG, Barrow RE, et al. Metabolic and hormonal changes of severely burned children receiving long-term oxandrolone treatment. Ann Surg 242:384-389, discussion 390-391, 2005.

12. Jeschke MG, Chinkes DL, Finnerty CC, et al. Pathophysiologic response to severe burn injury. Ann Surg 248:387-401, 2008.

   The authors defined the magnitude and severity of the metabolic and physiologic derangements of severe burn injury. It became the basis of future metabolic studies of severe burn injury.

13. Jeschke MG, Gauglitz GG, Kulp GA, et al. Long-term persistence of the pathophysiologic response to severe burn injury. PLoS One 6:e21245, 2011.

   The authors defined the length of time the metabolic and physiologic derangements of severe burn injury last. It underscores the group's contribution to defining severe burn injury and the ramifications of injury long-term.

14. Williams FN, Herndon DN, Suman OE, et al. Changes in cardiac physiology after severe burn injury. J Burn Care Res 32:269-274, 2011.

   In this article, the authors defined the length of time pediatric patients demonstrated supraphysiologic cardiac function after severe burn injury.

STUDY AUTHOR REFLECTIONS

David Herndon, MD, FACS

Fifty years ago, severe burn injury was a death sentence to those with greater than 50% total body surface area injuries. We battled severe muscle catabolism, sepsis, multi-organ dysfunction, and profound metabolic derangements. Advances in resuscitation, surgical technique, early excision and grafting, exercise, and antimicrobial therapies have improved our outcomes dramatically. Our current task is to find pharmacologic and nonpharmacologic therapies to further improve morbidity and mortality. Anabolic and anticatabolic agents such as insulin, growth hormone, oxandrolone, and propranolol have shown such promise in improving outcomes for our patients so that they can thrive and once again contribute to society. We have been able to show significant improvements in whole-body composition, essentially reversing protein catabolism with the use of oxandrolone in pediatric patients. This is a change so pervasive that it changes the genetic makeup in these patients. In the adult observational study, we found a link to improved survival for those receiving therapy. Although survival is no longer the exception but the rule, our current responsibility to our patients is to continue studying the physiologic and metabolic changes to injury in multicenter, randomized, controlled trials, looking at all populations and all walks of life, to provide the best tools for survival, rehabilitation, and continued growth.

CHAPTER 40

Pulsed Dye Laser Therapy and Z-plasty for Facial Burn Scars: The Alternative to Excision

Donelan MB, Parrett BM, Sheridan RL. Ann Plast Surg 60:480-486, 2008

Reviewed by Shiara Ortiz-Pujols, MD

> [Therapy] with pulsed dye laser for hypertrophic facial burns in combination with focal z-plasty tension relief when indicated has demonstrated the potential to greatly decrease the need for scar excision surgery[1]

Research Question Does the combination of pulsed dye laser (PDL) therapy and tension-relieving Z-plasties obviate the need for excision of hypertrophic scars?

Funding Unknown

Study Dates 2000 to 2007

Publishing Date May 2008

Location Shriners Burn Hospital, Boston, MA

Design A retrospective chart review of the results of PDL therapy and Z-plasty versus excision for facial burns

Subjects All consecutive patients with hypertrophic facial burns who were treated with PDL from 2000 to 2007

Exclusion Criteria None

Sample Size   Fifty-seven patients were treated with PDL for facial hypertrophic scars. All of these patients had facial burns that initially healed well with flat epithelium within 4 to 5 weeks of the burn. These patients then developed hypertrophic scars.

Overview of Design   A retrospective chart review of the results, indications, and timing of a combination of PDL and tension-relieving Z-plasties for the treatment of hypertrophic facial scars in all consecutive patients who were treated with PDL from 2000 to 2007.

Intervention   Patients were treated with the 595 nm Candela Vbeam PDL in an overlapping manner for the duration of 1.5 ms for each session. After laser therapy, patients were treated twice daily with Aquaphor healing ointment for 1 week. Multiple laser treatments were performed in 2-week intervals. Focal Z-plasties were performed within the scar tissue when tension was thought to contribute to the hypertrophy.

Follow-up   Variable; follow-up period not specified depending on the extent of the burn and the number of treatments

Endpoints   Clinical improvement in the appearance, erythema, and texture of hypertrophic scars

Results   Fifty-seven patients were treated with PDL therapy over a 7-year period. Twenty patients (35%) were treated with intralesional corticosteroids before laser therapy. The average number of PDL treatments per patient was 3.7 treatments (range 1 to 15 treatments). Thirty-four patients (60%) were also treated with Z-plasties.

Analysis Strategy   Patients were divided into three groups according to the time from burn to initial laser treatment: group I (less than 1 year), group II (1 to 4 years), and group III (greater than 5 years) (Fig. 40-1).

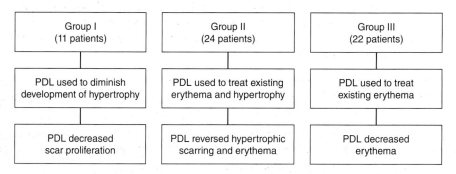

Fig. 40-1   Treatment with PDL therapy in three different groups. *PDL,* Pulsed dye laser.

In all groups, treatment with PDL therapy resulted in clinical improvement of scars with decreased erythema and a softer texture of the scars.

Criticisms/Limitations This study did not discuss the assessment tools used to measure the improvement in the appearance of the scars. Furthermore, it did not discuss the decision algorithm used to determine when to use Z-plasties to augment PDL therapy.

Relevant Studies Hypertrophic scars after burns can be a significant source of morbidity because of pruritus, neuropathic pain, stiffness and contracture, loss of thermoregulation, and decreased protection from mechanical trauma.[1] Several different approaches are used in the management of hypertrophic scarring, which include observation, massage, moisturizing agents, compression garments, silicone sheeting, steroid injections, fat grafting, and direct excision.[2-8] Laser therapies have emerged as an attractive and low morbidity modality for the treatment of hypertrophic scars.[9-22]

However, there have not yet been studies on the long-term success of these therapies, particularly regarding the recurrence of scars. In a large, prospective, before-after study, laser treatment was found to be effective in the objective and subjective improvement of hypertrophic burn scars, but the median follow-up time was less than 5 months after treatment.[22] Similar to the study of Donelan et al, an improvement in the appearance of the scars was seen soon after laser therapy.[23] However, the questions of optimal timing, duration, and type of therapy, as well as an assessment of the efficacy of long-term therapy, have not been widely explored. In a follow-up study by the same authors,[24] 147 patients treated with laser therapy were followed for up to 25 months after therapy and showed sustained improvement in the appearance of the scars. Even 2 years after laser treatment, burn patients had lasting improvements in the texture, thickness, and stiffness of their hypertrophic scars.

There is still much to learn about the physiology of how laser therapy affects scar maturation. Nevertheless, much data are available that substantiate the use of laser therapy in the management of hypertrophic burn scars.[25-29] Dr. Donelan's work was one of the first papers to show the potential of laser therapy in the management of hypertrophic facial scars after burns, with the promise of obviating the need for surgical excision for many people with this condition.

Summary PDL therapy with or without Z-plasties is an effective and viable option in the treatment of hypertrophic facial scars.

Implications This study set the groundwork for further exploration of conservative therapies for the management of hypertrophic facial scars that can potentially offer equivalent if not superior therapy to excision.

REFERENCES

1. Donelan MB, Parrett BM, Sheridan RL. Pulsed dye laser therapy and z-plasty for facial burn scars: the alternative to excision. Ann Plast Surg 60:480-486, 2008.
2. Berman B, Viera MH, Amini S, et al. Prevention and management of hypertrophic scars and keloids after burns in children. J Craniofac Surg 19:989-1006, 2008.
3. Patel PA, Bailey JK, Yakuboff KP. Treatment outcomes for keloid scar management in the pediatric burn population. Burns 38:767-771, 2011.
4. Steinstraesser L, Flak E, Witte B, et al. Pressure garment therapy alone and in combination with silicone for the prevention of hypertrophic scarring: randomized controlled trial with intraindividual comparison. Plast Reconstr Surg 128:306e-313e, 2011.
5. O'Brien L, Jones DJ. Silicone gel sheeting for preventing and treating hypertrophic and keloid scars. Cochrane Database Syst Rev 9:CD003826, 2013.
6. Sultan SM, Barr JS, Butala P, et al. Fat grafting accelerates revascularisation and decreases fibrosis following thermal injury. J Plast Reconstr Aesthet Surg 65:219-227, 2012.
7. Klinger M, Caviggioli F, Klinger FM, et al. Autologous fat graft in scar treatment. J Craniofac Surg 24:1610-1615, 2013.
8. Gentile P, De Angelis B, Pasin M, et al. Adipose-derived stromal vascular fraction cells and platelet-rich plasma: basic and clinical evaluation for cell-based therapies in patients with scars on the face. J Craniofac Surg 25:267-272, 2014.
9. Bowes LE, Nouri K, Berman B, et al. Treatment of pigmented hypertrophic scars with the 585 nm pulsed dye laser and the 532 nm frequency-doubled Nd:YAG laser in the Q-switched and variable pulse modes: a comparative study. Dermatol Surg 28:714-719, 2002.
10. Cho SB, Lee SJ, Chung WS, et al. Treatment of burn scar using a carbon dioxide fractional laser. J Drugs Dermatol 9:173-175, 2010.
11. Haedersdal M, Moreau KE, Beyer DM, et al. Fractional nonablative 1540 nm laser resurfacing for thermal burn scars: a randomized controlled trial. Lasers Surg Med 41:189-195, 2009.
12. Waibel J, Beer K. Ablative fractional laser resurfacing for the treatment of a third-degree burn. J Drugs Dermatol 8:294-297, 2009.
13. Lee Y. Combination treatment of surgical, post-traumatic and post-herpetic scars with ablative lasers followed by fractional laser and non-ablative laser in Asians. Lasers Surg Med 41:131-140, 2009.
14. Ghalambor AA, Pipelzadeh MH. Low-level CO_2 laser therapy in burn scars: which patients benefit most? Pak J Med Sci 22:158-161, 2006.
15. Waibel J, Wulkan AJ, Lupo M, et al. Treatment of burn scars with the 1,550 nm nonablative fractional erbium laser. Lasers Surg Med 44:441-446, 2012.
16. Gaida K, Koller R, Isler C, et al. Low-level laser therapy—a conservative approach to the burn scar? Burns 30:362-367, 2004.
17. Eberlein A, Schepler H, Spilker G, et al. Erbium:YAG laser treatment of post-burn scars: potentials and limitations. Burns 31:15-24, 2005.
18. Erol OO, Gurlek A, AgaogluG, et al. Treatment of hypertrophic scars and keloids using intense pulsed light. Aesthetic Plast Surg 32:902-909, 2008.
19. Shumaker PR, Kwan JM, Landers JT, et al. Functional improvements in traumatic scars and scar contractures using an ablative fractional laser protocol. J Trauma Acute Care Surg 73(2 Suppl 1):S116-S121, 2012.
20. Alam A, Warycha M. Complications of lasers and light treatments. Dermatol Ther 24:571-580, 2011.

21. Clayton JL, Edkins RE, Cairns BA, et al. Incidence and management of adverse events after the use of laser therapies for the treatment of hypertrophic burn scars. Ann Plast Surg 70:500-505, 2013.
22. Hultman CS, Edkins RE, Wu C, et al. Prospective, before-after cohort study to assess the efficacy of laser therapy on hypertrophic burn scars. Ann Plast Surg 70:521-526, 2013.
23. Hultman CS, Edkins RE, Lee CN, et al. Shine on: review of laser- and light-based therapies for the treatment of burn scars. Dermatol Res Pract 2012:243651, 2012. [Epub June 20, 2012]
24. Hultman CS, Edkins RE, Friedstat JS, et al. Laser resurfacing and remodeling of hypertrophic burn scars: the results of a large, prospective, before-after cohort study, with long term follow-up. Ann Surg 260:519-532, 2014.
25. Jin R, Huang X, Li H, et al. Laser therapy for prevention and treatment of pathologic excessive scars. Plast Reconstr Surg 132:1747-1758, 2013.
26. Lister TS, Brewin MP. Prevention or treatment of hypertrophic burn scarring: a review of when and how to treat with the pulsed dye laser. Burns 40:797-804, 2014.
27. Anderson RR, Donelan MB, Hivnor C, et al. Laser treatment of traumatic scars with an emphasis on ablative fractional laser resurfacing: consensus report. JAMA Dermatol 150:187-193, 2014.
28. Vrijman C, van Drooge AM, Limpens J, et al. Laser and intense pulsed light therapy for the treatment of hypertrophic scars: a systematic review. Br J Dermatol 165:934-942, 2011.
29. Parrett BM, Donelan MB. Pulsed dye laser in burn scars: current concepts and future directions. Burns 36:443-449, 2010.

STUDY AUTHOR REFLECTIONS

Matthias B. Donelan, MD, FACS

With the introduction of new technologies to manipulate scars, my approach to the treatment of scars has changed dramatically over the past decade. The amount of damage that can be done by the ill-advised and simplistic excision of "scars" is truly incredible.

One way to understand this concept is by applying models of logic developed by Aristotle. A syllogism is an argument formed by two statements, in which the conclusion must be true if the two statements are true. For example, "every virtue is laudable; kindness is a virtue; therefore kindness is laudable." On the other hand, sophistry is the use of reasoning or arguments that sound correct but are actually false. For patients with scars, one could incorrectly argue, "having less scars is good; excising scars results in less scars; therefore excising scars is good."

One idea I have shared a lot lately in lectures just to shake up people's minds is, "Every scar has the right to live." I did it first as a joke, but I am beginning to think in this new era, it may become an axiom. I hardly ever excise a burn scar in my practice anymore. It just does not seem to make sense with all the ways we can rehabilitate them; they are "original equipment."

My LAWS and AXIOMS of scar management are as follows.

Donelan's top 10 LAWS of scar management:
1. Scars are an essential part of healing, so scars are your friends.
2. Scars are living things and respond to their environment.
3. Relaxed scars are happy scars, so tight is never right.
4. Be patient and understand scars and they will reward you.
5. Scar excision is an oxymoron.
6. There is nothing like original equipment, so rehabilitate scars.
7. Rehabilitated scars look normal and not contrived.
8. The Z-plasty causes profound and salubrious changes.
9. Do not be a slave to aesthetic units.
10. Excise scars as a last resort and not as a first option.

Donelan's AXIOMS of burn scar management:
- Successful burn reconstruction is based on an overall strategy and basic principles and not specific surgical techniques.
- Reconstructive surgery must strive to make patients clearly better and not just deformed in a different way.
- Do not sacrifice overall facial appearance for the excision of scars.
- Reconstructive surgeons do not have a "right" to all the other areas of a patient's body.
- Gratuitous donor sites are not an insignificant iatrogenic deformity.

CHAPTER 41

The Superficial Musculo-aponeurotic System (SMAS) in the Parotid and Cheek Area

Mitz V, Peyronie M. Plast Reconstr Surg 58:80-88, 1976

Reviewed by Cindy Wu, MD

> *There is a "superficial muscular and aponeurotic system" (SMAS) in the parotid and cheek areas . . . A careful study of the SMAS may lead to its proper use during surgical procedures on the face. Thus, in this paper, we consider both the anatomy and the potential surgical applications of the SMAS.[1]*

Research Question What is the anatomy of the superficial muscular and aponeurotic system (SMAS), and what are its surgical applications?

Funding None

Study Dates None

Publishing Date 1976

Location Paris, France

Subjects The authors studied 15 fresh cadavers. In 7 cadavers ages 50 or older, 14 hemifacial preparations were performed. Three heads were then serially sectioned into 1 cm thick cuts in one of three planes: sagittal, frontal, and horizontal. Before sectioning, the heads were injected with Radiocorrodan to opacify arteries and veins and then studied radiographically. Another three heads were similarly injected and sectioned into 0.1 mm cuts. Histologic specimens were stained with Masson's trichrome stain (muscles = red or black, connective tissue = green). Particular attention was paid to the border zones: temporozygomatic, mandibular, nasolabial, and pretragal areas. The dissection showed the general features of the SMAS. The injections allowed precise dissection in an avascular plane. The ultra-radiographic plates demonstrated the fibrous layers. Macroscopic and microscopic sections demonstrated the delicate structure of the SMAS and its relationship with each fibromuscular layer.

Exclusion Criteria   None

Sample Size   15

Overview of Design   An anatomic study of the SMAS in cadavers

Intervention   Dissection and characterization of the SMAS

Follow-up   Not applicable

Endpoints   To describe the facial anatomy and discuss its surgical relevance in face-lift surgery

Results

Description of the SMAS.   The SMAS divides the subcutaneous fat into two layers. In the superficial compartment fat lobules are enclosed by fibrous septa running from the SMAS to the dermis. In the deep compartment the fat is abundant, lies between the deep facial muscles, and is not divided by fibrous septa. The SMAS is thick in the parotid-masseteric area and thin and discontinuous in the cheek area. The SMAS is in continuity with the posterior part of the frontalis muscle and with the platysma muscle (Fig. 41-1).

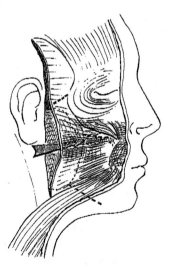

Fig. 41-1   Schema of the SMAS. The *arrow* goes deep to the SMAS, which extends from the *frontalis* to the *platysma* muscle. (From Mitz V, Peyronie M. The superficial musculo-aponeurotic system (SMAS) in the parotid and cheek area. Plast Reconstr Surg 58:80-88, 1976.)

Macroscopic and microscopic structures of the SMAS.   In the parotid area the SMAS is a condensed mesh distinct from the parotid fascia. It is adherent in the pretragal area for 1 to 2 cm and then becomes separated from the parotid fascia. Microscopic slides show that the SMAS can be composed of one to three layers between the parotid fascia proper and the skin. Sometimes the muscular fibers are obvious within the fibrous layer; hence the term *musculoaponeurotic system.*

In the cheek area the SMAS is thinner microscopically. Underneath the dermis, the SMAS is a continuous fibrous net sending several extensions out to the dermis and constantly covers the facial muscles. The SMAS composes all the attachments from these muscles to the dermis.

Relationship of the SMAS to other facial structures.   Contrary to what Gray wrote, "the superficial fascia (tela subcutanea) of the head invests the facial muscles and carries the superficial blood vessels and nerves," the motor branches of the facial nerve lie deep to the SMAS and not within it.

When describing the nerve anatomy in the parotid area, only sensory nerves (the branches of the anterior cervical plexus) are located between the dermis and SMAS. Facial nerve branches run deep into the parotid gland, protected by the fascia and external lobe of the gland. In the cheek area the facial motor nerves run deeper than the SMAS and reach facial muscles through their deeper aspect. Only sensory nerves go through the SMAS. An important layer of fat between the dermis and SMAS, this subcutaneous fat is completely separated from Bichat's fat pad by the SMAS.

The SMAS invests and extends into the external part of the superficial facial muscles and includes the risorius, frontalis, platysma, and peripheral part of the orbicularis oculi muscle.

The facial artery and vein lie deep to the SMAS. Their perforating branches go through it and the subdermal vascular network lies superficial to it. Thus the SMAS forms the deep border of the neurovascular and musculocutaneous complex.

In the pretragal area the SMAS and parotid fascia are united in a dense layer of connective tissue. Here a surgical dissection of the SMAS is possible and safe. Anterior to this, the SMAS is completely independent of this parotid fascia. However, because it is thin and covers the motor nerve branches, its surgical dissection anteriorly becomes difficult and dangerous.

In the temporozygomatic area the SMAS adheres to the periosteum by thin expansions. The temporal frontal branch of the facial nerve lies deep to the SMAS. Sensory nerve branches run between the SMAS and the dermis. However, this space overlying the external part of the zygomatic arch is very narrow, and thus dissection of the SMAS here is difficult and dangerous. A better plane of dissection is between the SMAS and the skin.

In the mandibular area the SMAS is close to the platysma muscle. Here the safe plane of dissection is deep to the platysma and SMAS because the mandibular branch of the facial nerve runs deeper there. This plane is cited by some who use and elevate the platysma during rhytidoplasty.[2]

In the mastoid area the SMAS is intimately attached to the dermis and fibrous tissue around the insertions of the sternocleidomastoid muscle. It is difficult to isolate the SMAS around the ear.

At the nasolabial fold, the SMAS is deep and thin and separated from the dermis by a large amount of fat. Several thin muscle expansions run forward, slanting from the SMAS to the dermis. This fold appears to be a cutaneous fold where the SMAS ends as a distinct layer rather than a fold caused by the insertions of specific muscles.

Criticisms/Limitations   None

Relevant Studies   Gray[3] described the superficial fascia precisely, but he did not indicate that the fascia was tensed upward by the frontalis muscle and downward by the platysma muscle. He also did not point out any value in its surgical dissection.

Poirier et al[4] discussed Gegenbaur's and Futamura's description of the superficial muscular layers of the face, but they do not assess either the relationship or function of the SMAS.

Podwyssovsky[5] described the insertions of the facial muscles into the deep dermis through perpendicular attachments connected by the SMAS.

Saban[6] wrote, "The superficialis fascia, which covers the body, ends therefore at the neck; its extension above the facial muscles would hinder all expression . . ."

Farisse et al[7] looked at the histology of the parotid fascia but did not clearly assess the SMAS. Also, its muscular connections are not described.

Couly et al[8] described a cervicofacial fascia without pointing out the musculature and dermal relationship of the SMAS. They only considered this fascia a sliding system on the subcutaneous fat and periosteum.

Summary   The SMAS is a fibromuscular network located between the facial muscles and the dermis, one which covers the facial motor nerves. Such a double attachment between the muscles deep and the skin superficially through the SMAS does not hinder the expressive function of those muscles but rather transmits it.

The SMAS is stretched superiorly and inferiorly by the frontalis and platysma muscles. It is attached posteriorly to the tragus and mastoid area. Such a peripheral stretching explains how the SMAS could be an amplifier of facial muscle contractions; the more it is tensed, the less energy is necessary for the muscle to transmit its action.

The SMAS transmits facial muscle action through two directions: a longitudinal network parallel to the skin plane and a perpendicular direction toward the facial skin through fibrous connections from the SMAS to the dermis.

The surgical application of the SMAS is in meloplasty (rhytidectomy). The classic approach of undermining the skin superficial to the SMAS destroys the fibrous connections between it and the dermis. Deep to the SMAS, the dissection plane is safe in the parotid area but not anteriorly. The SMAS dissection allows stronger pullback of the fascia and skin together.

Mitz and Peyronie[1] caution that facial nerve injury can occur in three situations:
1. When the SMAS is thin
2. When the superficial lobe of the parotid is short and does not protect the nerves
3. When the retrofascial dissection is carried too far anteriorly (beyond the anterior border of the parotid)

To avoid nerve injury, the dissection should start in front of the tragus between the SMAS and parotid fascia. The dissection should stop 1 cm below the zygomatic arch (to prevent injury to the frontal branch of the facial nerve) and 1 cm below the inferior margin of the mandible (marginal mandibular nerve). Once the SMAS is freed up from the parotid fascia, it becomes possible to lift the face more easily and strongly than the skin only.

Implications   This was the first translational paper of the SMAS that accurately describes its anatomy and surgical relevance. The anatomic findings are histologically confirmed. The authors also review previous literature and compare their findings with others. Mitz and Peyronie were the first to understand the function of the SMAS as it relates to the muscles of facial expression, fat compartments, and the dermis. This allowed them to develop this "dissection guide" for face lifts at the end of their paper. It is on their landmark work that modern face-lift techniques have been built.

REFERENCES

1. Mitz V, Peyronie M. The superficial musculo-aponeurotic system (SMAS) in the parotid and cheek area. Plast Reconstr Surg 58:80-88, 1976.
2. Guerrero-Santos J, Espaillat L, Morales F. Rhytidoplasty with sectioning and lifting of the platysma muscle [abstract]. In Abstracts of the Sixth International Congress of Plastic and Reconstructive Surgery, Paris: Masson, 1975.
3. Gray H. Anatomy of the Human Body, 25th ed. Philadelphia: Lea & Febiger, 1949.

   This is the anatomy textbook that many medical students had used. Gray described the superficial fascia precisely, but did not indicate that the fascia was tensed upward by the frontalis muscle and downward by the platysma muscle. He also did not point out any value in its surgical dissection.
4. Poirier A, Charpy A, Cunéo B. Abrégé d'Anatomie. Paris: Masson, 1908.

   These three authors were the first to describe the superficial muscular layers of the face. However, they did not assess either the relationship or the function of the SMAS.
5. Podwyssovsky. In Testut L, Latarjet A. Traité d'Anatomie Humaine: Anatomie Descriptive, Histologie, Développement. Paris: O Doin, 1948.

   The author described the insertions of the facial muscles into the deep dermis through the perpendicular attachments connected by a SMAS.
6. Saban P. In Grasse PP, ed. Traite de Zoologie. Paris: Masson, 1972.

   The author believed that the SMAS or the "'superficialis fascia which covers the body, ends therefore at the neck; its extension above the facial muscles would hinder all expression . . .''
7. Farisse J, Bonnoit J, Di Marino V, et al. [Surgical anatomy of the parotid region] C R Assoc Anat 147:254-261, 1970.

   The authors examined the histology of the parotid fascia but did not clearly assess the SMAS. Its muscular connections were not described.
8. Couly C, Hureau J, Vaillant JM. [The superficial cephalis fascia] Ann Chir Plast 20:171-182, 1975.

   The authors described a cervicofacial fascia without pointing out the musculature and dermal relationship of the SMAS. They only considered this fascia to be a sliding system on the subcutaneous fat and periosteum.

EDITORIAL PERSPECTIVE

C. Scott Hultman, MD, MBA, FACS

The discovery of the functional importance of the superficial muscular and aponeurotic system (SMAS) in the 1970s proved that not all human anatomy had been defined by 1543, when the Brabantian surgeon Andreas Vesalius published *De humani corporis fabrica (On the Fabric of the Human Body)*. Recognized as the fascial bridge connecting the platysma in the neck to the galea in the scalp, the SMAS had eluded famous anatomists such as Leonardo Da Vinci, Henry Gray, and Frank Netter. That the SMAS would remain hidden, nearly in plain sight, for centuries should come as no surprise. This fascial structure proved to be one of the most powerful assets a surgeon could deploy to rejuvenate the face and neck.

Anatomy itself does not change, but our understanding of the anatomic relationships continues to evolve. As we enter the twenty-first century, applied anatomy continues to inspire plastic surgeons, revealing intricate relationships between perfusion, innervation, and drainage of the human body. Instead of using a scalpel for exposure, we now have PET scans, functional MRIs, high-resolution ultrasound, and fluorescent angiography, all of which open up new windows to the interaction of the normal with the abnormal, within and between our organ systems. The final frontier surely exists at a cellular or subcellular level, where nanotechnology will allow us to truly reengineer form and function.

The following articles and/or books below have been pivotal in this area:

Furnas DW. The retaining ligaments of the cheek. Plast Reconstr Surg 83:11-16, 1989.
The author described the anatomy and function of the retaining ligaments of the cheek. These ligaments are important surgical landmarks in facial dissection.

Futamura R. Uber die entwicklung der facialis muskulatur des menschen. Anat Hefte 30:433-516, 1906.

Gegenbaur C. Lehrbuch der Anatomie des Menschen, vol 2, ed 4. Leipzig: Wilhelm Engleman, 1890.

Mendelson BC, Freeman ME, Wu W, et al. Surgical anatomy of the lower face: the premasseter space, the jowl, and the labiomandibular fold. Aesthetic Plast Surg 32: 185-195, 2008.
The authors described the premasseter space, an avascular plane containing important structures through which sub-SMAS dissection can be performed easily. They concluded that the premasseteric plane should be considered the preferred dissection plane for lower face lifts.

Mendelson BC, Muzaffar AR, Adams WP. Surgical anatomy of the midcheek and malar mounds. Plast Reconstr Surg 110:885-896; discussion 897-911, 2002.
The authors performed a cadaver study and identified a gliding plane space over the zygomatic body. In addition to the anatomic boundaries of this area, this gliding plane allows the characteristic facial aging changes and is an explanation of malar mounds. As a result, the authors discussed surgical methods to reverse these aging changes.

Moss CJ, Mendelson BC, Taylor GI. Surgical anatomy of the ligamentous attachments in the temple and periorbital regions. Plast Reconstr Surg 105:1475-1490; discussion 1491-1498, 2000.

This study described the deep ligamentous attachments of the superficial fascia in the temple and periorbital regions. The precise anatomy of this region is helpful in avoiding critical neurovascular structures in forehead and facial rejuvenation.

Rohrich RJ, Pessa JE. The fat compartments of the face: anatomy and clinical implications for cosmetic surgery. Plast Reconstr Surg 119:2219-2227; discussion 2228-2231, 2007.

The authors performed a cadaveric study and characterized the fat compartments of the face. Based on this study, our understanding of facial aging has changed in that we now believe that the face does not age as a confluent or composite mass. Shearing between adjacent compartments may be an additional factor in soft tissue malposition. Restoring youthful facial volume involves harmoniously blending the junction between fat compartments.

Rohrich RJ, Pessa JE. The retaining ligament of the face: histologic evaluation of the septal boundaries of the subcutaneous fat compartments. Plast Reconstr Surg 121:1804-1809, 2008.

The authors described the retaining ligaments that separate fat compartments. They originate from the underlying fascia and insert onto the dermis. This septal system provides an interconnecting framework that protects against shearing forces, providing a "retaining system" for the face. An extrapolation of this concept is that as facial aging occurs three dimensionally, the separate fat compartments change relative to one another in both volume and position.

Testut L, Latarjet A. Traité d'Anatomie Humaine: Anatomie Descriptive, Histologie, Développement. Paris: G Doin, 1948.

CHAPTER 42

Spreader Graft: A Method of Reconstructing the Roof of the Middle Nasal Vault Following Rhinoplasty

Sheen JH. Plast Reconstr Surg 73:230-239, 1984

Reviewed by Cindy Wu, MD

> *Submucosal placement of strips of cartilage along the anterior border of the septum—the spreader graft—has proved to be an effective method for reconstructing the roof of the middle vault. It is recommended in all primary rhinoplasty patients in whom resection of the roof of the upper cartilaginous vault is a necessary part of the surgical plan.[1]*

Research Question Middle vault collapse in patients undergoing primary and secondary rhinoplasty manifests as an "inverted V" deformity that represents the delineation of the bony vault from the collapsed middle vault. These patients have a narrow (<15 degrees) internal nasal valve, which is the angle formed between the septum and the upper lateral cartilages. Is there a technique to reconstruct a narrow middle vault?

Funding None

Study Dates Early 1980s

Publishing Date 1984

Location Los Angeles, CA

Subjects Patients undergoing primary and secondary rhinoplasty

Exclusion Criteria Not defined

Sample Size Unclear but included three case reports

Overview of Design   This was a technique paper that included three case reports.

Intervention   Spreader grafts were used in patients undergoing primary and secondary rhinoplasty. The cartilage graft is placed along the dorsal edge of the septum that provides width to the dorsal roof and increases the internal valve angle by moving the lateral wall away from the septum. A closed, endonasal rhinoplasty approach is used. A transfixing incision is made to expose the septal angle. This incision extends 1 cm posterior to the angle. Next, mucoperichondrial dissection is performed. Septal cartilage is harvested. A 5 mm wide subperichondrial pocket is made just cephalad past the caudal arch of the bony pyramid. The spreader grafts are carved out and placed into the pocket. A mattress suture through both grafts at the dorsal edge of the septum secures its position.

Follow-up   Not described

Endpoints   Improved nasal function (specifically, the effect of spreader grafts on the internal valve) and aesthetic appearance

Results
Primary rhinoplasty.   Patients with the "narrow nose syndrome" have visible fall-in of the lateral walls and abnormal valving on inspiration. This should prompt the surgeon to plan a broader dorsal roof as part of the surgical plan. Other characteristics that are predisposed to middle vault collapse include short nasal bones, thin skin, weak cartilages, or a combination of these traits. In the patient with short nasal bones, the short bony vault does not adequately support the relatively long middle vault. The lateral walls fall in, even with the support of the broad dorsal edge of the septum. Even patients with average length nasal bones with thin skin will have the appearance of cave-in of the lateral walls and delineation of the caudal edges of the nasal bones after dorsal resection, which is seen as an inverted V deformity. Weak cartilages are also predisposed to middle vault collapse. After resection of the roof when cartilages are no longer held away from the septum by the broad dorsal edge, flaccid cartilages will droop medially, resulting in a narrow middle vault.

Secondary rhinoplasty.   Middle vault collapse occurs because of avulsion of the upper lateral cartilages from the nasal bone or by resection of the roof, resulting in the collapse of the lateral nasal walls, discontinuity of the dorsal aesthetic lines, and airway obstruction.

Case reports.   Sheen then proceeds to describe three case reports in which spreader grafts were used: case 1—short nasal bones; case 2—too narrow middle vault; and case 3—secondary rhinoplasty (Fig. 42-1).

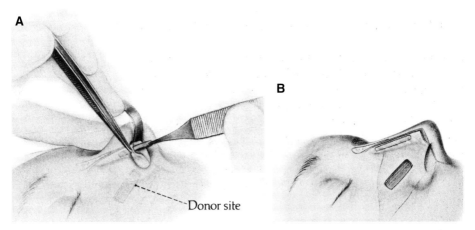

Fig. 42-1 A, A donor site at the vomer ensures the integrity of the graft pocket. **B,** The graft extends under the bony arch to the caudal border of the upper lateral cartilage. The graft's anterior edge is flush with the septum. (From Sheen JH. Spreader graft: a method of reconstructing the roof of the middle nasal vault following rhinoplasty. Plast Reconstr Surg 73:230-239, 1984.)

Criticisms/Limitations   Dr. Sheen stated: "This paper is not a study, but rather a clinical report and description of an original technique developed by a single clinician. It does not purport to be otherwise. Representing hundreds of cases (later thousands), three representative cases were chosen to illustrate three categories of patients. Although there was no 'results section,' results were shown for every patient in the illustrations. Functional results were mentioned in each case report. True, air flow studies were not presented, but the focus of the article was to offer a new surgical technique for a significant clinical problem."

Relevant Studies

Skoog T. A method of hump reduction in rhinoplasty. A technique for preservation of the nasal roof. Arch Otolaryngol 83:283-287, 1966.
> *In this article Skoog describes a technique of composite dorsal hump removal and reconstruction, in which the bony and cartilaginous dorsum are removed en bloc, contoured to achieve adequate dorsal reduction, and then replaced as a free graft.*

Sheen JH. Aesthetic Rhinoplasty, 2nd ed. St Louis: CV Mosby, 1987.
> *This is Sheen's textbook on aesthetic rhinoplasty, which he describes in detail on how to harvest, shape, and place spreader grafts.*

Byrd HS, Hobar PC. Rhinoplasty: a practical guide for surgical planning. Plast Reconstr Surg 91:642-654; discussion 655-656, 1993.
> *This article provides a comprehensive method of nasofacial analysis for preoperative rhinoplasty planning.*

Byrd HS, Meade RA, Gonyon DL Jr. Using the autospreader flap in primary rhinoplasty. Plast Reconstr Surg 119:1897-1902, 2007.

This article describes the use of autospreader grafts, which are the transverse portions of the scored upper lateral cartilages that are turned medially to serve as a spreader graft between the upper lateral cartilages and the septum. This method accomplishes two goals: increasing the internal nasal valve angle and decreasing the dorsal hump without harvesting septal cartilage.

Gunter JP, Rohrich RH, Adams WP Jr, eds. Dallas Rhinoplasty: Nasal Surgery by the Masters, 2nd ed, vols I and II. St Louis: Quality Medical Publishing, 2007.

This is a comprehensive textbook on rhinoplasty. Highly renowned rhinoplasty surgeons contributed to this essential rhinoplasty reference.

Gruber RP, Melkun ET, Woodward JF, et al. Dorsal reduction and spreader flaps. Aesthet Surg J 31:456-464, 2011.

This article reviews the authors' 15-year experience with this technique and provides a detailed description of their internal nasal valve reconstruction.

Rohrich RJ, Ahmad J. Rhinoplasty. Plast Reconstr Surg 128:49e-73e, 2011.

This is a comprehensive CME article on rhinoplasty. It discusses preoperative assessment, goals of treatment, advantages and disadvantages to treatment, key elements of surgery, perioperative management, avoidance and management of complications, and expected outcomes.

Murrell GL. Correlation between subjective and objective results in nasal surgery. Aesthet Surg J 34:249-257, 2014.

This article reports the objective and subjective outcomes of 119 functional rhinoplasty patients using a scientifically validated patient questionnaire and preoperative and postoperative rhinomanometry measurements. There was a statistically significant subjective and objective functional improvement in 98.9% and 95.6% of patients, respectively, whereas 94.4% of patients had both subjective and objective statistically significant functional improvement. A statistically significant correlation between subjective and objective improvements was noted.

Summary and Implications   Spreader grafts solve a very common rhinoplasty problem and should be considered the procedure of choice for internal nasal valve collapse in primary and secondary rhinoplasties.

REFERENCE

1. Sheen JH. Spreader graft: a method of reconstructing the roof of the middle nasal vault following rhinoplasty. Plast Reconstr Surg 73:230-239, 1984.

STUDY AUTHOR REFLECTIONS

Jack H. Sheen, MD

The genesis of the idea for spreader grafts is interesting. In my rhinoplasty training, nasal appearance (primarily reduction) was everything. In fact, nasal function was not stressed at all; it was considered in the purview of ear, nose and throat. It was not until well into my practice doing burgeoning numbers of rhinoplasties that I started to observe and make connections between nasal function and nasal aesthetics. What brought my attention to the middle vault was a patient with a straight septum and normal airways, who complained of difficulty breathing. On examination I observed that his middle vault collapsed on inspiration. His nasal bones were exceedingly short and simply did not support the nasal walls when he breathed in. When I placed Q-tips high in the vestibule, he breathed perfectly. This led to a series of "eureka" moments. I realized that several aesthetic and functional problems relating to the middle vault could be corrected by spreading the roof both in selected primary and secondary cases in which the roof had been resected. Thus the idea for spreader grafts was hatched.

In my practice spreader grafts proved to be an invaluable technique, producing noses with smooth contours and well-functioning airways—results that were satisfying to me and my patients.

CHAPTER 43

A Placebo-Controlled Surgical Trial of the Treatment of Migraine Headaches

Guyuron B, Reed D, Kriegler JS, Davis J, Pashmini N, Amini S. Plast Reconstr Surg 124:461-468, 2009

Reviewed by Cindy Wu, MD

> *This study confirms that surgical deactivation of peripheral migraine headache trigger sites is an effective alternative treatment for patients who suffer from frequent moderate to severe migraine headaches that are difficult to manage with standard protocols.[1]*

Research Question   Does surgical deactivation of trigger points (frontal, temporal, and occipital) improve migraine headaches compared with sham surgery?

Funding   Deborah Reed is a consultant for and has received grant/research support from Allergan, is a consultant and paid speaker, and has received grant/research support from GlaxoSmith Kline. Julie S. Kriegler is a consultant and paid speaker for Pfizer, GlaxoSmithKline, Merck, and Endo. None of the other authors has any disclosures.

Study Dates   Not stated

Publishing Date   2009

Location   Cleveland, OH

Subjects   Patients with moderate-to-severe migraine headaches triggered from a single or predominant site

Exclusion Criteria   Not stated

Sample Size   76

Overview of Design   Patients with migraines that were triggered by a single or predominant site were interviewed by a physician on the research team. After completion of both a daily migraine headache for a 1-month period and a comprehensive migraine headache information form, they were examined by two headache neurologists. The diagnosis of migraine was confirmed by the International Classification of Headache Disorders II criteria. Patients were also asked to complete the Medical Outcomes Study 36-Item Short Form Health Survey, Migraine-Specific Quality of Life, and Migraine Disability Assessment questionnaires before treatment. They were placed into three groups: frontal, temporal, and occipital guided by the most prevalent site of migraine origin and a positive response (>50% decrease in migraine intensity, duration, frequency, and the migraine index, all four of which were considered the endpoint) to the injection of 25 units of onabotulinumtoxinA (Botox). In each group, one third received sham surgery, and two thirds were randomly assigned and received actual surgery. Operations were performed only when migraine headaches recurred after the disappearance of the Botox effect.

Intervention   For the frontal group, surgery involved resection of the glabellar muscles (corrugator supercilii, depressor supercilii, and procerus) encasing the supraorbital and supratrochlear nerves through an upper blepharoplasty incision. A small amount of fat from the medial compartment filled the muscle defect to shield the nerves.

For the temporal group, endoscopic removal of a segment (2.5 cm) of the zygomaticotemporal branch of the temporal nerve was performed through two 1.5 cm incisions approximately 7 to 10 cm from the midline of the scalp in the right and left hair-bearing temples.

For the occipital group, the patient was anesthetized, placed in the prone position, and a 4 cm incision was made in the midline occipital area. A segment of semispinalis capitis muscle medial to the greater occipital nerve, approximately 1 cm wide by 2.5 cm long, was removed. A subcutaneous flap was interposed between the nerve and muscle to isolate it from the surrounding muscles and to avoid impingement of the nerve.

All procedures were performed in an outpatient facility, with average surgery times of less than 1 hour. Patients were permitted to resume ordinary activities in 1 week and heavy exercise in 3 weeks.

Follow-up   Patients were seen after their initial recovery and at 1, 3, 6, 9, and 12 months after surgery. Four outcome measures were assessed: (1) complete elimination of migraine headaches, (2) significant improvement in frequency, intensity, duration, or migraine index, (3) the difference between the baseline and 12-month follow-up measures, and (4) the difference between the average measures at 1 year and baseline.

Table 43-1 Patient Results Comparing Actual Surgery to Sham Surgery

	Surgery Group at 12 Months	Sham Surgery Group at 12 Months
Complete elimination ($p < 0.0001$)	28/49 (57.1%)	1/26 (3.8%)
No change ($p = 0.02$)	8/49 (16.5%)	11/26 (42.3%)
Significant improvement in frequency, intensity, duration, or migraine index ($p = 0.014$)*	41/49 (83.7%)	15/26 (57.7%)
Difference between baseline and 12-month follow-up	All of the measures were significantly improved	Only some of the measures were improved

Data from Guyuron B, Reed D, Kriegler JS, et al. A placebo-controlled surgical trial of the treatment of migraine headaches. Plast Reconstr Surg 124:461-468, 2009.
*Improvements were not dependent on the trigger site.

Endpoints All patients maintained a daily headache diary and completed monthly migraine headache questionnaires that assessed the frequency, intensity, and duration of their headaches. At the beginning of the study and at the end of 1 year, patients completed the Medical Outcomes Study 36-Item Short Form Health Survey, Migraine-Specific Quality of Life, and Migraine Disability Assessment questionnaires.

Results Only 1 of 76 patients failed to complete the 1-year follow-up. The mean age was 44.9 years. All preoperative baseline scores were comparative between the treatment and sham groups. Sham group patients were offered actual surgery after the completion of the 1-year follow-up. Of these 26 patients, 22 had undergone actual surgery.

Patients who experienced migraine headaches both with and without aura had greater improvement in intensity scores at 12 months compared with those who always experienced migraines with aura or without aura (Table 43-1). This bordered statistical significance ($p = 0.057$). Otherwise, there was no significant difference between the groups on any of the other variables. The extent of improvement in the frequency, intensity, Migraine Disability Assessment score, and Migraine-Specific Quality of Life scores was significantly higher in the actual versus the sham group ($p < 0.05$).

The outcome measures obtained at 3, 6, 9, and 12 months were averaged and compared with the baseline values (Table 43-2). The average of the outcome measures over 12 months was significantly improved from the baseline values in the actual surgery group ($p < 0.01$). The only significant factor affecting improvement was actual surgery ($p = 0.016$) with an adjusted odds ratio of 3.97.

Table 43-2   Overall Change From Baseline to 12 Months By Location and Type of Surgery

Variable	Actual Surgery*	Sham Surgery*	p
Number	49	26	
Elimination	28/49 (57.1%)	1/26 (3.8%)	<0.001
Significant improvement	41/49 (83.7%)	15/26 (57.7%)	0.014
Frequency, MH/mo	7.4 ± 5.8 (<0.001)	3.5 ± 5.4 (0.003)	$p_G = 0.005$
Frontal	6.3 ± 6.7 (<0.001)	1.5 ± 3.3 (0.18)	$p_L = 0.17$
Temporal	7.8 ± 74.8 (<0.001)	4.1 ± 6.8 (0.11)	
Occipital	8.7 ± 6.1 (<0.001)	5.7 ± 5.6 (0.04)	
Intensity (visual analog scale, 1-10)	3.0 ± 3.5 (<0.001)	1.3 ± 2.9 (0.03)	$p_G = 0.03$
Frontal	2.5 ± 3.5 (0.005)	2.1 ± 3.1 (0.51)	$p_L = 0.34$
Temporal	2.4 ± 3.8 (0.001)	0.46 ± 2.7 (0.17)	
Occipital	4.2 ± 3.4 (<0.001)	1.3 ± 3.2 (0.45)	
Duration, days	0.30 ± 0.46 (<0.001)	0.87 ± 4.5 (0.34)	$p_G = 0.43$
Frontal	0.24 ± 0.36 (0.01)	−0.18 ± 0.94 (0.57)	$p_L = 0.13$
Temporal	0.21 ± 0.47 (0.07)	0.10 ± 0.33 (0.40)	
Occipital	0.54 ± 0.55 (0.009)	3.37 ± 7.7 (0.34)	
Migraine headache index	21.6 ± 29.6 (<0.001)	9.7 ± 23.9 (0.05)	$p_G = 0.07$
Frontal	15.4 ± 19.1 (0.003)	12.2 ± 15.4 (0.03)	$p_L = 0.29$
Temporal	18.9 ± 21.8 (0.001)	7.8 ± 36.5 (0.54)	
Occipital	37.1 ± 48.4 (0.03)	8.5 ± 15.1 (0.18)	
MIDAS	1.5 ± 1.5 (<0.001)	0.77 ± 1.3 (0.007)	$p_G = 0.05$
Frontal	1.3 ± 1.5 (0.001)	0.2 ± 1.0 (0.56)	$p_L = 0.32$
Temporal	1.6 ± 1.6 (<0.001)	1.3 ± 1.2 (0.01)	
Occipital	1.5 ± 1.5 (0.01)	0.86 ± 1.7 (0.22)	
MSQEM	36.0 ± 45.8 (<0.001)	10.8 ± 39.0 (0.17)	$p_G = 0.02$
Frontal	24.0 ± 41.9 (0.02)	0.4 ± 29.6 (0.97)	$p_L = 0.12$
Temporal	36.5 ± 44.6 (0.002)	16.6 ± 52.1 (0.37)	
Occipital	56.0 ± 51.0 (0.005)	18.1 ± 33.2 (0.20)	
MSQPRE	18.7 ± 22.0 (<0.001)	−13.1 ± 22.1 (0.006)	$p_G = 0.29$
Frontal	−18.8 ± 19.7 (<0.001)	−16.0 ± 30.7 (0.13)	$p_L = 0.85$
Temporal	−15.3 ± 21.6 (0.006)	−14.4 ± 11.6 (0.006)	
Occipital	−24.5 ± 26.9 (0.013)	−7.1 ± 19.8 (0.39)	
MSQRES	−27.8 ± 23.3 (<0.001)	−13.3 ± 20.9 (0.003)	$p_G = 0.01$
Frontal	25.7 ± 23.2 (<0.001)	−11.8 ± 29.6 (0.24)	$p_L = 0.83$
Temporal	−29.1 ± 22.5 (<0.001)	−16.3 ± 17.3 (0.02)	
Occipital	−29.2 ± 26.9 (0.005)	−11.4 ± 9.1 (0.02)	
SFPH	−4.9 ± 8.7 (0.003)	−2.1 ± 8.7 (0.23)	$p_G = 0.20$
Frontal	5.9 ± 6.9 (0.002)	1.5 ± 7.0 (0.51)	$p_L = 0.87$
Temporal	−5.4 ± 11.4 (0.056)	−0.89 ± 8.4 (0.76)	
Occipital	−2.1 ± 5.6 (0.24)	−8.7 ± 8.6 (0.4)	

From Guyuron B, Reed D, Kriegler JS, et al. A placebo-controlled surgical trial of the treatment of migraine headaches. Plast Reconstr Surg 124:461-468, 2009.

*The p values inside the parentheses adjacent to each measure represent the comparison between baseline and 12 months using paired analysis.

Continuous data are represented as mean ± SD.

p_G, Comparison between actual and sham surgery (p value computed from two-sample t test and verified by Wilcoxon rank test); p_L, comparisons among the trigger sites; *MH*, migraine headaches; *MIDAS*, Migraine Disability Assessment Score; *MSQEM*, Migraine-Specific Quality of Life, emotional; *MSQPRE*, Migraine-Specific Quality of Life, preventive; *MSQRES*, Migraine-Specific Quality of Life, restrictive; *SFPH*, Medical Outcomes Study 36-Item Short Form Health Survey, physical.

Adverse events.   All patients reported some degree of paresthesia in the immediate postoperative period. Only one patient had persistent numbness at 1 year. There were no neuromas. Temporal hollowing occurred in 10 of 19 (53%) patients in the temporal group. There was temporary intense pruritus in two patients. One patient had slight asymmetrical eyebrow movement. Temporary hair loss or thinning occurred in one patient. One patient had residual corrugator supercilii function, which was associated with residual migraines. Postoperative neck stiffness occurred in one patient at 1 year in the occipital group. There were no adverse events noted in the sham surgery group.

Criticisms/Limitations   How do the authors explain the 26 patients who underwent sham surgery who had complete elimination of their migraine headaches at 1 year? How do they explain the 8 of 49 patients who underwent actual surgery who had no change in their migraine headaches? The authors explain that this could be because these patients had more than one trigger point.

How did the authors identify the primary trigger site? The authors point out "when the failed cases were analyzed, it appears that the predominant migraine headache trigger site was incorrectly assigned in some instances." It is likely that pinpointing the primary trigger point is made more difficult if the pain from one site is almost equal in intensity to another site and "masks" the true trigger point. Alternatively, treatment with Botox or surgery may change the primary trigger site over time.

Also, it would be interesting to see the outcomes of the 22 of 26 sham surgery patients, who returned for actual surgery, because these subjects would serve as internal controls.

Relevant Studies

Moskowitz MA. The neurobiology of vascular head pain. Ann Neurol 10:157-168, 1984.

Zwart JA, Bovim G, Sand T, et al. Tension headache: botulinum toxin paralysis of temporal muscles. Headache 34:458-462, 1994.

Hobson DE, Gladish DF. Botulinum toxin injection for cervicogenic headache. Headache 37:253-255, 1997.

Relja M. Treatment of tension-type headache by local injection of botulinum toxin [abstract]. Eur J Neurol 4(Suppl 2):S71-S72, 1997.

Binder W, Brin MF, Blitzer A, et al. Botulinum toxin type A (BTX-A) for migraine: an open label assessment. Mov Disord 13(Suppl 2):241, 1998.

Johnstone SJ, Adler CH. Headache and facial pain responsive to botulinum toxin: an unusual presentation of blepharospasm. Headache 38:366-368, 1998.

Wheeler AH. Botulinum toxin A, adjunctive therapy for refractory headaches associated with pericranial muscle tension. Headache 38:468-471, 1998.

Relja M, Korsic M. Treatment of tension-type headache by injections of botulinum toxin type A: double-blind, placebo-controlled study. Neurology 52:A203, 1999.

Schulte-Mattler WJ, Wieser T, Zierz S. Treatment of tension-type headache with botulinum toxin: a pilot study. Eur J Med Res 4:183-186, 1999.

Guyuron B, Varghai A, Michelow BJ, et al. Corrugator supercilii resection and migraine headaches. Plast Reconstr Surg 106:429-434; discussion 435-437, 2000.
  The authors performed this study based on the two observations that the incidental discovery of Botox injection is beneficial in some patients and that similar relief is experienced in those who had undergone resection of the corrugator supercilii muscles. They found that 79.5% of patients had elimination or improvement of migraines after corrugator resection, and the benefits lasted over a mean of 47 months.

Silberstein S, Mathew N, Saper J, et al. Botulinum toxin type A as a migraine preventative treatment. For the BOTOX Migraine Clinical Research Group. Headache 40:445-450, 2000.
  This was a double-blind, vehicle-controlled trial of 123 patients with migraine headaches. Compared with control subjects, those treated with 25 units of Botox had significantly improved migraine symptoms at 1 month, which demonstrated the efficacy of the pericranial injection of Botox for the improvement of migraine symptoms.

Dirnberger F, Becker K. Surgical treatment of migraine headaches by corrugator muscle resection. Plast Reconstr Surg 114:652-657; discussion 658-659, 2004.
  As a response to the 2000 article of Guyuron et al, the authors (Dirnberger, a plastic surgeon, and Becker, a neurologist), conducted a study of 60 patients with migraine headaches who underwent corrugator supercilii resection. Seventeen (28.3%) reported total relief from migraine, 24 (40%) reported an essential improvement, and 19 (31.7%) reported minimal or no change. After 3 months, the results in all patients could be declared permanent. All side effects, including paresthesia in the frontal region, resolved in all patients within 3 to 9 months.

Guyuron B, Kriegler J, Davis J, et al. Comprehensive surgical treatment of migraine headaches. Plast Reconstr Surg 115:1-9, 2005.

After it was shown that surgical deactivation of one peripheral migraine trigger site was effective, Guyuron et al then proceeded to ask whether deactivation worked at all other trigger points. In this study 100 patients underwent surgical deactivation of the frontal, temporal, and occipital trigger points. In comparison with 25 control subjects, the 92% of surgically treated patients had a 50% or greater decrease in symptoms.

Guyuron B, Kriegler J, Davis J, et al. Five-year outcome of surgical treatment of migraine headache. Plast Reconstr Surg 127:603-608, 2011.

The authors reported the 5-year results of patients in their 2005 study. Sixty-one of 69 patients (88%) experienced a positive response to the surgery after 5 years. Twenty patients (29%) reported complete elimination of migraine headache, 41 (59%) noticed a significant decrease, and 8 (12%) experienced no significant change. When compared with the baseline values, all measured variables at 60 months improved significantly (p <0.0001).

Kung TA, Guyuron B, Cederna PS. Migraine surgery: a plastic surgery solution for refractory migraine headache. Plast Reconstr Surg 127:181-189, 2011.

This article is a comprehensive overview of the history of migraine headache surgery. It first details the pathogenesis of migraine headache, the inadequacy of pharmacologic agents to treat migraines, the successful use of Botox as support for peripheral triggers, and ends with a review of the literature.

Kung TA, Pannucci CJ, Chamberlain JL, et al. Migraine surgery practice patterns and attitudes. Plast Reconstr Surg 129:623-628, 2012.

This was a Web-based survey that asked the 3747 members of the American Society of Plastic Surgeons about their attitude toward migraine surgery. Of the 193 returned surveys, 34 respondents (18%) had performed surgical treatment of migraine headaches and more than 80% reported improvement in patient symptoms. Of those who had not performed migraine surgery, 60% stated they would be interested if appropriate patients were referred to them by a neurologist.

Menghyan TL, Chim H, Guyuron B. Outcome comparison of endoscopic and transpalpebral decompression for treatments of frontal migraine headaches. Plast Reconstr Surg 129:113-119, 2012.

This study compared the efficacy of transpalpebral versus endoscopic approach for surgical decompression of frontal migraine headaches. Endoscopic decompression had a higher success rate and higher symptom elimination rate than the transpalpebral approach. The authors recommended the endoscopic approach as the first choice for frontal migraine headache surgery when anatomically possible.

Summary   Surgical deactivation of peripheral migraine trigger points is an effective treatment for moderate-to-severe migraine headaches that are difficult to manage with standard protocols.

The high incidence of improvement in the sham group could be related to altered neurosensory function that resulted from incision and undermining around the trigger point.

When the failed cases were analyzed, it revealed that the primary trigger site was not properly assigned, which indicated that more than one trigger point contributed to the migraine headaches.

Implications   This prospective, placebo-controlled, double-blinded trial was the culmination of previous research initiated by Guyuron et al. Botox became more widely used to treat forehead rhytids, and patients would see incidental improvements in their migraine headaches. Practitioners began targeted Botox treatment to pericranial muscles for migraine relief. This, along with reports that corrugator supercilii resection incidentally improved migraine symptoms, led Guyuron et al to ask whether corrugator resection helped eliminate migraine symptoms. In 2000 Guyuron et al showed that 79.5% noted the elimination or improvement of migraines after corrugator resection and that the benefits lasted over a mean of 47 months. After they proved that surgical deactivation worked at one trigger point, Guyuron et al then proceeded to ask whether deactivation would work at other trigger points. In 2005, 100 patients who had improvement of symptoms after Botox injection underwent surgical deactivation of trigger points. In comparison with 25 control subjects, the 92% of surgically treated patients had a 50% or greater decrease in symptoms. After they proved that surgery works to deactivate all peripheral trigger points, Guyuron et al then conducted the current study to determine whether the improvement was from the actual procedure versus a placebo effect. The origin of headache surgery, whose timeline began with the use of Botox for blepharospasm and was then applied to treat glabellar rhytids and peripheral migraine trigger points, is an elegant evolution of translational research and an example of how plastic surgeons can innovate in collaboration with ophthalmology and neurology colleagues.

REFERENCE

1. Guyuron B, Reed D, Kriegler JS, et al. A placebo-controlled surgical trial of the treatment of migraine headaches. Plast Reconstr Surg 124:461-468, 2009.

STUDY AUTHOR REFLECTIONS

Bahman Guyuron, MD, FACS

The development of a surgical treatment for migraine headaches, as a result of the reports from patients who were undergoing forehead rejuvenation, has been the most rewarding event in my 34 years of plastic surgery practice for several reasons. First, millions of patients do not benefit from preventive or abortive migraine treatments and have an utterly poor quality of life that could be altered drastically by surgical interventions. Second, many of the patients who undergo surgery not only feel better, but they also look better or can breathe more comfortably through the nose if the septum and turbinates are part of the migraine trigger sites. Furthermore, in an era when the field of plastic surgery is primarily identified as the specialty that deals mostly with the frivolous use of filler and suction lipectomy, recognition of life-changing procedures will contribute to securing the respect that our specialty deserves. The wide incorporation of migraine surgery will serve such an enormous role.

CHAPTER 44

Subfascial Endoscopic Transaxillary Augmentation Mammaplasty

Graf RM, Bernardes A, Auersvald A, Damasio RC. Aesthetic Plast Surg 24:216-220, 2000

Reviewed by Cindy Wu, MD

> *Breast augmentation with an S-shape incision for transaxillary access is utilized to introduce the implant, in a submuscular or subglandular and, recently (since October 1998), in a subfascial location . . . Patient satisfaction was high, especially regarding the axillary incision. There have been no capsular contractions to date.[1]*

Research Question None

Funding None

Study Dates August 1998 to January 1999

Publishing Date 2000

Location A private clinic in Curitiba, Brazil

Subjects Sixty-two patients underwent endoscopic augmentation: 49 submuscular, 5 subglandular, and 8 subfascial; ages ranged from 15 to 48 years.

Exclusion Criteria None

Sample Size 62

Overview of Design A retrospective review of a single surgeon's experience

Intervention None

Follow-up 3 years

Endpoints   Any complications

Results   There were no capsular contractures and a very high patient satisfaction rate. One hematoma was treated with US-guided drainage, and two malpositions were treated with transaxillary endoscopic repositioning.

Conclusion   Endoscopic transaxillary mammaplasty is a safe alternative to breast augmentation and gives better and more natural results.

The subfascial plane has recently been the authors' choice for breast augmentation because at the upper pole, the implant resembles a submuscular implant without sharp demarcation, whereas at the lower pole, the breast looks like a subglandular implant without flattening as occurs in submuscular implants. The end result is a more natural breast shape with the subfascial implant.

Criticisms/Limitations   There was no control group. A reasonable control group would have been patients who underwent submuscular, subglandular, or subfascial augmentation by inframammary or periareolar incision.

There was no patient or physician aesthetic analysis of subfascial augmentation compared with submuscular or subglandular augmentation. Without a validated scale, it is difficult to conclude that subfascial augmentation gives a "more natural" appearing breast augmentation than the other two planes.

There was a small sample size (8/62) of patients who underwent subfascial augmentation.

Related Studies

Ho LC. Endoscopic assisted transaxillary augmentation mammaplasty. Br J Plast Surg 46:332-336, 1993.
This was the first description of endoscopic transaxillary augmentation.

Johnson GW, Christ JE. The endoscopic breast augmentation: the transumbilical insertion of saline-filled breast implants. Plast Reconstr Surg 92:801-808, 1993.
This was the first description of the use of an endoscope for saline augmentation with a transumbilical approach. The transumbilical approach is not commonly used today, but endoscopic transaxillary augmentation is still performed.

Benito-Ruiz J. Transaxillary subfascial breast augmentation. Aesthet Surg J 23:480-483, 2003.
The author published his own cadaveric dissection findings in the subfascial plane along with his clinical outcomes in 16 patients after 1-year follow-up. There were no postoperative complications, no capsular contractions, and no loss of nipple sensa-

tion. He stated that compared with submuscular placement, this technique involved less risk of hematoma, less pain, and faster recovery, and injury to the intercostobrachial nerve was less likely. Also, there was no change in implant shape with muscle contracture.

Graf RM, Bernardes A, Rippel R, et al. Subfascial breast implant: a new procedure. Plast Reconstr Surg 111:904-908, 2003.

Graf first performed subfascial augmentation in 1998 but did not publish the technique until the paper was reviewed in this chapter. After this, she published "Techniques in Cosmetic Surgery," which included 3-year follow-up on 263 patients who underwent subfascial augmentation. None of the patients had implant distortion or palpable edges. Six (2.3%) had Baker class II capsular contracture, three (1.1%) had a unilateral hematoma requiring reoperation, and eight (3%) had unilateral implant malposition requiring reoperation. There were no infections.

Benito-Ruiz J. Subfascial breast implant. Plast Reconstr Surg 113:1088-1089; author reply 1089, 2004.

The author confirmed the ease of subfascial dissection in his own cadaveric study. He stated that endoscopic assistance was unnecessary: that blunt dissection, packing, and then hemostasis with a lighted retractor have helped him avoid endoscopy. He supported the several advantages to this approach: ease of insertion in the subglandular plane, a natural result, no animation deformity, faster recovery compared with submuscular placement, lower risk of intercostobrachial nerve damage resulting from more superficial dissection, and the use of the axillary approach for grade 1 ptosis.

Tebbetts JB. Does fascia provide additional, meaningful coverage over a breast implant? Plast Reconstr Surg 113:777-779; author reply 779-780, 2004.

The author countered Graf's notion that subfascial augmentation avoids animation deformity and stated that the dual-plane technique reduces both static and dynamic distortions because of the thicker coverage of the pectoralis muscle (1 cm thick pectoralis muscle versus 0.1 to 0.5 mm thickness of the fascia). He also stated that the intact elevation of the fascia is difficult even for the most technically skilled surgeons. "Absent 1) the quantitative data documenting fascial thickness, 2) proof that fascia is intact over implant edges, and 3) data comparing submammary to subfascial pocket locations long term with respect to implant edge visibility and traction rippling. Surgeons have no scientific proof whatsoever that a layer of fascia, known to be highly variable and difficult to predictably raise intact, provides any meaningful coverage over a breast implant." Graf subsequently replied that the fascia is thicker superiorly, and therefore it is possible to raise intact medially, superiorly, and laterally. Although the fascia is not a thick tissue, it is inelastic compared with the skin or muscle and therefore protects the overlying soft tissue from atrophy over time. She referenced ongoing tensiometry studies. Although it is true that no current data confirmed fascia thickness and it varied among patients, cadaveric dissections revealed a thickness of 0.2 cm centrally and 1 mm superiorly, laterally, and medially. It also had more resistance than the mammary gland or subcutaneous tissue. Considering the trade-offs of the submuscular pocket location, the additional coverage that the fascia provides, the greater tensile strength of this fascia and therefore less deformity, and with the use of smaller implants (235 to 250 cc), they concluded that the subfascial implant pocket location can, in the majority of cases, lead to optimal implant coverage, as supported by their long-term results.

Hunstad JP, Webb LS. Subfascial breast augmentation: a comprehensive experience. Aesthetic Plast Surg 34:365-373, 2010.

This was a retrospective review of 61 subfascial augmentations with 2- to 24-month follow-up. The authors reported their 3-year experience with subfascial augmentation and reported a high degree of patient and surgeon satisfaction with few complications, a low rate of capsular contracture, no evidence of breast animation with arm movement, excellent lower pole coverage, and a brief recovery period.

Summary and Implications   Graf was the first to describe the subfascial technique and bring it to the United States. This method combined the advantages of both the submuscular and subglandular approaches and added another dimension to breast augmentation planning. Her transaxillary endoscopic approach also gave plastic surgeons another access point for breast augmentation.

REFERENCE

1. Graf RM, Bernardes A, Auersvald A, et al. Subfascial endoscopic transaxillary augmentation mammaplasty. Aesthetic Plast Surg 24:216-220, 2000.

STUDY AUTHOR REFLECTIONS

Ruth Graf, MD, PhD

A key way that this procedure fits into my body of work is that I am always optimization oriented. I always look for approaches that offer less surgical trauma and reduced scarring while providing results that are equal or superior to results with more traditional approaches. After performing this procedure more than 700 times with minimal complications and seeing it adopted by more and more surgeons worldwide, I find that it is an easy procedure to perform with electrocautery and offers reproducible results.

In terms of how it fits into the plastic surgery literature in general, optimal results with minimal invasion, scarring, and the risk of complications are always the continually advancing goals. The subfascial pocket is an option for patients who desire more natural-looking results, because the fascia provides enough coverage to soften the implant outline, the S scar hidden in the fold of the axilla is nominal and discrete, and unlike with submuscular placement, we do not see implant displacement from arm movement.

From another perspective—because breast augmentation with implants is one of the most performed plastic surgeries worldwide and because of the inevitable necessity of periodic replacement of those implants, surprisingly little attention has been paid until now regarding how future implants will be accommodated with adequate support and coverage. The ability to use the subfascial plane for one of those sequential implantations offers another excellent pocket option in that lifetime scenario.

CHAPTER 45

Treatment of Glabellar Frown Lines With C. Botulinum-A Exotoxin

Carruthers JD, Carruthers JA. J Dermatol Surg Oncol 18:17-21, 1992

Reviewed by Cindy Wu, MD

Because C. botulinum-A exotoxin therapy of glabellar frown lines treats the underlying cause of these lines, it is more effective than soft tissue augmentation although this improvement is temporary. Treatment with C. botulinum-A exotoxin is a simple, safe procedure [1]

Research Question   Does C. botulinum-A exotoxin improve glabellar frown lines? C. botulinum-A exotoxin had previously been used for the treatment of blepharospasm, strabismus, and hemifacial spasm, with incidental improvement of glabellar frown lines. Therefore the authors investigated whether targeted treatment of the corrugator muscles with C. botulinum-A exotoxin improved glabellar rhytids.

Funding   None; C. botulinum-A exotoxin was obtained from the Smith-Kettlewell Institute of Visual Sciences, San Francisco, CA, as part of a multicenter trial of C. botulinum toxin therapy of strabismus, benign essential blepharospasm, hemifacial spasm, and spastic lower eyelid entroprion. After September 1990, it was obtained from Allergan Pharmaceuticals, Irvine, CA.

Study Dates   Not reported

Publishing Date   1992

Location   Vancouver, British Columbia, Canada

Subjects   Patients ages 34 to 51 years; average age was 41.4 years, all of whom had undergone a full ophthalmologic examination.

Exclusion Criteria   None described

Sample Size   18 white patients (17 women and 1 man)

Overview of Design   Subjects with glabellar rhytids were injected with C. botulinum-A exotoxin and followed for up to 6 years to determine toxin longevity (in months) and the number of repeated injections needed. Repeat injections were performed on average every 4 to 11 months.

Intervention   Subjects were treated in the seated position. After cleaning the glabella with an alcohol wipe, the subject was asked to frown and maintain this expression during the procedure. Injection was performed with a 30-gauge needle on a tuberculin syringe. The toxin was injected along the entire vertical length of the rhytid in a deep subdermal plane. The toxin was injected on withdrawal and evenly distributed along the rhytid. The other method of injection was directly into the corrugator muscle belly after contraction. The dilution of C. botulinum-A exotoxin was as follows: a 100-unit vial of freeze-dried ($-4°$ C) onabotulinumtoxinA (Botox) was reconstituted with 1 mL of preservative-free normal saline solution, making each 0.1 mL = 10 units. Carruthers described: "The compound in solution is highly unstable and must be used within several hours of preparation." Each corrugator was injected with the initial dose of 10 to 12.5 units per rhytid, and the final dose was 10 to 20 units per rhytid or per corrugator. Bilateral rhytids were treated.

Follow-up   After the 3-month follow-up period had passed, the frequency of injections was every 4 months for most patients. One patient required six injections, with an 11-month duration between injections.

Endpoints   The results were measured by both an objective analysis of cutaneous appearance (smooth, no furrow visible, minimal line, residual but improved line, or no response) and a subjective patient analysis (scale of 0 to 7 where 7 was the highest correlation with patient expectations).

Results   Ninety percent of patients who had multiple injections (Table 45-1) needed a second injection within 3 months of the first injection (Table 45-2). All patients had their first injection into the rhytid itself. Six had one or more subsequent injection sessions into the corrugator muscle.

Objective analysis.   The cutaneous appearance gauge was smooth—no furrow visible, minimal line, residual but improved line, or no response. Responders: six had brows that became completely smooth, two had residual minimal lines, and eight still had a discernible crease, but it was less deep. One patient did not respond to follow-up requests; one patient was lost to follow-up.

Subjective analysis results can be found in Table 45-3.

Table 45-1 Number of Patients Having Single or Multiple Injection Sessions

Number of Patients	Number of Injections
8	1
3	3
2	9
1	2
1	4
1	6
1	7
1	8
0	5

Data from Carruthers JD, Carruthers JA. Treatment of glabellar frown lines with C. botulinum-A exotoxin. J Dermatol Surg Oncol 18:17-21, 1992.

Table 45-2 Time Between Injection Sessions in Patients Who Have Undergone Six or More Sessions

Number of Injections (Patients)	Interval Between Sessions (Months)
9 (2)	9 and 4
8 (1)	10
7 (1)	7
6 (1)	11

Data from Carruthers JD, Carruthers JA. Treatment of glabellar frown lines with C. botulinum-A exotoxin. J Dermatol Surg Oncol 18:17-21, 1992.

Table 45-3 Subjective Patient Response to C. Botulinum Toxin Injection for Brow Furrows*

Scale	Patients (N = 18)
7	5
6	5
5	3
4	2
3	0
2	0
1	0
0	2
Lost to follow-up	1

Data from Carruthers JD, Carruthers JA. Treatment of glabellar frown lines with C. botulinum-A exotoxin. J Dermatol Surg Oncol 18:17-21, 1992.
*Based on a scale, 0 to 7, where 7 was an exact correlation between subjective expectations and perceived beneficial results.

Table 45-4   Complications of C. Botulinum Toxin Injection Treatment of Glabellar Frown Lines

Complications	N
Transient headache	2
Transient numbness	1
Ptosis	
Brow	1
Lid	1

Data from Carruthers JD, Carruthers JA. Treatment of glabellar frown lines with C. botulinum-A exotoxin. J Dermatol Surg Oncol 18:17-21, 1992.

Complications from the treatment can be found in Table 45-4.

Collagen injections.   Eight patients received both Botox and collagen injections: six had collagen injection before Botox, one was allergic to collagen, and five preferred the Botox effect. Two had collagen injection after Botox: one preferred the combination of Botox and collagen, and one preferred collagen because she was concerned about the systemic toxicity of Botox.

Reasons for the discontinuation of Botox.   Most patients (10/18) wanted to continue Botox because they liked not being able to frown with the attendant positive self-image and because of the simplicity of treatment. The most frequent reason for discontinuation was because the patient moved away (3/18).

Criticisms/Limitations   The objective and subjective analyses were not validated scales. The authors did not screen out patients for pregnancy, allergy, neuromuscular disorders, and aminoglycoside use, and they were not clear about why they chose the six patients to have injections into the corrugator muscle during the subsequent sessions. (All of the patients had injection directly into the rhytid during the first session.)

Related Studies   This landmark study was the foundation for future studies by Carruthers and Carruthers. In 2002 they published the first large, multicenter, double-blind, randomized, placebo-controlled study of the efficacy and safety of botulinum toxin type A in the treatment of glabellar lines in the Botox Glabellar Lines I Study Group. In this paper 246 patients with moderate-to-severe glabellar frown lines were enrolled. The 203 patients who received Botox had a significantly greater reduction of glabellar lines according to all measures compared with placebo (all measures, every follow-up visit; $p < 0.022$). This effect was maintained until day 120. The adverse events (5.4%) mostly were mild blepharoptosis in the Botox-treated group.

After collecting an additional 10 patients, they published their results in a plastic surgery journal in 2003, which confirmed their previous results in a second large, multicenter, clinical trial in the Botox Glabellar Lines II Study Group.

Carruthers J, Stubbs HA. Botulinum toxin for benign essential blepharospasm, hemifacial spasm and age-related eyelid entroprion. Can J Neurol Sci 14:42-45, 1987.

> *This article described the use of Botox for the treatment of blepharospasm, hemifacial spasm, and entroprion. Because of the incidental findings of rhytid elimination in patients treated with Botox for blepharospasm, the authors used Botox to treat other facial rhytids.*

Tsui JK, Wong NLM, Wong E, et al. Production of circulating antibodies to botulinum A toxin in patients receiving repeated injections for dystonia [abstract]. Ann Neurol 23:181, 1988.

Scott AB. Clostridial toxins as therapeutic agents. In Simpson LL, ed. Botulinum Neurotoxin and Tetanus Toxin. New York: Academic Press, 1989.

Smith Kettlewell Institute of Visual Sciences. Botulinum toxin (Oculinum®) study: IND-723. Patients treated as of 31 December 1989. San Francisco: Smith Kettlewell Institute of Visual Sciences, 1990.

Therapeutics and Technology Assessment Committee of the American Academy of Neurology. The clinical usefulness of botulinum toxin-A in treating neurologic disorders. Report of the Therapeutics and Technology Assessment Committee of the American Academy of Neurology. Neurology 40:1332-1333, 1990.

Borodic GE. Botulinum A toxin for (expressionistic) ptosis overcorrection after frontalis sling. Ophthal Plast Reconstr Surg 8:137-142, 1992.

Blitzer A, Brin MF, Keen MS, et al. Botulinum toxin for the treatment of hyperfunctional lines of the face. Arch Otolaryngol Head Neck Surg 119:1018-1022, 1993.

American Academy of Neurology Therapeutics and Technology Assessment Subcommittee. Training guidelines for the treatment of neurologic disorders. Report of the Therapeutics and Technology Assessment Subcommittee of the American Academy of Neurology. Neurology 44:2401-2403, 1994.

Keen M, Blitzer A, Aviv J, et al. Botulinum toxin A for hyperkinetic facial lines: results of a double blind, placebo-controlled study. Plast Reconstr Surg 94:94-99, 1994.

Lowe NJ, Maxwell A, Harper H. Botulinum A exotoxin for glabellar folds: a double-blind, placebo-controlled study with an electromyographic injection technique. J Am Acad Dermatol 35:569-572, 1996.

Silberstein S, Matthew N, Saper J, et al. Botulinum toxin type A as a migraine preventative treatment. For the BOTOX Migraine Clinical Research Group. Headache 40:445-450, 2000.

> *This was a double-blind, vehicle-controlled trial of 123 patients with migraine headaches. Compared with control subjects, those treated with 25 units of Botox had significantly improved migraine symptoms at 1 month, which demonstrated the efficacy of pericranial injection of Botox for the improvement of migraine symptoms.*

Naumann M, Lowe NJ. Botulinum toxin type A in treatment of bilateral primary axillary hyperhidrosis: randomised, parallel group, double blind, placebo controlled trial. BMJ 323:596-599, 2001.

Carruthers JA, Lowe NJ, Menter MA, Gibson J, Nordquist M, Mordaunt J, Walker P, Eadie N; BOTOX Glabellar Line I Study Group. A multicenter, double-blind, placebo-controlled study of the efficacy and safety of botulinum toxin type A in the treatment of glabellar lines. J Am Acad Dermatol 46:840-849, 2002.

> *This article described the first large, multicenter, double-blind, randomized, placebo-controlled study of the efficacy and safety of botulinum toxin type A in the treatment of glabellar lines in the Botox Glabellar Lines I Study Group. In this study 246 patients with moderate-to-severe glabellar frown lines were enrolled. The 203 patients who received Botox had a significantly greater reduction of glabellar lines according to all measures compared with placebo (all measures, every follow-up visit; p <0.022). This effect was maintained until day 120. The adverse events (5.4%) were mostly of mild blepharoptosis in the Botox-treated group.*

Carruthers JA, Lowe NJ, Menter MA, Gibson J, Eadie N; BOTOX Glabellar Line II Study Group. Double-blind, placebo-controlled study of the safety and efficacy of botulinum toxin type A for patients with glabellar lines. Plast Reconstr Surg 112:1089-1098, 2003.

> *After collecting an additional 10 patients, they published their results in a plastic surgery journal in 2003, which confirmed their previous results in a second large, multicenter clinical trial in the Botox Glabellar Lines II Study Group.*

Summary   Botox inhibits acetylcholine release at the neuromuscular junction, preventing neuromuscular transmission after a 3- to 5-day latency period with a variable but average 3-month duration.

In patients who have undergone this therapy for a long time, Botox can last for 7 to 11 months. In a large series of patients with blepharospasm treated over 8 years, patients required 6-month intervals after the first 3 years. The authors hypothesized that this may be the result of a "retraining" effect because patients cannot frown during this period of chemodenervation. Repeated injection into a small area may be damaging the muscle or its innervation.

The side effects of central brow and eyelid ptosis are transient. The ptosis rate in this current study was 11% (2/18), which is consistent with the 11% ptosis rate reported in a series of benign essential blepharospasm injections.

Botox is less likely than collagen, fat, or silicone to cause embolic damage to the retina.

An immune reaction to Botox does not seem to occur.

Botox is a safe and effective treatment for glabellar frown lines.

Implications   Botox, which was originally described to treat blepharospasm, has also been shown to be useful for aesthetic indications. This led the Food and Drug Administration to approve Botox for the treatment of glabellar rhytids. As a result, Botox became widely popular for the off-label treatment of other facial rhytids. The ease of treatment, minimal down time, and wide patient tolerance made Botox and facial fillers the most popular nonsurgical procedure in plastic surgery in 2012.

REFERENCES

1. Carruthers JD, Carruthers JA. Treatment of glabellar frown lines with C. botulinum-A exotoxin. J Dermatol Surg Oncol 18:17-21, 1992.
2. Cosmetic Surgery National Data Bank: statistics 2012. Aesthet Surg J 33(2 Suppl):1S-21S, 2013. *These are the national statistics of all cosmetic procedures performed in the United States for 2012. It shows that Botox and fillers were the number one cosmetic and nonsurgical procedure in 2012.*

EDITORIAL PERSPECTIVE

C. Scott Hultman, MD, MBA, FACS

The introduction of C. botulinum toxin therapy represents one of the most substantial innovations in the history of plastic surgery. Although Botox functions as a "substitute good" for surgical procedures such as brow lift, facial rejuvenation with this product can be performed at a fraction of the cost, with a better safety profile than surgery, sometimes with better results, and by nonsurgeons. Patients are willing to accept this "inferior service" because of improved value, which is the ratio of quality to cost. As such, Botox is now a commodity, subject to market pressures of supply and demand.

The good news for plastic surgeons is that because innovation is our core competency, we can incorporate this disruptive force into our own practices, yielding results not previously possible.

Peter Drucker, founder of Modern Management Theory, declared, "Knowledge has to be improved, challenged, and increased constantly, or it vanishes." The process of innovation can be incremental or disruptive. When big companies fail, they often do so not because they neglected innovation or made mistakes, but because they did everything right. Established, successful businesses usually focus on sustaining innovations, incremental changes that yield a slightly higher profit margin through improved efficiency or quality. These changes help the company sustain market position by maintaining the rate of improvement of a product or service, which results in increased production or improved attributes, thereby making the product or service better in ways that are already valued by the consumer.[2]

However, these companies are vulnerable to disruptive innovations that often emerge in the nebulous, low-margin fringes of the market. Disruptive innovation improves a product or service in ways that the market does not expect, first by attracting a different set of consumers and later by lowering prices to attract the existing conventional market. The final result is that disruptive innovation creates new markets, networks, and values, and displaces older technologies. Such is the strategy of new entrants, who must first capture a small market share by competing with substitute goods or services, usually with a low profit margin. A paradigm shift occurs, which the consumer changes what she or he wants or needs.[2]

Recent examples include adoption of the MP3 music file, which forever altered distribution channels in the music industry, as well as the introduction of smartphones, which simultaneously affected the three industries that produce cell phones, cameras, and laptops. The development of office-based surgery, when done in an accredited facility by board-certified surgeons, threatens the incumbent positioning of hospital-based operating rooms by disrupting the channels of distribution (where the procedure is performed). Patients benefit from equivalent outcomes, rigorous safety standards, dramatically lower costs, and improved experience.[2]

As innovators, we must embrace change. This is really the only way to manage the future.

CHAPTER 46

The Vascular Territories (Angiosomes) of the Body: Experimental Study and Clinical Applications

Taylor GI, Palmer JH. Br J Plast Surg 40:113-141, 1987

Reviewed by Ida Janelle Wagner, MD

The blood supply is shown to be a continuous three-dimensional network of vessels not only in the skin but in all tissue layers. The anatomical territory of a source artery in the skin and deep tissues was found to correspond in most cases, giving rise to the angiosome concept . . . This primary supply is reinforced by numerous small indirect vessels, which are spent terminal branches of arteries supplying the deep tissues . . . Our arterial roadmap of the body provides the basis for the logical planning of incisions and flaps. The angiosomes defined the tissues available for composite transfer.[1]

Research Question   What are the cutaneous territories of source arteries, and how do these superficial territories anastomose with the deeper territories of the muscle and fascia?

Funding   Not delineated

Study Dates   1972 to the first work started; 2-year study

Publishing Date   1987

Location   Melbourne, Australia

Subjects   200 fresh cadaver studies over the whole review; 6 complete cadavers and 4 cadaver limbs

Exclusion Criteria   Elderly, cardiovascular disease, metastatic disease, and greater than two surgical scars

Sample Size   6 complete cadavers and 4 limbs

Overview of Design   The review portion of the paper describes over 200 cadaveric studies that began in 1972 and involves dissection, injection, and radiography of defined areas. The projects were initially designed around a specific patient and/or surgical questions and eventually included different tissue types and tissue composites. During this work, the concept of the *angiosome* was developed. The methods evolved in three stages: the first, dissection, followed by injection techniques, and finally radiography, which was used to define the paths and dissemination of cutaneous perforators.

In this study dye injections were performed on cadavers, with radiologic investigations of six whole bodies (three adult men and three adult women), two upper limbs, and four lower limbs. An average of four vascular territories was examined in each cadaver. The process evolved in four stages: (1) preliminary investigations, (2) whole-body studies, (3) examination of isolated limbs, and (4) cross-section studies.

Preliminary investigation included (1) selecting a tissue preservative that was compatible with lead oxide–gelatin injections; (2) designing an x-ray platform that would support the body weight of a full cadaver and provide a uniform grid on which to place the skin envelope; and (3) determining the locations of incisions on the skin envelope to preserve important areas at the groin, axillae, neck, and limb joints. Incision patterns were tested on latex models of whole bodies.

The sequence of steps performed in total-body studies is as follows: inject preservative, inject lead oxide, suspend cadavers in a fluid bath to avoid pressure point formation, 10% formalin injection to preserve viscera, and dissection 1 day later. The dissection was begun with skin; an integument "carpet" was placed on the x-ray platform and x-rayed and a photographic composite was created. Deep tissues were then x-rayed. Cutaneous perforators were tagged and traced to underlying source vessels. Studies of viscera were also performed for comparison of patterns of vascular distribution. Isolated limb studies were performed as described previously. Cross-section studies were performed to define the course of vessels between the deep fascia and the skin. This involved forming strips of integument along axes of cutaneous arteries. The strips were then x-rayed on their sides to provide a cross-sectional view.

Intervention   Dye was injected into source arteries, noting the staining patterns of skin and underlying tissues. Radiographic studies of vascular territories were performed after the injection of lead oxide into the source vessels.

Follow-up   Not applicable

Results   Ink injection, dissection, perforator mapping, and radiographic studies were performed. One hundred nine radiographs of each cadaver were completed, and 374 mapped perforators were defined and traced to source vessels. The results described the anatomic distribution of these cutaneous perforators and their angiosomes. They also classified direct and indirect vessels and described the relationship between cutaneous perforators and the connective tissue framework.

With the dissection and perforator mapping principles and trends identified, the "Most striking feature was the relationship of the vessels to the connective tissue framework of the body—they followed it closely where it was rigid and travelled within it where it was loose." "Few vessels crossed mobile tissue planes, they crossed where planes were fused." "Vessels radiated from fixed to mobile areas," "where mobility existed between tissues vessels coursed parallel to the surface for long distances, usually separated from the plane of mobility by a sheet of connective tissue."[1]

The cutaneous blood supply was classified. Two cutaneous blood supplies were defined: primary and secondary. The primary cutaneous supply is delivered by direct vessels. Direct vessels form a source artery and proceed directly to the skin, providing a cutaneous blood supply. They emerge from the deep fascia where it is anchored to bone, which appears as a groove at the muscle border on a lean person. The size and density of direct vessels were then described. Indirect vessels are the secondary cutaneous supply. Indirect vessels are also the terminal branches of vessels that are mainly meant to supply the muscle, and they serve to join the primary blood supply to the skin.

The cutaneous blood supply is described as a "three dimensional mesh of vessels . . . subdivided into anatomical vascular territories [outlined] by the perimeter of choke arteries." Source arteries and their branches form a continuous network, and the connections between local networks are sometimes true anastomoses (between vessels of equal diameter) and sometimes connections between vessels of smaller diameter (choke vessels). The arterial caliber was found to be inversely proportional to the number of connections.

The authors defined the angiosome concept as a "composite unit of skin and deep tissue supplied by a source artery." They outlined both cutaneous and deep tissue angiosomes. Interestingly, angiosomes are sometimes, but more commonly not, limited by muscle boundaries. Many muscles span multiple angiosomes. They observed a correlation between dermatomes and angiosomes on the head and upper body, but this correlation is less so in the extremities.

Criticisms/Limitations
- The technology is limited to 1987—this study could possibly be performed with CT and digital photographic composites, which would enhance the accuracy and allow more study subjects.
- These anatomic studies are quite labor intensive, and combined with the difficulty in obtaining fresh cadavers, yield limited numbers of dissections.

Relevant Studies   The work of Manchot and Salmon[2-6] predated that of the authors. Manchot had previously defined 40 cutaneous territories, all without the aid of x-ray studies. Salmon defined over 80 territories across the entire body and source arteries of individual muscles. The authors built on this work by further describing cutaneous blood flow territories of source arteries, defining deeper territories, and describing the anastomotic relationship between the two.

Discussion   Manchot's work defined 40 cutaneous territories without the use of x-ray studies. This work excluded the head, neck, hands, and feet and was limited to the cutaneous vasculature. Salmon defined more than 80 cutaneous territories throughout the entire body. Neither work addressed the blood supply to deep tissues. Taylor et al were the first to describe the vascular territories of deep tissue and to delineate the relationships between these deep tissues and the cutaneous territories. They describe these relationships as angiosomes, "composite blocks of tissue which span between the skin and bone." Furthermore, they describe the relationships between the adjacent angiosomes that are interconnected in each tissue layer by reduced caliber choke arteries. This is clinically relevant for flap planning. The authors note, "When a flap is based on the vessels of one angiosome, tissues of the adjacent angiosome can be captured with safety." Choke vessels dilate when a skin flap is delayed. The authors also describe the relationship between vasculature and connective tissue, noting that blood vessels follow septa and fascial planes.

The authors describe this paper as an attempt to synthesize their work with the work of others, notably Salmon and Manchot, in an attempt to build on that initial work with the goal of providing data clinically useful in flap and incision planning. To that end, they make specific recommendations for raising skin flaps. In the scalp or extremities, the fascia is included because the vessels hug the fascia. For skin flaps on the torso, the fascia does not need to be included, because the vessels enter the skin at an early stage. These vessels do not run within the fascia but adjacent to it, and the inclusion of the fascia allows the surgeon to prevent a tedious perforator dissection. The authors outline the necessary data for the survival of a skin flap, which include "the caliber and length upon which the flap is based, the caliber and span of the adjacent capture arteries, the caliber and length of the connecting choke vessels, and adequate venous return." The authors point out an area of concern: when the superficial venous return of an island skin flap is disconnected and the flap is forced to rely on drainage from the deep venous system, problems may arise. They note that this is commonly seen with island neurovascular flaps raised from a digit. The observation of vessel length gives information regarding what type of flap it may support. If the vessels are long, the flap may be long, but if the vessels are short, the flap will be constrained to a smaller area because the vessels do not have a large territorial reach.

Regarding musculocutaneous flaps, attention should be paid to the connection of blood vessels to the flap. When skin and deep fascia are bound strongly to the underlying muscle, the skin is well supplied. When the skin is loosely bound, the blood supply is more fragile.

Summary   This paper provides a comprehensive review of the authors' work and that of their predecessors and contemporaries, which incorporates their findings with those of others and outlines the relevance of all three. In addition, the authors present new work that defines the angiosome concept and the anatomic distribution of angiosomes throughout the body. The authors' goal is to provide a three-dimensional arterial road map of the body.

Implications   This paper is the first to introduce the novel concept of angiosomes— composite units of skin and underlying structures supplied by a given artery. Angiosomes provide a roadmap of the arterial surface of the body and are clinically relevant when planning for incisions and flaps. Before this work, flaps were vulnerable to ischemia because of the ignorance of their supplying arterial distribution.

Previous anatomic studies had been carried out by Manchot and Salmon[2-6]; however, these failed to gain notoriety because they were not published in English. These works were not translated into English until 1983 and 1987, respectively. Manchot identified cutaneous perforators and their underlying source vessels without the benefit of radiology because it had yet to be invented. Salmon expounded on Manchot's work by using x-rays combined with radiopaque injections to map cutaneous and muscle circulation throughout the body.

What new information do Taylor et al impart? The goals of their paper are threefold: (1) to reappraise the work of Manchot and Salmon by performing their own studies of cutaneous circulation with radiography and injections, (2) to correlate their work with that of Manchot and Salmon, and (3) to integrate their findings into those of others' work. Their results agree with those of Manchot and Salmon and they are more extensive.

Conclusion   The authors build on the previous work of Manchot and Salmon, wherein they describe the angiosome concept and define the relationships between superficial and deep cutaneous and muscular blood supply.

REFERENCES

1. Taylor GI, Palmer JH. The vascular territories (angiosomes) of the body: experimental study and clinical applications. Br J Plast Surg 40:113-141, 1987.
2. Salmon M. Artères de la Peau. Paris: Masson et Cie, 1936.
3. Salmon M. Artères des Muscles des Membres e du Tronc. Paris: Masson et Cie, 1936.
4. Salmon M. Arteries of the Skin. Translated from the French. Taylor GI, Tempest M, eds. London: Churchill Livingstone, 1988.
5. Manchot C. Die Hautarterien des Menschlichen Körpers. Leipzig: Vogel, 1889.

6. Manchot C. The Cutaneous Arteries of the Human Body. Translated by Ristic J, Morain WD. New York: Springer-Verlag, 1983.
7. Rozen WM, Phillips TJ, Ashton MW, et al. A new preoperative imaging modality for free flaps in breast reconstruction: computed tomographic angiography. Plast Reconstr Surg 122:38e-40e, 2008.
8. Suami H, Taylor GI, Pan WR. The lymphatic territories of the upper limb: anatomical study and clinical implications. Plast Reconstr Surg 119:1813-1822, 2007.
9. Hong MK, Hong MK, Taylor GI. Angiosome territories of the nerves of the upper limbs. Plast Reconstr Surg 118:148-160, 2006.
10. Rozen WM, Ashton MW, Taylor GI. Reviewing the vascular supply of the anterior abdominal wall: redefining anatomy for increasingly refined surgery. Clin Anat 21:89-98, 2008.
11. Taylor GI. The angiosomes of the body and their supply to perforator flaps. Clin Plast Surg 30:331-342, 2003.
12. Taylor GI, Corlett RJ, Dhar SC, et al. The anatomical (angiosome) and clinical territories of cutaneous perforating arteries: development of the concept and designing safe flaps. Plast Reconstr Surg 127:1447-1459, 2011.
13. Houseman ND, Taylor GI, Pan WR. The angiosomes of the head and neck: anatomic study and clinical applications. Plast Reconstr Surg 105:2287-2313, 2000.
14. Dhar SC, Taylor GI. The delay phenomenon: the story unfolds. Plast Reconstr Surg 104:2079-2091, 1999.
15. Daniel RK, Taylor GI. Distant transfer of an island flap by microvascular anastomoses: a clinical technique. Plast Reconstr Surg 52:111-117, 1973.

EDITORIAL PERSPECTIVE

C. Scott Hultman, MD, MBA, FACS

Over the past four decades, Ian Taylor's work with angiosomes has revealed why flaps work, how they can be modified, and has provided surgeons with the anatomic knowledge needed to develop new techniques in tissue transfer, such as perforator flaps.[1,7-14] Discovering the secrets of how angiosomes contribute to tissue perfusion deserves a place with skin grafting, craniofacial surgery, myocutaneous flaps, and microsurgery as the five greatest innovations of plastic surgery in the twentieth century.

We cannot forget about, however, another important milestone in Taylor's career. Many would argue that Ian Taylor's most important contribution to plastic surgery was the first publication, in 1973, of a "distant transfer of an island flap by microvascular anastomoses," which we know today as a "free flap."[15] An iliofemoral groin flap was successfully transferred to a right lower extremity defect in a 21-year-old man who had an open fracture–crush injury from a motor vehicle collision. In that article, Harry Buncke was inspired to comment, "The successful transplantation of a block of tissue by reanastomosing the microvascular pedicle has untold experimental and clinical possibilities." So impressed was Frank McDowell, the Editor of *Plastic and Reconstructive Surgery* at the time, that he felt compelled to write, "After this paper was in press, your editor was in China and learned of a second case of free transfer of an island flap, on March 26, 1973 by Dr. Yang Don-Yoa . . . and a third case on or about March 28, 1973 by Dr. Bernard O'Brien. All of this appears to be a case of an idea whose time has come. The future of it should be most interesting."

Of course, microsurgery and free tissue transfer began decades earlier with Joseph Murray's twin kidney transplant in 1956, Harold Kleinart's revascularization of a partial digital amputation in 1963, Nakayama's free jejunal autograft for cervical esophageal reconstruction in 1964, and John Cobbett's first toe-to-thumb transfer in 1968. By 1973, the stage was set for an explosion of innovation in microsurgery. Any tissue with a defined blood supply—bone, fascia, muscle, skin, or fat—could be transferred to nearly any defect in the body.

My discourse about angiosomes, the first free flap, and Ian Taylor would not be complete unless I shared a clinical case from my residency. Dr. Taylor came to Atlanta to serve as the William G. Hamm Visiting Professor (an endowed Professorship currently held by my close friend Bert Losken), where tradition dictated that the esteemed surgeon would scrub in and assist us with a complex case at Grady (where credentialing, licensure, and patient confidentiality did not seem to apply for some reason). Our chief resident selected a patient with a large mastectomy defect who needed delayed breast reconstruction, but had multiple contraindications for a pedicled transverse rectus abdominis myocutaneous (TRAM) flap: a body mass index well over 40, insulin-dependent diabetes mellitus, previous chest radiation, a midline laparotomy scar from an open cholecystectomy, and total abdominal hysterectomy with bilateral salpingo-oophorectomy.

Dr. Taylor was excited about this challenging case and explained that the final flap would be quite tenuous because of so many confounding variables in this high-risk patient. He did not seem to be overly worried that perfusion of zone 2 of the TRAM flap would have crossed over at least two angiosomes from its inflow, the superior epigastric vessels. He only became frustrated in the operating room when our circulating nurse kept asking him if he "wanted" her to raise his mask back up over his nose, over which it had fallen and was now resting comfortably on his upper lip. "Not really," he answered, explaining that this was the tradition in Australia, especially at his hospital where he had performed this operation over a thousand times.

The case went well until later that night after Dr. Taylor had boarded a plane for Melbourne when the patient developed severe venous congestion in zone 2 in the contralateral skin across the midline scar. My chief resident performed a maneuver that saved the day, one that I have never since seen and hope never to see again. Unable to find a nearby vein to assist with "super-drainage" of the TRAM flap (the thoracodorsal vessels had been ligated from the previous axillary node dissection), our fearless and undeterred chief cannulated the previously divided end of the deep inferior epigastric vein with an 18-gauge intravenous catheter, heparinized the patient, and performed manual drainage of the flap every 2 to 4 hours. It worked despite incredible odds against success. My explanation, and perhaps Taylor would concur, was that the venous congestion from zone 2 had to cross only one "venosome"—a scarred midline—to get to the freedom of that catheter, salvaging the flap and avoiding the use of leeches, which at Grady were kept stocked in the pharmacy. We may not have had a very good inventory of tissue expanders or breast implants, but we had an unlimited supply of *Hirudo medicinalis.*

CHAPTER 47

Vacuum-Assisted Closure: A New Method for Wound Control and Treatment: Clinical Experience

Argenta LC, Morykwas MJ. Ann Plast Surg 38:563-576; discussion 577, 1997

Reviewed by Anne E. Argenta, MD

Wounds were treated until completely closed, were covered with a split-thickness skin graft, or a flap was rotated into the health, granulating would bed. The technique removes chronic edema, leading to increased localized blood flow, and the applied forces result in the enhanced formation of granulation tissue. Vacuum-assisted closure is an extremely efficacious modality for treating chronic and difficult wounds.[1]

Introduction This is the second part of a two-part landmark study in the plastic surgery literature that introduced the concept of negative-pressure therapy for wound care. The first paper reviewed the basic science and animal studies establishing safety and efficacy of negative-pressure therapy.[2] This paper presented the first clinical data.[1]

Research Question As the field of plastic surgery has evolved, wound healing has remained the foundation of our specialty. The search for ways to optimize wound healing is ongoing. This paper represents the paradigm shift in our approach to wound healing, introducing negative-pressure therapy for a variety of difficult wounds. This case series is the first reported use of the vacuum-assisted closure (VAC) device in humans.

Funding Developmental Technology Fund of North Carolina Baptist Hospital, Winston-Salem, NC, and Kinetic Concepts, Inc., San Antonio, TX

Study Dates 1990s

Publishing Date June 1997

Location Wake Forest University Baptist Medical Center, Winston-Salem, NC

Overview of Design A prospective case series

Subjects Any patient with a wound not amenable to primary closure was eligible for the trial of VAC therapy. Etiology, location, and chronicity of wounds were variable.

Exclusion Criteria Wounds with active malignancy, active osteomyelitis, or exposed vessels or viscera

Sample Size 300 patients

Overview This paper begins with a brief description of the VAC device, which uses an open cell polyurethane ether foam matrix attached to a noncollapsible tube. In turn, the tube is attached to a collection canister and computerized vacuum pump, which supplies negative pressure through the tubing. The foam is placed in the wound, covering the entire wound surface. An adhesive cover seals the apparatus in the wound. After the tubing is sealed to the foam, there is an equal distribution of subatmospheric pressure force across the wound, creating a controlled closed wound. The device has the setting option to deliver negative pressure continuously or intermittently.

The wounds in this study were arbitrarily divided into one of three categories: chronic (>1week old; for example, pressure sores and stasis ulcers), subacute (12 hours to 7 days old; for example, dehisced wounds and open amputations), and acute (<12 hours old; for example, gunshot wounds and acute avulsions). At the initial evaluation, the wounds were aggressively debrided until all nonviable tissue was removed. VAC therapy was then initiated, and VAC dressings were changed every 48 hours, which allowed regular wound inspection and measurements. VAC therapy was continued until the wounds were completely epithelialized, until the patient and wound were stable enough to allow a lesser surgical procedure for wound closure, until the patient refused treatment, or until the patient died. The first 50 patients were treated as inpatients for close monitoring under the care of the plastic surgery service. As patients and physicians became more comfortable with VAC therapy, patients were allowed to continue therapy as outpatients. The study period spanned approximately 6 years.

Intervention Wound debridement of nonviable tissue, application of VAC therapy, and a secondary procedure in some patients

Endpoints Complete epithelialization of wound; stabilization of wound and patient, which allowed a lesser surgical procedure for wound closure; patient refusal of therapy; and patient died

Results One hundred seventy-five wound treated fell into the chronic wound category and included pressure sores, diabetic ulcers, venous stasis ulcers, and radiation ulcers. Patients in this category were often debilitated nonsurgical candidates, who failed multiple other regimens. One hundred seventy-one of these patients responded favorably to VAC therapy, which was defined as the removal of edema, production of granulation tissue, and softening of surrounding tissues. In those patients with pressure sores (n = 141), 32% of wounds healed completely in 2 to 16 weeks, whereas 60% of wounds healed between 50% and 80% and subsequently underwent skin grafting or local flap coverage. The time course required for VAC therapy directly corresponded with the size of the wound. Six patients died for reasons unrelated to VAC therapy during the course of their treatment; two patients' wounds were improving, whereas the remaining four wounds showed no signs of healing. For those patients with venous stasis ulcers (n = 31), VAC therapy was used until a granulating wound bed was obtained. A split-thickness skin graft was then applied, and the VAC was placed to immobilize the graft. Ninety percent of these wounds healed with the first graft attempt.

Ninety-four patients fell into the subacute wound category, which included 36 dehisced wounds and 37 wounds with exposed orthopedic hardware or bone. Of these wounds, 28% healed completely, whereas the remaining 72% contracted to smaller wounds that were controlled with skin grafting, secondary closure, or small local flaps. In general, the subacute wounds granulated more rapidly than the chronic wounds.

Thirty-one patients fell into the acute wound category, including avulsions, contaminated wounds, and gunshot wounds. These wounds granulated more rapidly than either the chronic or subacute wounds. Thirty patients were treated to healing by VAC therapy alone or in conjunction with grafting or local flaps. One patient died of a pulmonary embolus during therapy.

Regarding complications, two patients developed late infections because granulation covered the nonviable bone, stressing the importance of debridement on all nonviable tissue before the initiation of VAC therapy. One patient developed an enteric fistula when the foam was placed over compromised bowel.

Limitations As with most studies introducing novel therapies, this case series provided mostly descriptive results without a randomized control comparison and strict inclusion and exclusion criteria. There was a significant amount of heterogeneity within and between the study groups, as well as a lack of standardization in the treatment regimen. For example, some patients underwent VAC therapy with the continuous setting, whereas others were subjected to the intermittent setting. Little objective data of wound size measurements and the rate of contracture or granulation were supplied. The authors themselves acknowledge in the discussion that VAC therapy at the time of this publication was in early development, and they encouraged collaboration with readers on a multicenter, randomized, controlled trial.

Impact Since the introduction of this paper to the medical community 16 years ago, VAC therapy has revolutionized wound care and crossed boundaries into all other surgical specialties. It is difficult to enter any hospital ward—whether the plastic surgery floor, orthopedic or general surgery floor, or medical ICU—without finding a patient on VAC therapy. The device has become the standard of care for battlefield injuries in Iraq and Afghanistan. To date more than 9 million wounds worldwide have been treated with negative-pressure wound therapy.

Many of the limitations presented in this initial paper have been further investigated. Numerous randomized, controlled trials have since been published, which demonstrated the safety, efficacy, and superiority of VAC therapy over "standard" wound care, including wet-to-dry dressings, gels, and silver sulfadiazine (Silvadene).[3-6] The proposed mechanisms of VAC therapy that are speculated on in this paper, such as the acceleration of healing by the removal of edema and the stimulation of mitosis through cell deformation, have been further studied and confirmed.[7] Quality of life studies have demonstrated higher levels of satisfaction for both patients and providers with VAC therapy over standard dressings.[8]

This study's impact in stimulating future wound healing research is unparalleled. This paper and its basic science counterpart are the second and third most cited articles in the plastic surgery literature,[9] with almost 4000 citations currently. Furthermore, it is routinely cited in the orthopedic, vascular, general, and neurosurgical literature.

It is significant that concepts derived from VAC therapy have been recently adapted for uses beyond soft tissue wound healing. Applying the principles of negative-pressure therapy, Argenta and Morykwas developed a modified device for application in the setting of traumatic brain injuries and cardiac reperfusion injury. In the first paper in the journal *Neurosurgery* ever first authored by a plastic surgeon, they demonstrated that mechanical tissue resuscitation with controlled subatmospheric pressure modulates the levels of excitatory amino acids and lactate in traumatic brain injury, decreases water content and volume of the injured brain, improves neuronal survival, and speeds functional recovery in an animal model.[10] Likewise, in the *Journal of Cardiothoracic Surgery,* they showed that the treatment of reperfusion injury in infarcted myocardium with negative-pressure therapy for a controlled period of time during reperfusion greatly reduced myocardial death after acute infarction.[11] Human trials in both areas are underway.

REFERENCES

1. Argenta LC, Morykwas MJ. Vacuum-assisted closure: a new method for wound control and treatment: clinical experience. Ann Plast Surg 38:563-576; discussion 577, 1997.
2. Morykwas MJ, Argenta LC, Shelton-Brown E, et al. Vacuum-assisted closure: a new method for wound control and treatment: animal studies and basic foundation. Ann Plast Surg 38:553-562, 1997.
3. Braakenburg A, Obdeijn MC, Feitz R, et al. The clinical efficacy and cost effectiveness of the vacuum-assisted closure technique in the management of acute and chronic wounds: a randomized controlled trial. Plast Reconstr Surg 118:390-397; discussion 398-400, 2006.

4. Vuerstaek JD, Vainas T, Wuite J, et al. State of the art treatment of chronic leg ulcers: a randomized controlled trial comparing vacuum-assisted closure (V.A.C.) with modern wound dressings. J Vasc Surg 44:1029-1037, 2006.

5. Armstrong DG, Lavery LA; Diabetic Foot Study Consortium. Negative pressure wound therapy after partial diabetic foot amputation: a multicentre, randomized, controlled trial. Lancet 366:1704-1710, 2005.

6. Ford CN, Reinhard ER, Yeh D, et al. Interim analysis of a prospective, randomized trial of vacuum-assisted closure versus the healthpoint system in the management of pressure ulcers. Ann Plast Surg 49:55-61; discussion 61, 2002.

7. Morykwas MJ, Simpson J, Punger K, et al. Vacuum-assisted closure: state of basic research and physiologic foundation. Plast Reconstr Surg 117(7 Suppl):121S-126S, 2006.

8. Karatepe O, Eken I, Acet E, et al. Vacuum assisted closure improved the quality of life in patients with diabetic foot. Acta Chir Belg 111:298-302, 2011.

9. Loonen MP, Hage JJ, Kon M. Plastic Surgery Classics: characteristics of 50 top cited articles in four Plastic Surgery Journals since 1946. Plast Reconstr Surg 121:320e-327e, 2008.

10. Argenta LC, Zheng Z, Bryant A, et al. A new method for modulating traumatic brain injury with mechanical tissue resuscitation. Neurosurgery 70:1281-1295, 2012.

11. Argenta LC, Morykwas MJ, Mays JJ, et al. Reduction of myocardial ischemia-reperfusion injury by mechanical tissue resuscitation using sub-atmospheric pressure. J Card Surg 25:247-252, 2012.

STUDY AUTHOR REFLECTIONS

Louis C. Argenta, MD, FACS

Publication of this paper took more than 2½ years during which time the first four submissions were rejected. Fortunately, during that period, the concept was widely accepted and advanced across all surgical disciplines at Wake Forest so that by the time the paper was published, the number of reported cases had grown from 100 to 300. Throughout this entire period, Mike Morykwas and our research personnel refined our understanding of the basic science of the technique, allowing wider and more aggressive clinical application to more difficult cases. Without the unending encouragement, hard work, and curiosity of my colleagues and residents, this work would never have evolved into the successful technology we use today. Progress evolves slowly in medicine. As our mentors would say, "press on."

CHAPTER 48

Facial Augmentation With Structural Fat Grafting

Coleman SR. Clin Plast Surg 33:567-577, 2006

Reviewed by Rafi Fredman, MD, FACS

> *Fat grafts can be placed in such a fashion that they are long lasting, completely integrated, and natural appearing . . . We now approach rejuvenation and adjustment of facial proportion with a better understanding of the need for the restoration or adjustment of facial volume.*[1]

Research Questions   The Coleman technique for fat grafting provides a systematic and reproducible method for the transplantation of autologous fat, emphasizing the respect for handling tissues and basic sound surgical technique to produce reliable and consistent clinical results. However, several questions remain. What is the efficacy of fat grafting to the face? What is the best process for harvest and application of fat grafts? What are the best clinical uses for fat grafting, in addition to aesthetic indications?

Funding   Not stated

Study Dates   Early 2000s

Publishing Date   2006

Location   New York University School of Medicine, New York, NY

Overview of Design   Technical paper case reports

Methods   Coleman fat grafting technique

Harvesting.   A harvesting site is selected based on the availability or desired body contouring because no correlation between the donor site and graft longevity has been demonstrated. A blunt Lamis infiltrator is inserted through small incisions to deliver the solution for local anesthesia and hemostasis. A 10 mL Luer-Lok syringe attached to a two-hole Coleman harvesting cannula with a blunt tip is inserted through the same incisions, and with slight negative pressure and curreting action, fatty tissue is drawn into the syringe barrel.

Refinement and transfer.   Nonviable components (oil, blood, local) should be discarded to maximize proper volume estimation. A Luer-Lok plug replaces the cannula and the plunger is removed from the syringe. The syringe is centrifuged for 3 minutes at 3000 rpm. The oil layer is decanted, the aqueous component is drained, and porous paper is used to remove the remaining oil. The fat is then transferred to a 1 mL Luer-Lok syringe.

Placement.   A blunt type I Coleman infiltration cannula and a 3 mL syringe are used for local anesthesia and hemostasis, after which the cannula is attached to the 1 mL Luer-Lok syringe containing harvested fat. The blunt cannula is advanced through natural tissue planes, and fat is injected as the cannula is withdrawn. No fat is injected during cannula advancement to avoid fat clumping, thereby maximizing the proximity of transplanted fat to the blood supply, improving graft integration into the host tissue, and minimizing any contour irregularities.

Postoperative care.   To decrease edema, Tegaderm (3M, St. Paul, MN) is placed over the infiltrated areas and left in place for 3 to 4 days. Cold should be applied for 72 hours and the infiltrated areas should be elevated. Light touch increases lymphatic drainage and may decrease edema, but deep massage should be avoided.

Complications.   Swelling is common. Damage to underlying structures, intravascular emboli, infection, fat migration, and donor-site complications are rare complications.

Cases.   Four patients are presented who underwent fat grafting to the face for aesthetic complaints. Favorable results were obtained after the use of the Coleman technique to transplant autologous fat to various locations on the face, including the periorbital region, lips, and mandibular border. The key to accurate grafting is familiarity with the technique, knowledge of attractive facial topography, and understanding the goals of the patient.

Relevant Studies   More than 100 years have passed since Eugene Hollander first described the use of fat transfer in the treatment of patients with lipoatrophy of the face.[2] Initially, fat grafting did not gain popularity because of the novelty of using adipose tissue in surgery, the uncertainty of the properties of adipose tissue, and an early report of negative outcomes.[3] An interest in fat grafting resurged in the 1990s, leading to Coleman's development of a reproducible grafting technique and setting the stage for its successful adaptation to many avenues in plastic and reconstructive surgery.

Long before fat grafting became popular, alongside improvements in laparoscopic and microsurgical techniques, the omental flap was described as a useful tool in the reconstruction of extremity and craniofacial defects.[4] Recognized as a versatile tissue for reconstruction, the omentum contains a large amount of easily pliable tissue, a long and reliable vascular pedicle, a high amount of lymphoid tissue, and growth factors and stem cells. The omentum is an effective choice for three-dimensional defect reconstruction with intrinsic properties that lead to improved local conditions and wound healing.

Fat grafting has many aesthetic applications, and gluteal reshaping serves as a good example of fat grafting in aesthetic plastic surgery. In gluteal reshaping, fat is injected to help shape and contour the gluteus and to add volume to the buttocks. Gluteal reshaping with fat injections is a preferred method of augmentation and when compared with gluteal implants provides greater versatility, precision, and finely tuned augmentation with a quicker postoperative recovery and fewer complications.[5]

In 1987 the American Society of Plastic Surgeons placed a ban on fat grafting to the breast because of fears that fat necrosis, fatty cysts, and changes in breast architecture could be confused with malignancy. This delayed the emergence of lipotransfer as a tool in breast reconstruction until 2009, when improved imaging technology permitted the ban to be lifted. Small-to-moderate–volume fat grafting to the breast for aesthetic augmentations became common; however, large-volume transfer, especially to scarred or irradiated breasts, was still problematic. Khouri et al[6] were instrumental in developing a technique of "megavolume" fat grafting to the breast, which optimized recipient-site conditions to allow large-volume fat grafting to problematic breasts. They showed that the preoperative use of external volume expansion improved recipient-site local conditions through microangiogenesis while increasing interstitial space. Improved blood supply creates a more supple skin envelope, especially in irradiated breasts, while increased interstitial space allows the injection of a larger volume of fat into an oxygen-rich environment. Their results were consistent with other studies showing that fat grafting to the breast does not hinder imaging.[6] Brava-assisted megavolume fat grafting to the breasts provides a safe and effective reconstructive option for cosmetic augmentation, congenital defects, scarred breasts (iatrogenic), and implant-to-autogenous conversion.

Considering the regenerative properties of adipose tissue, it is no surprise that autologous fat grafting has proved useful in the management of cicatricial tissue. Klinger et al[7] showed in their study of nearly 700 patients with retractile and painful scars that autologous fat grafting to scarred tissue resulted in significantly improved functionality, aesthetics, pain, and scar elasticity. Histologic changes showed regeneration of dermis and subcutaneous tissue, with improved quality of dermal and hypodermic elements. Structures previously injured after burns and other trauma may have new collagen deposition, reorganization of the extracellular matrix, and local neoangiogenesis, in addition to a thicker fat layer.

The success of fat grafting in cicatricial tissue has resulted in an introduction of fat grafting to the world of burn reconstruction to improve the contour, elasticity, and quality of skin. Sultan et al[8] were the first to explore the mechanism of this effect by using a murine model of thermal injury to investigate the effect of fat grafting on burn scars. In a fat-grafted burn scar, a more rapid revascularization at the burn site was identified with Doppler scanning, CD31 staining, and enzyme-linked immunosorbent assay, which showed a significant increase in vasculogenic proteins (vascular endothelial growth factor and stromal cell–derived factor 1). Fat grafting also resulted in decreased fibrosis as seen by Sirius red staining and a significant decrease in fibrotic markers (transforming growth factor beta and matrix metalloproteinase 9). As more research emerges detailing the complex interactions between multiple cell types (adipose stem cells, adipocytes, and necrotic adipocytes) that are likely integral to the regenerative ability of adipose tissue in burn scars and with additional clinical trials, fat grafting may provide a long-lasting solution and improved quality of life for patients suffering from burns.[9]

An eloquent use of fat grafting was developed by Khouri et al,[10] who suggested percutaneous aponeurotomy and lipofilling as a regenerative alternative to flap reconstruction. Adapted from the technique of releasing Dupuytren contractures by nicking the cord and palmar aponeurosis, fat is injected into the contracted area after which small gaps are placed in the scarred tissue (percutaneous mesh expansion). "Meshing" the restrictive tissue will cause the grafted fat to pool in small gaps, allowing optimal survival of the fat grafts, which then transform the restrictive cicatrix into a regenerative matrix. To correct volume deficits, nicks are made in multiple planes ("Rigottomies") to achieve three-dimensional expansion. This technique adheres to basic plastic surgery principles: releasing a contracture, grafting of a created defect, and graft splinting (the use of extension splints or Brava). The authors incorporate percutaneous aponeurotomy and lipofilling into their technique of Brava-assisted megavolume fat grafting to the breast by mesh expanding the lower pole of the breast to release congenital bands.[6] When faced with a wide range of reconstructive problems, this method provides a valuable alternative to flap reconstruction.

The stromal vascular fraction (SVF) of lipoaspirate contains a large number of adipose-derived stem cells (ADSCs), which have the ability to regenerate local tissue after fat grafting. Platelet-rich plasma (PRP) is blood plasma enriched with platelets that contain regenerative growth factors and cytokines. PRP stimulates fat regeneration and induces microangiogenesis in fat grafts.[11] A study investigating fat grafts treated with SVF or PRP showed that both SVF-enhanced and PRP-enhanced fat grafts produce significantly better maintenance of contour and three-dimensional volume compared with fat graft alone after 1-year follow-up.[11]

Coleman's fat grafting technique centered on the use of centrifugation to separate suction-acquired lipoaspirate components before injection. The increased use of ultrasound-guided lipoaspiration, the application of fat grafting to both small-volume and large-volume transfers, and the increased understanding of adipose stem cells have required additional data regarding processing methods and their effect on graft retention. Rubin et al used a murine model to compare fat grafting harvest methods (ultrasound-assisted lipoaspiration versus conventional suction-assisted lipoaspiration) and processing methods (centrifuge, filtration, and cotton gauze rolling).[3] Both harvest methods produced the same fat graft yield, SVF, and in vivo graft retention. Of the processing methods, cotton gauze rolling resulted in the lowest residual oil and aqueous fractions and a significantly higher SVF and improved fat graft retention when compared with centrifugation and may be most appropriate for small-volume fat grafting in cosmetically sensitive areas (the face). Filtration (500 or 800 µm pores) is comparable with centrifuge in fat graft yield, SVF, and graft retention and therefore may be useful for large-volume grafting (buttocks and breast).[3]

Coleman described fat grafting as a singular procedure, and yet technologic and innovative advances necessitate variation in technique and strategy for different problems. Advances in understanding the regenerative properties of adipose tissue have presented an additional element. Fat grafting strategies must incorporate and combine the need for regenerative effects and replacing deficient volumes.[12] Methods of harvesting, cell processing, transplantation, and recipient-site management are chosen based on whether the recipient tissue is healthy or pathologic and whether large-volume or small-volume grafts are required.

Summary   Fat grafting provides a reliable and favorable modality for facial rejuvenation and contouring. A reproducible technique is discussed, which paved the way for further innovation that will elucidate optimal methods for the most consistent results.

Implications   With the broad application of fat grafting to many areas of plastic surgery, modification of the fat grafting technique is both practical and useful to create a strategy for optimal results.

REFERENCES

1. Coleman SR. Facial augmentation with structural fat grafting. Clin Plast Surg 33:567-577, 2006.
2. Billings E Jr, May JW Jr. Historical review and present status of free fat graft autotransplantation in plastic and reconstructive surgery. Plast Reconstr Surg 83:368-381, 1989.
3. Fisher C, Grahovac TL, Schafer ME, et al. Comparison of harvest and processing techniques for fat grafting and adipose stem cell isolation. Plast Reconstr Surg 132:351-361, 2013.

4. Upton J, Mulliken JB, Hicks PD, et al. Restoration of facial contour using free vascularized omental transfer. Plast Reconstr Surg 66:560-569, 1980.
5. Mendieta CG. Gluteal reshaping. Aesthet Surg J 27:641-655, 2007.
6. Khouri RK, Khouri RK Jr, Rigotti G, et al. Aesthetic applications of Brava-assisted mega-volume fat grafting to the breasts: a 9-year, 476-patient, multicenter experience. Plast Reconstr Surg 133:796-807; discussion 808-809, 2014.
7. Klinger M, Caviggioli F, Klinger FM, et al. Autologous far graft in scar treatment. J Craniofac Surg 24:1610-1615, 2013.
8. Sultan SM, Barr JS, Butala P, et al. Fat grafting accelerates revascularisation and decreases fibrosis following thermal injury. J Plast Reconstr Aesthet Surg 65:219-227, 2012.
9. Ranganathan K, Wong VC, Krebsbach PH, et al. Fat grafting for thermal injury: current state and future directions. J Burn Care Res 34:219-226, 2013.
10. Khouri RK, Smit JM, Cardoso E, et al. Percutaneous aponeurotomy and lipofilling: a regenerative alternative to flap reconstruction? Plast Reconstr Surg 132:1280-1290, 2013.
11. Gentile P, De Angelis B, Pasin M, et al. Adipose-derived stromal vascular fraction cells and platelet-rich plasma: basic and clinical evaluation for cell-based therapies in patients with scars on the face. J Craniofac Surg 25:267-272, 2014.
12. Del Vecchio D, Rohrich RJ. A classification of clinical fat grafting: different problems, different solutions. Plast Reconstr Surg 130:511-522, 2012.

EXPERT COMMENTARY

John A. van Aalst, MD, FACS

The ready availability of fat makes it an ideal tissue source for grafting and tissue engineering purposes. However, improvements in harvest techniques need to move hand-in-glove with an improved understanding of the behavior of the stem cell populations that are the active components within these grafts. Harvest site location, amount harvested and implanted, differences in patient sex, age, including menopausal status, and recipient site influence the success of fat grafting. Understanding these factors and improving the synergy between clinical use and scientific understanding will enable plastic surgeons to improve outcomes for our patients.

CHAPTER 49

A Prospective Analysis of 100 Consecutive Lymphovenous Bypass Cases for Treatment of Extremity Lymphedema

Chang DW, Suami H, Skoracki R. Plast Reconstr Surg 132:1305-1314, 2013

Reviewed by Saif Al-Bustani, MD, DMD

> *Lymphovenous bypass can effectively reduce the severity of lymphedema, particularly in patients with early-stage lymphedema affecting the upper extremities.*[1]

Research Question   Is lymphovenous bypass efficacious in the treatment of extremity lymphedema secondary to cancer treatment?

Funding   In part by the Kyte Research and Education Fund and the National Institutes of Health through MD Anderson's Cancer Center Support Grant

Study Dates   December 2005 to December 2012

Publishing Date   November 2013

Location   MD Anderson Cancer Center, Houston, TX

Subjects   Patients with lymphedema secondary to treatment for cancer

Exclusion Criteria   None

Sample Size   100 total lymphedematous extremities: 89 were upper and 11 were lower.

Overview of Design   This is a prospective study of 100 consecutive patients with extremity lymphedema undergoing lymphovenous bypass. Preoperatively and 3, 6, and 12 months after lymphedema bypass, qualitative assessment and quantitative volumetric analysis were performed by a lymphedema therapist. Verbal questions were used for the qualitative assessment, whereas an optoelectronic limb volumeter was used for quantitative analyses. Volume measurements were performed three times and were averaged. After it became institutionally available, indocyanine green fluorescent lymphography was used to preoperatively classify the severity of the lymphedema and to plan the operative sites for the lymphovenous bypass based on patent lymphatic vessels in 65 patients.

Intervention   Indocyanine green lymphography was accomplished by injecting indocyanine green intradermally into each finger or toe web. Patent lymphatic pathways and incision sites were then marked based on those images. Intradermal isosulfan blue dye injections distal to the incision sites were used intraoperatively to identify lymphatic vessels. Bypasses were performed by anastomosis of the identified lymphatic vessels to adjacent venules of similar size. The entire operation was performed with microscope magnification. The average number of bypasses per limb was 5.6. All patients were instructed to wear compression garments 4 weeks after surgery.

Follow-up   The mean follow-up time for patients with upper extremity lymphedema was 30.4 months, with a range of 3 to 84 months. The mean follow-up time for patients with lower extremity lymphedema was 18.2 months, with a range of 1 to 36 months.

Endpoints   For the upper extremity:
1. Symptom improvement per patient report
2. Quantitative improvement of limb volumes
3. Quantitative improvement of limb volumes broken down by lymphedema stage 1 or 2 versus 3 or 4
4. Postoperative complications

For the lower extremity:
1. Symptom improvement per patient report
2. Quantitative improvement of limb volumes

Results   For the upper extremity, mean lymphedema duration was 3.5 years. The mean preoperative volume differential compared with the unaffected arm was 32%. The mean operative time was 4 hours. Ninety-six percent of patients reported symptom improvement (lighter, softer, and less painful). Symptom improvement did not always correlate with quantitative improvement. Seventy-four percent of patients had quantitative improvements. Mean volume differential reductions were 33% at 3 months, 36% at 6 months, and 42% at 12 months. Those reductions were statistically significant. Patients with stage 1 or 2 lymphedema (as determined by the MD Anderson lymphedema classification based on indocyanine green lymphangiographic imaging) had a higher mean number of bypasses and significantly better reductions than their advanced-stage counterparts. There were no complications or worsening of lymphedema.

For the lower extremity, mean lymphedema duration was 6.6 years. The mean preoperative volume differential compared with the unaffected leg was 37.6%. Four of seven patients reported symptom improvement. Only two patients had postoperative volume measurements, both of whom had bilateral lymphovenous bypasses. One had a volume differential reduction of 42% at 1 year and 33% at 3 years for the right leg and only a 7% reduction at 3 years for the left leg. The second patient had symptom improvement but no quantitative improvement.

Criticisms/Limitations   No comparison was made with a control group (for example, conservative/compression therapy group). The average follow-up was only 2.5 years. The sample size for lymphedematous lower extremities was very small and did not allow meaningful conclusions. Finally, this study did not mention the percentage of patients with symptom improvement but no measurable quantitative improvement in the upper extremity group.

Relevant Studies   From a historical perspective, there have been scattered reports of lymphovenous anastomoses as early as 1962 by Cockett and Goodwin, Mistling and Skyring, and Sedlacek. However, those procedures were on large vessels.[2] Degni[3] may be credited for the first microvascular lymphovenous anastomosis in the early 1970s, with a reported series in lower extremity lymphedema. Interestingly, O'Brien et al[2] published the first series of 22 lymphedematous upper extremities managed with lymphovenous anastomoses by means of an operating microscope. Their preoperative preparation included objective measurements, lymphography, and venography of the affected extremities. It is noteworthy that one third of the patients evaluated were not offered surgery based on lymphography showing inadequate vessels, which likely represented stages 3 and 4 lymphedema with the current study's classification system. Loupe 4× magnification was used to make incisions and locate appropriate vessels, whereas an operating microscope was used to perform the anastomoses. Vessels were approximately 0.5 mm in diameter, and one to seven anastomoses were performed per extremity. The average operative time was 6 to 8 hours. Overall, average volume reduction was 19%. Fifty-five percent experienced an average volume reduction of 38%. There was also a considerable reduction in the rate of cellulitis of the affected extremities after surgery. Subjectively, two thirds of patients reported improved symptoms (arms were softer, lighter, and clothing fit better). Later in 1990, O'Brien et al[4] published their long-term experience with 90 patients undergoing lymphovenous anastomoses. Thirty-eight patients had reduction surgery, in addition to the microlymphatic procedure. The average follow-up was 4.2 years (up to 13.8 years). Forty-two percent of the microlymphatic procedure alone group showed objective improvement, which was defined as a 10% reduction in volume from preoperative measurements. Interestingly, 45% of patients worsened, but the authors attributed that to the natural progression of late-stage disease. In contrast, 60% of the microlymphatic and reduction surgery group showed objective improvement, whereas only 24% worsened.

One may credit technologic improvements in the detection of the appropriate lymphatic vessels for anastomosis and refined supermicrosurgery techniques to the differences in results between the current study and the study of O'Brien et al.[4] In the current study, the authors noted that the mean number of lymphovenous anastomoses per extremity was higher when indocyanine green lymphography was used compared with Chang's prior[5] study without it (5.6 versus 3.5). They also subjectively observed that patients who underwent lymphovenous bypass with indocyanine green lymphography had better outcomes than those without it.

The use of indocyanine green–enhanced near-infrared lymphography for the intraoperative identification of patent lymphatic vessels for lymphovenous anastomosis was first reported by Ogata et al[6] in 2007. This is the same technology used by Chang et al in the current study. Similarly, the photodynamic eye system was used to obtain the images. The advantages of this approach included simplicity requiring only an intradermal injection, surgeon administration of the study, improvement in efficiency, and reduction in operative time because incisions are guided by obtained images, ease of image interpretation, portability of the system, ease of indocyanine green handling and storage, low toxicity of indocyanine green, and permissibility of repeat injection and imaging.[6] The disadvantages included limited depth (although this may be optimal for lymphovenous anastomosis) and small areas of imaging at a time.[6]

Various modifications of the current lymphovenous bypass techniques have been described in the literature. Yamamoto et al[7] reported the use of navigation lymphatic supermicrosurgery with indocyanine green lymphography. A near-infrared illumination system–integrated microscope can now be used in finding and dissecting the lymphatic vessel and in evaluating the quality of the anastomosis under direct live microscopic indocyanine green lymphography. Another modification is the description of Yamamoto et al[8] of a ladder-shaped lymphovenous anastomosis by the use of multiple side-to-side lymphatic anastomoses combined with a side-to-side venous anastomosis. This maximizes the use of available lymphatic vessels in one field.

The authors of the current study alluded to vascularized lymph node transfer for lower extremity lymphedema, because it may be less amenable to lymphovenous bypass because of its length, dependence, and higher venous pressure.[1] Cheng et al[9] described the successful transfer of vascularized submental lymph node flaps to the ankles of six patients with seven lymphedematous lower extremities. With a mean follow-up of 8.7 months, the mean reduction of leg circumference was 64% above the knee, 63.7% below the knee, and 67.3% above the ankle.

Prophylactic lymphovenous anastomosis has been suggested in the literature, and it may play a significant role in the prevention of lymphedema secondary to cancer treatment. Lymphadenectomy and lymphovenous bypass may be performed simultaneously, and that may represent a treatment direction in the future.[10]

Summary Lymphovenous bypass can effectively reduce the severity of lymphedema both subjectively and objectively, especially in early-stage upper extremity lymphedema. Indocyanine green fluorescence lymphography aids in the identification of the appropriate candidates for lymphovenous bypass and the optimal surgical sites for bypass and perhaps could be used to objectively assess the change in lymphedema after lymphedema surgery.

Implications Lymphovenous bypass is an evolving treatment modality for lymphedema secondary to cancer treatment. This study demonstrates the authors' significant and successful experience with new and perhaps superb technology in indocyanine green fluorescence lymphography.

REFERENCES

1. Chang DW, Suami H, Skoracki R. A prospective analysis of 100 consecutive lymphovenous bypass cases for treatment of extremity lymphedema. Plast Reconstr Surg 132:1305-1314, 2013.
2. O'Brien BM, Sykes P, Threlfall GN, et al. Microlymphaticovenous anastomoses for obstructive lymphedema. Plast Reconstr Surg 60:197-211, 1977.
3. Degni M. New technique of lymphatic-venous anastomosis (buried type) for the treatment of lymphedema. VASA 3:479-483, 1974.
4. O'Brien BM, Mellow CG, Khazanchi RK, et al. Long-term results after microlymphaticovenous anastomoses for the treatment of obstructive lymphedema. Plast Reconstr Surg 85:562-572, 1990.
5. Chang DW. Lymphaticovenular bypass for lymphedema management in breast cancer patients: a prospective study. Plast Reconstr Surg 126:752-758, 2010.
6. Ogata F, Narushima M, Mihara M, et al. Intraoperative lymphography using indocyanine green dye for near-infrared fluorescence labeling in lymphedema. Ann Plast Surg 59:180-184, 2007.
7. Yamamoto T, Yamamoto N, Numahata T, et al. Navigation lymphatic supermicrosurgery for the treatment of cancer-related peripheral lymphedema. Vasc Endovascular Surg 48:139-143, 2014.
8. Yamamoto T, Kikuchi K, Yoshimatsu H, et al. Ladder-shaped lymphaticovenular anastomosis using multiple side-to-side lymphatic anastomoses for a leg lymphedema patient. Microsurgery 34:404-408, 2014.
9. Cheng MH, Huang JJ, Nguyen DH, et al. A novel approach to the treatment of lower extremity lymphedema by transferring a vascularized submental lymph node flap to the ankle. Gynecol Oncol 126:93-98, 2012.
10. Koshima I, Narushima M, Yamamoto Y, et al. Recent advancement on surgical treatments for lymphedema. Ann Vasc Dis 5:409-415, 2012.

STUDY AUTHOR REFLECTIONS

David W. Chang, MD, FACS

Lymphedema is a chronic, debilitating condition that causes physical and psychological morbidity and affects up to 250 million people worldwide. In the United States and other developed countries, cancer and its treatments are the most common causes of lymphedema.

Unfortunately, no definitive treatment for lymphedema currently exists. Physiologic methods, such as vascularized lymph node transfer or lymphatic bypass (LVB; also known as *lymphaticovenular bypass*), attempt to restore lymphatic drainage by reconstructing conduits for unimpeded flow. The advent of microsurgery and more recently supermicrosurgery has had a major impact on the evolution of these physiologic procedures, which have gained popularity to help reduce the severity of lymphedema.

One recent technologic advance in lymphovenous bypass procedures is the use of indocyanine green fluorescence lymphangiography to map lymphatic vessels. Indocyanine green fluorescence lymphangiography enables surgeons to locate and make incisions precisely over functional lymphatic vessels for the lymphovenous bypass, substantially reducing operating time, and may significantly improve the outcomes of LVB surgeries.

In the this study, we prospectively evaluated our experience with LVB in 100 consecutive patients with extremity lymphedema secondary to cancer treatment to assess its efficacy and to better understand the lymphedema evaluation process and the optimal patient selection for the LVB procedure. We have found that LVB can be effective in reducing lymphedema severity, particularly in patients with early-stage, upper extremity lymphedema with a reasonable amount of intact functioning lymphatic vessels and minimal tissue fibrosis. In these patients, mean volume differential reductions of 61% after LVB were noted at 12 months. In patients with late-stage lymphedema with few functioning lymphatic vessels and significant tissue fibrosis, the results were not as impressive; only 17% mean volume differential reductions at 12 months after LVB.

Currently, there is no cure for lymphedema. Worldwide interest in the use of microsurgical procedures to treat lymphedema is gaining momentum. However, there is no consensus on the indications for which procedure to perform, when to intervene, or how to comparatively grade outcomes. We need further research and a better understanding of lymphatic anatomy and lymphedema pathophysiology. In addition, more prospective and controlled studies are needed to objectively evaluate the outcomes of various treatment methods.

CHAPTER 50

Near-Total Human Face Transplantation for a Severely Disfigured Patient in the USA

Siemionow M, Papay F, Alam D, Bernard S, Djohan R, Gordon C, Hendrickson M, Lohman R, Eghtesad B, Coffman K, Kodish E, Paradis C, Avery R, Fung J. Lancet 374:203-209, 2009

Reviewed by Ida Janelle Wagner, MD, and Kimberly S. Jones, MD

Unlike solid organ transplantation, which is potentially life-saving, facial transplantation is life-changing. Although episodes of acute skin rejection continue to pose a serious threat to face transplant recipients, all cases have been controlled with conventional immunosuppressive regimens, and no cases of chronic rejection have been reported.[1]

We show the feasibility of reconstruction of severely disfigured patients in a single surgical procedure using composite face allotransplantation. Therefore, this should be taken in consideration as an early option for severely disfigured patients.[1]

Editor's Note: As this book was going to press, Khalifian et al[2] published a comprehensive review of the world's total experience with facial transplantation, 28 cases, in the *Lancet,* the same journal that had published the first North American transplant as a case report. Both articles complement each other exceedingly well and are therefore included, as a tie, as the fiftieth study that all plastic surgeons should know.

Research Questions Is face transplant a reasonable alternative to traditional reconstructive methods after severe facial disfigurement? Does face transplant offer a benefit to these patients over traditional reconstructive methods?

Funding   Cleveland Clinic

Study Dates   August 2004 to December 2008 (June 2009)

Publishing Date   July 15, 2009

Location   Cleveland, OH

Subject   A 45-year-old woman with severe facial disfigurement after a gunshot wound to the face, refractory to multiple reconstructive attempts

Exclusion Criteria   Significant medical or psychiatric illness in the recipient

Sample Size   1

Overview of Design   This paper describes the preoperative planning, intraoperative experience, and 6-month postoperative course of the first face transplant in the United States.

Intervention   Face transplant

Follow-up   6 months

Endpoints   6 months after surgery

Results   A composite allograft consisting of bone, soft tissue, nerve, and parotid gland was transplanted from a 45-year-old brain-dead donor to a 45-year-old recipient, who was matched for age, sex, race, and skin complexion. The allograft had excellent take, with no postoperative episodes of clinically apparent rejection. Multiple functions were restored to the recipient, including speech, sense of smell, and the ability to eat solid food, drink from a cup, and breathe through the nose without a tracheostomy.

Criticisms/Limitations   This procedure is the first of its kind and therefore has a sample size of one. There are insufficient data to compare the results with any others in this case report.

Description   Siemionow et al described their experience with the first face transplant in the United States, which was the most complex of its time. The procedure was performed in December 2008 after a 4-year waiting period, during which institutional review board approval, organ donor status approval, and extensive patient and surgical team preparation were undertaken.

The team conduced 20 years' worth of basic science studies to prove the possibility of a face transplant. After institutional review board approval, they performed six dry runs with cadavers to learn the intricacies and nuances of donor procurement, preparation of the recipient, and graft inset. Recipient selection was another time-intensive part of the process, because the recipient had to be medically fit, psychologically adapted, and intelligent and insightful enough to completely understand the risks and benefits of such a procedure—something that no one, not even the surgeons, could know at the time but only speculate on.

A multidisciplinary approach was essential to the success of the project. The face transplant team included bioethicists, psychiatrists, transplant biologists, speech therapists, physical therapists, organ procurement specialists, eight attending surgeons, and one surgical fellow.

The procedure took 22 hours and was a technologic and psychosocial success. The allograft was composed of the total nose, lower eyelids, upper lip, infraorbital floor, bilateral zygomas, anterior maxilla with incisors, total alveolus, hard palate, and bilateral parotid glands. The allograft was pedicled on the bilateral common facial arteries, external jugular veins, and left posterior facial vein. It was innervated via the facial nerve, which was anastomosed via interposition nerve grafts bilaterally. The patient came to accept her new face within several weeks after the procedure and ranked her feelings of self-esteem and attractiveness higher and higher as time progressed. She gained significant functional improvement—she went from feeding tube dependent to having the ability to chew and swallow solid food and drink liquid from a cup. Her sense of smell returned and her speech became intelligible. She lost her tracheostomy and breathed through her nose.

Postoperative immunosuppression regimens consisted of induction with thymoglobulin and tapered steroids, followed by tacrolimus, mycophenolate mofetil, and prednisone. At 6 months after surgery, there were no episodes of clinical rejection, and one episode of rejection seen on a routine skin biopsy was successfully treated with a single bolus of methylprednisolone. The patient underwent significant postoperative psychological treatment along with speech and physical therapy

Discussion   Siemionow and colleagues spent 20 years in the laboratory research-ing both the technical feasibility of performing face transplants and the immunologic safety of chronic immunosuppression.

This work, along with 4 years of preparation for this patient in particular, paid off with an excellent outcome and tremendous support for the patient in all areas—psychiatric, patient advocate, ethical, medical, speech, and physical therapy. The procedure was meticulously conceptualized, planned, and practiced with cadaver dry runs. During the 4 years from institutional review board application in 2004 to face transplant surgery in December 2008, three other partial face transplants were performed in France and China. However, this procedure was the most extensive undertaking of its kind at the time, transplanting not only facial soft tissues but also bone, parotid gland, and facial functional units. It was also the first face transplant performed in the United States.

Since then, several centers have emerged as leading face transplant centers. These in-clude Brigham and Women's Hospital, with a team led by Bohdan Pomahač, and the University of Maryland, led by Eduardo Rodriguez (Rodriguez has since become the chairman of Plastic Surgery at New York University). Rodriguez's team performed the world's first full face transplant in March 2012. This was a complex graft that included the midface and double jaws. It used multimodal technology that had not been previ-ously applied in the face transplant.

To be considered a candidate for face transplant, this patient had to have previously undergone multiple failed attempts at reconstruction. She had 23 surgeries before her transplant, including multiple free flaps. The authors concluded that although face transplantation was novel and complex, it should be entertained as an early therapy for patients with severe facial deformity. Given the technical feasibility of the procedure and the tremendous benefit it has to restore a patient's life, what good does it serve the patient to have to make them undergo many failed procedures so that face transplant remains a last resort?

Since the publication of this paper in 2009, a total of 27 face transplants have been performed worldwide. The terminology has subsequently changed to *vascularized composite allograft*. Siemionow has since published on lessons learned since the 2009 procedure. In 2013 the Department of Health and Human Services recognized vascu-larized composite allografts as organs, which allowed faces to be included in the Na-tional Organ Procurement and Transplantation Network. This facilitates patient listing and procurement and hopefully will increase the number of face allotransplants performed. Long-term studies are now available,[2,3] and there are now enough patients to begin comparing the data between them.[4] Outcomes of face transplant are significant for functional recovery, including the restoration of sensation, smell, eating, smiling, and speaking. Motor function recovery has not been as robust as sensory recovery and is delayed, taking 8 to 24 months, compared with the restoration of sensation by 8 months. Interestingly, sensation was restored even without coaptation of sensory nerves. Chronic pain was improved as a result of the removal of scar tissue in the recipient. In addition, psychological outcomes showed improved self-esteem, quality of life, and decreased anxiety and depression.[5,6]

Ethical considerations have shifted from an initial concern over the identity and risks of lifelong immunosuppression therapy to a more focused discussion on face transplantation in blind individuals. Often the initial traumatic injury impairs vision. The Boston group has argued in favor of face transplant in the blind, finding that motor and sensory recovery is comparable with that of sighted patients.[7] A report from the first U.S. face transplant patient suggests that her limited vision impairs both her ability to participate in rehabilitation therapy and to take her immunosuppressive therapy.

Complications data have become available. The first face transplant patient experienced side effects from immunosuppressive therapy that included impaired renal function, cervical carcinoma, hypertension, hyperlipidemia, cholangitis, and opportunistic infections. Other reported complications included opportunistic infections, massive intraoperative hemorrhage, renal insufficiency, acute respiratory distress syndrome, and jugular vein thrombosis.[8,9] There have been three deaths—the first was from a failure to comply with immunosuppression therapy, the second was from severe infection after combined face and bilateral hand transplantation. The third death was from squamous cell carcinoma of the hypopharynx. The mortality rate for face transplantation is 11%.

A cost analysis reported by Siemionow et al[10] in 2011 compared the cost of multiple failed reconstructive procedures to the cost of one face transplant with data from the first U.S. face transplant patient. The cost of multiple reconstructions was $353,480, and the cost of the face transplant was $349,959. Worldwide, face transplant is more expensive than solid organ transplant: 85.581€ for heart transplant and 64.247€ for liver transplant versus 102.227€ to 170.071€ for face transplant. The average cost for face transplant in Europe was less than in the United States (129.798€ versus 163.548€).

Face transplantation is a young and exciting field. As a discipline, it has overcome major hurdles and has provided a select group of patients with a renewed quality of life. Challenges ahead include affecting a culture shift in which a face transplant is accepted as a first-line therapy for severe facial deformity, thus sparing a patient the pain and cost of years of failed reconstructions. The transition of the face transplant from an experimental procedure to the standard of care will help obtain routine insurance coverage for this procedure. Cost containment is another concern—both the cost of the procedure and the cost of lifetime immunosuppression—which has been projected to be between $370,000 and $518,000.[11] Safer immunosuppression therapy or even finding a way to supplant it with bone marrow or other cellular therapies is an ultimate goal. Finally, clinicians must consistently report new transplants and their outcomes on the International Registry on Hand and Composite Tissue Transplantation. Face transplantation may not be lifesaving, but it is an effective, life-changing procedure that offers new hope of normal form and function.

Summary   The findings presently indicate that face transplantation is a feasible method of facial reconstruction after severe facial disfigurement and that the benefits of restoring a patient's life in society may outweigh the risks of lifetime immunosuppression therapy and allograft failure.

Implications   The public has readily accepted the face transplant as a viable alternative for patients with severe facial trauma who have become social recluses as a result of their deformities. Severe facial disfigurement is in its own way social death, and face transplantation brings these patients back to life. In light of that tremendous benefit, the risk of lifelong immunosuppression fades. Current research is investigating the immunity that may be bestowed on the recipient by bone marrow in the graft. This work has been effective in rodent models but has yet to show a result in humans.

REFERENCES

1. Siemionow M, Papay F, Alam D, et al. Near-total human face transplantation for a severely disfigured patient in the USA. Lancet 374:203-209, 2009.
2. Khalifian S, Brazio PS, Mohan R, et al. Facial transplantation: the first 9 years. Lancet. 2014 April 25. [Epub ahead of print]
3. Petruzzo P, Testelin S, Kanitakis J, et al. First human face transplantation: 5 years outcomes. Transplantation 93:236-240, 2012.
4. Shanmugarajah K, Hettiaratchy S, Butler PE. Facial transplantation. Curr Opin Otolaryngol Head Neck Surg 20:291-297, 2012.

5. Coffman KL, Siemionow MZ. Face transplantation: psychological outcomes at three-year follow up. Psychosomatics 54:372-378, 2013.
6. Chang G, Pomahac B. Psychosocial changes 6 months after face transplantation. Psychosomatics 54:367-371, 2013.
7. Carty MJ, Bueno EM, Lehmann LS, et al. A position paper in support of face transplantation in the blind. Plast Reconstr Surg 130:319-324, 2012.
8. Sedaghati-Nia A, Gilton A, Liger C, et al. Anaesthesia and intensive care management of face transplantation. Br J Anaesth 111:600-606, 2013.
9. Edrich T, Cywinski JB, Colomina MJ, et al. Perioperative management of face transplant, a survey. Anesth Analg 115:668-670, 2012.
10. Siemionow M, Gatherwright J, Djohan R, et al. Cost analysis of conventional facial reconstruction procedures followed by face transplantation. Am J Transplant 11:379-385, 2011.
11. Siemionow M, Gharb BB, Rampazzo A. Successes and lessons learned after more than a decade of upper extremity and face transplantation. Curr Opin Organ Transplant 18:633-639, 2013.

STUDY AUTHOR REFLECTIONS

Maria Siemionow, MD, PhD, DSc

Face transplantation became a clinical reality after the world's first institutional review board approval was granted to our team on Nov. 15, 2004. During the past 10 years, 28 face transplantations were performed worldwide in six countries including France, China, United States, Spain, Turkey, and Poland. The reported outcomes are encouraging despite the complexity of the transplant procedure. Because of the differences in patients' disfigurement, the selection criteria, and the limited number of cases with long-term outcomes, it is still impossible to provide a comparative analysis. The deaths of three patients within the case series bring the mortality rate up to 10.7%—an unexpected and sobering outcome that is raising some debates and concerns.

As with any innovative treatment or procedure, the success and failure rates will balance over time, and with a larger number of cases, the risks and benefits of face transplantation will be thoroughly assessed. This will be facilitated by international registry data. Thus it is imperative that all centers performing face transplantation report their cases. After an assessment of the risks and benefits, it is our obligation and privilege to introduce innovative procedures and therapies to the armamentarium of reconstructive surgery. The ultimate goal, however, is the safety of our patients.

Index